BLACKPOOL HEALTH
PROFESSIONALS LIBRARY

KT-552-041

CONSULTANT PHYSICIANS WORKING WITH PATIENTS

The duties, responsibilities and practice of physicians
in general medicine and the specialties

THIRD EDITION

PART 1 **Duties and responsibilities**

PART 2 **Work in the specialties**

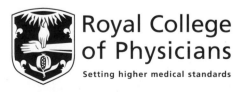

Royal College
of Physicians

Setting higher medical standards

Blackpool, Fylde and Wyre NHS
Library

TV04063

Cover
Photograph: COLIN CUTHBERT/SCIENCE PHOTO LIBRARY
Design: Merriton Sharp

BARCODE No.	TVO4063	
CLASS No.	610.695	
BIB CHECK	--	PROC CHECK
	NAL CHECK	
OS	SYSTEM No.	T
LOAN CATEGORY	NL	

ROYAL COLLEGE OF PHYSICIANS OF LONDON
11 St Andrews Place, London NW1 4LE
Registered Charity No 210508

Copyright © 2005 Royal College of Physicians

ISBN 1 86016 229 0

Text design by Royal College of Physicians Publications Unit
Typeset by Dan-Set Graphics, Telford, Shropshire

Printed in Great Britain by Sarum ColourView Group, Salisbury, Wiltshire

Contents

PART 2: WORK IN THE SPECIALTIES

Foreword

Consultant physicians working for patients is a respected and authoritative source of information for hospital physicians and managers working in the NHS. The two previous editions emphasised the importance of working arrangements and relationships, facilities and manpower, as well as the competence of healthcare professionals in ensuring high quality healthcare. This edition reflects new influences and their impact on practice and service.

The College has always emphasised the importance of close partnership with patients, and this is firmly brought out in the new title: *Consultant physicians working **with** patients.*

Changes in the organisation and delivery of healthcare include foundation hospitals, payment by results and steps to unify care across primary, secondary and social care. All impact on the work of physicians. Primary care trusts now lead in commissioning healthcare services, but consultant physicians have always had a leading role in the development and improvement of hospital-based clinical services and must engage with primary care colleagues in the commissioning process.

Changes in education and training, brought about through the Postgraduate Medical Education and Training Board (PMETB) and Modernising Medical Careers, compounded by the effects of the European Working Time Directive, are further major influences.

The reformed General Medical Council's new requirements for licensing and revalidation is a significant change in the regulation of the medical profession. The College has an essential role in maintaining public confidence by reinforcing the central place of clinical and professional standards in the revalidation process.

Consultants have a wide range of responsibilities to maintain and improve the quality of patient care. Part 1 of *Consultant physicians working with patients* reaffirms the duties and responsibilities of consultant physicians in the modern health service. It emphasises other professional activities, among them teaching, training, research, management, clinical governance, audit and appraisal, and sets out the supporting staff and facilities that are required to meet those responsibilities.

Increasing attention to patient experience and health outcomes, and promotion of patient choice are now high priorities for the NHS but, despite expansion of training and recruitment, shortages of qualified healthcare professionals and continuing pressures on the service still threaten standards of patient care. Enforced changes in work practice, particularly shift work and attendant loss of the medical team structure, and changes in medical training, may pose a further threat to quality of care.

Part 1 of the document also addresses the needs of emergency medical patients, emphasising the development of acute medicine as a new specialty. It sets out recommendations for the delivery of acute medical services with standards to improve the continuity of care of medical inpatients.

Part 2 comprises statements from the specialties that the College represents. The statements set out the clinical needs of patients, highlighting the opportunities for education and support to enable patients to participate fully in their own care. Each makes explicit recommendations for the resources, time, manpower and facilities that are required for high quality medicine. These statements are designed to inform and support clinicians and managers in planning the development, organisation and delivery of services, and in identifying and rectifying deficiencies. They have been prepared through the joint specialty committees with wide consultation. They may be regarded as position statements.

A further aim is to guide the preparation of job plans and annual appraisal. With the new consultant contract and the requirements of revalidation the exercise is now of utmost importance. The statements set out advice on clinical activity and clinical standards of care as well as detailing the range of supporting professional duties that underpin the work of consultant physicians.

Finally, each specialty sets out recommendations for its consultant workforce. It is widely accepted that the consultant workforce does need to be expanded to meet both current and foreseeable clinical needs. Estimates of the workforce expansion are set out in summary tables though the targets identified as desirable by each specialty may not be achievable in the short term.

Although the document contains specialised and technical information, we believe that it will also be of interest to non-clinical colleagues and to patients, carers and those who represent them, and other healthcare professionals working to deliver the highest quality medical care.

CAROL BLACK   MARY ARMITAGE   January 2005
President   *Clinical Vice-President*

Abbreviations

A&E	Accident and Emergency Department
CCST	Certificate of Completion of Specialist Training
CGST	Clinical governance support team
CHAI	Commission for Healthcare and Inspection
CME	Continuing medical education
COG	Clinical outcomes group
CPD	Continuing professional development
DGH	District general hospital
DH	Department of Health
DOPS	Directly observed procedural skills
EWTD	European Working Time Directive
GIM	General internal medicine
GP	General practitioner
GPSI	General practitioner with a special interest
HPA	Health Protection Agency
IOG	Improving outcomes guidance
JCHMT	Joint Committee for Higher Medical Training
MDT	Multidisciplinary team
MINAP	Myocardial Infarction National Audit Project
Mini-CEX	Mini clinical evaluation exercise
MRC	Medical Research Council
NCCG	Non-consultant career grade
NHS	National Health Service
NHSE	National Health Service Executive
NSF	National service framework
NTN	National training number
OoHMT	Out-of-hours medical team
PA	Programmed activity
PCT	Primary care trust
PGD	Patient group directive
PHLS	Public Health Laboratory Service
SAC	Specialist advisory committee
SHA	Strategic health authority
WTE	Whole time equivalent

PART 1

DUTIES AND RESPONSIBILITIES

1 Introduction

The aim of the Royal College of Physicians is to ensure the highest quality of patient care. Good standards of clinical care have always depended both on the hard work of those who work in the NHS, and on the resources available to run it. The first two editions of *Consultant physicians working for patients* highlighted the importance of working arrangements and relationships, as well as good facilities and adequate manpower.[1,2] These documents also emphasised the need for close partnership with patients, and the importance of that relationship is reflected in the title of this new edition: *Consultant physicians working **with** patients.*

Continuing pressures on the service, plus a shortage of qualified healthcare professionals, threaten high standards of patient care. Changes in health service organisation, and to the commissioning and delivery of healthcare, are having a major impact on the service, on the practice of physicians, and on the resources required to meet their responsibilities. The College has emphasised the need for physicians to be able to work flexibly and change their work practice to meet the requirements of modern medicine; this will be crucial in meeting the healthcare challenges of this and the next decade.

The Government has placed reform of our public services close to the top of its agenda. This agenda is underpinned by four key principles: devolution and delegation; national standards and accountability; flexibility and local initiatives; and choice. It is not difficult to identify how the drive to realise these principles is being reflected in a series of initiatives that impact on our health service, for example those that expand patient choice, encourage flexible deployment of health professionals, and refocus arrangements for healthcare commissioning.

Changes in the form and structure of the NHS are taking place to support the wider reforms. Twenty-eight strategic health authorities (SHAs), with the role of 'performance managing' the NHS, have replaced England's 95 health authorities. Each SHA will be expected to have a three-year strategic action plan designed to deliver local health improvements and meet national targets – targets such as those set out in the NHS plan[3] and integral to the delivery of national service frameworks.

In April 2000, just over 300 primary care trusts (PCTs) were established in England; these will take the lead in drawing up local delivery plans for the SHAs. Budgets for PCTs are set for a period of three years, providing opportunity for a longer-term approach to planning. Primary care trusts have a responsibility to work with local partners to improve health and to strengthen the primary, preventative aspect of healthcare, as well as working closely with the acute sector. In addition, care trusts are being established to allow closer integration of health and social care in the commissioning and delivery of primary and community healthcare.

A consistent theme in the core statements directing the strategic actions of these organisations is the requirement to develop a diverse and flexible workforce, equipped to take on the challenges of delivering modern healthcare. Associated with this is a desire to shift the balance of power away from central government to front-line NHS staff – staff with the knowledge and the devolved power to run and improve health services in their areas.

Both of these factors will have a considerable impact on how healthcare teams are staffed and organised at a local level. There is, therefore, considerable scope for imaginative and innovative structures, using the right mix of personnel with the appropriate skills and competencies. Doctors (GPs and specialists), with their experience of developing services and healthcare teams and listening to patients, will be well placed to contribute. They should be directly engaged in addressing issues of service design, access and delivery, whether in emergency care or elective care. Such engagement will not only reinforce the interdependency of hospital-based services and those delivered in the wider community, it will also bring the interests and concerns of patients closer to the acute trusts which serve them.

2 Medical professionalism

Physicians have expressed growing concern over what they perceive to be the erosion of professionalism and professional standards in UK medicine. Patients and the public are entitled to expect professionalism in medicine, yet it appears that in society at large the ideals that we equate with professionalism are in decline.

Medical professionalism has been defined as a combination of technical knowledge and skills, the upholding of strong ethical principles and values, and belief in the notion of medicine as a vocation, with the interest of the patient always paramount.[4] The acquisition of medical knowledge and competence is a vital step towards achieving this, but placing the provision of high quality clinical care and patient welfare at the heart of every action a doctor undertakes is equally important in adhering to the principles embodied in the concept of medical professionalism.

Factors threatening medical professionalism are numerous. Enforced changes in work practices, particularly shift work, are leading to a loss of continuity of care and to a diminution of personal responsibility. Modern medical training may be exacerbating the problem with the loss of the medical team structure and associated loss of the opportunity for senior leadership by example. The advent of the NHS 'blame culture' and rising consumerism in healthcare, coupled with a fall in public confidence in doctors due to the high profile failures of a few, are leading to a crisis in morale amongst the profession. Those expressing their distress to the College are asking how we can sustain our values in the face of these factors, which are compounded by the pressure of continuous organisational change. One way may be through the introduction of the concept of medical professionalism at the point of selection to medical school and its continuation throughout undergraduate training. Professional values should be a key feature of specialist registrar (SpR) management courses, and should be reinforced at each assessment and appraisal, at every stage of a doctor's career.

The College believes that it is necessary to redefine the concept of medical professionalism and to act in order to prevent its further erosion. Consequently, the College is taking forward preliminary work already done in this area with the aim of devising robust professional standards for national agreement. These will build on the standards set out by the General Medical Council (GMC) in *Good medical practice*, will support revalidation, and will aim to maintain the esteem in which the profession has always been held.[5]

3 Working with patients

Physicians have always placed clinical service to patients at the heart of their medical practice and have worked in partnership with patients over many years. The importance of involving patients in decisions about their treatment, and the benefits of facilitating self-care, are well established. Considering service users' views when planning and improving any clinical service is an essential part of modern healthcare. In Part 2, the clinical needs of patients are outlined for each specialty with a description of how the specialty can ensure patient-centred care, opportunities for education and patient choice. The roles of carers, patient support groups and expert patients are discussed, and the importance of information, support and empowerment for patients with chronic conditions is emphasised.

The NHS Plan identified 'the involvement of the public in health services in several capacities with the overall aim to give patients and the public a voice in national policy and local services' as a key issue.[3] The College is committed to encouraging patient and carer involvement in our activities, and established the Patient Involvement Unit (PIU) in September 2003 to promote this partnership (**www.rcplondon.ac.uk/college/PIU**).

PATIENT INVOLVEMENT UNIT

The College believes that if patients, carers and the medical profession work in collaboration they will have a powerful joint voice to bring their concerns to the attention of the Government. As experts on their illnesses, patients can do much to improve the quality of healthcare services and their involvement in strategies affecting care provision is essential. The Unit comes under the remit of the Professional Affairs Department, it has a full-time patient involvement manager, and the first College patient involvement officer was appointed in November 2003.

The main aim of the PIU is to identify areas where patients and doctors can build cooperative and mutually beneficial relationships. The College and Fellows and Members across the country have begun much excellent work to identify and recommend examples of partnership that are effective in improving healthcare.

The PIU was set up following the College Council's recognition of patient, carer and public involvement in College activities as a priority. A Patient and Carer Liaison Committee had been in place at the College for a number of years but in October 2002 Council recommended that a working group be convened to look at more innovative ways to involve patients and the general public. The working group recommended the creation of the Patient and Carer Network and the Patient and Carer Involvement Steering Group.

The Patient and Carer Network ensures that the interests of patients, carers and the wider public are fully integrated in the work of the College and helps the College develop and enhance its relationship with users of the NHS. The Network consists of approximately 75 patients, carers and members of the public who have been recruited from a range of backgrounds through adverts in the national press. The College can draw on this wide pool of skills and knowledge, derived from professional and personal experience, and gain a valuable insight into the needs of the communities in which Network members live, thus better informing its work.

The recruitment process highlighted the issues of major concern as communication, information, equity of access to – and coordination of – services, and involvement of patients and carers in decisions about their treatment and care.

Members join the Network for three years and undertake a number of activities, including membership of College working parties, committees and special project groups. The PIU aims to have two Network members on every College working party, committee or board by the end of 2005. Members provide comment on consultation documents, and take part in invited service reviews and general professional training visits. This is a new development for the College and proper evaluation is essential. Network members and the chair/organiser of the relevant activity complete evaluation forms to enable the PIU to review contributions and assess benefits, and to identify any problems to facilitate future work.

The PIU is the focus point for the Network to highlight relevant issues, and is a means by which patients, carers and the public can communicate with the College to bring attention to their needs and influence the College agenda. All patients and carers involved in College work will be registered with the PIU to enable them to receive appropriate information and support, and for the effectiveness of their involvement to be recorded.

The Patient and Carer Involvement Steering Group provides the strategic input into the PIU and assists with the development of overall College policy in respect of improving clinical standards for the benefit of patients, carers and the public. The Steering Group comprises six College staff and six lay representatives and works in close collaboration with the Patient and Carer Network. The chair is a lay member of the College Council.

The Steering Group advises on the most appropriate ways in which the PIU can help with College priority areas agreed by Council, such as the communications and education strategies, setting clinical standards, and wherever the partnership of physician and patient/ carer perspectives can be helpful in influencing national/Government policy.

4 Work of consultant physicians

EMPLOYMENT OF CONSULTANT PHYSICIANS AND JOB PLANS

Almost all consultants are employed by NHS trusts under nationally negotiated terms and conditions of service. In England, the 2003 consultant contract was agreed between the British Medical Association (BMA) and the Department of Health (DH), and individual consultant physicians now decide whether they wish to change to the new contract. In Wales, all consultants will change to the new contract under the agreement reached between BMA Cymru and the Welsh Assembly Government. The College does not advise on terms and conditions of service – it had no part to play in the negotiation of the new contract and no formal position regarding the final document. However, the College does give leadership and support to consultants in maintaining and improving the clinical service. The College has always given advice and, ultimately, approval for the content of new consultant job descriptions, through the network of regional and specialty advisers. In addition, the College has provided an independent representative on every advisory appointment committee to ensure that the appointee has the appropriate training and expertise to fulfil the commitments of the post.

The College has extensive data regarding the numbers of consultants and other career grades from the annual Census. This includes workload data and information about the balance between specialty work and general medical, mostly acute, workload. Through the work of our joint specialty committees, we are able to give advice about the workforce requirements and examples of job plans in each specialty in Part 2 of this document.

WORK TO MAINTAIN AND IMPROVE THE QUALITY OF HEALTHCARE

Supporting professional duties

There are many other duties of a consultant that lie outside direct clinical care, but that are essential professional commitments to maintaining and improving the clinical service. These supporting professional duties include teaching, mentoring, self-education, audit, appraisal, clinical governance, continuing professional development (CPD), revalidation, service development and research. These duties are time-consuming, they are expanding and can impact upon the time for clinical workload.

The job plan itemises the various tasks to be undertaken by an individual consultant; traditionally these duties were expressed in notional half days (NHD). In England, the 2003 contract changes the measure of consultants' work, now expressed as programmed activities (PAs), each representing four hours (three hours in premium time) of consultant time. In Wales, the aim is a working week of 37.5 hours made up of 10 sessions of three to four hours. Specifically, the contract framework sets out the number of PAs that new and established consultants should devote to direct clinical care, although clinical managers and consultants can agree flexible arrangements for the timing of work. Within a full-time framework of 10 PAs per week, it has been agreed that, in England, a full-time consultant will devote, on average, 7.5 PAs to direct clinical care and 2.5 PAs to supporting professional duties. Again, in Wales there are slightly different arrangements with, typically, seven sessions of direct clinical care and three for supporting professional activities. Physicians often have rotating commitments with other colleagues, and may agree an annualised job plan.

The role of educational supervisor of doctors in training requires an increasing commitment. For a consultant physician responsible for the educational supervision, appraisal and assessment of three or four trainees, this would be likely to amount to one session, reflected within the sessions for supporting professional activities. This is in keeping with the recommendation from the postgraduate deans of one hour per trainee per week. Those with a major and regular commitment to undergraduate teaching or to clinical research should have this formally recognised in their job plan with an appropriate number of PAs for supporting professional activities. The precise balance will be agreed as part of the annual job plan review and may vary taking into account circumstances where the agreed level of duties in relation to supporting professional activities, other NHS responsibilities and external duties is significantly greater or lower than the generally anticipated 2.5 (3 in Wales) programmed sessions for supporting professional acivities. Only in the most exceptional circumstances could the College envisage the key supporting professional duties being contained within less than 2.5 PAs; it is expected that they will frequently take more.

National duties

Consultants make a valuable contribution to the health service and British medicine through their work with national specialty societies, the Colleges and the BMA and in providing advice to Government departments – notably the DH – either directly or through many other bodies such as the National Institute for Clinical Excellence (NICE), the National Patient Safety Agency (NPSA) and others. The NHS Executive and the Welsh Assembly Government have stressed that trusts should support consultants in this. The 2003 contract details such work under external duties and outlines that these are undertaken as part of the job plan by agreement between the consultant and employing organisation. It recommends that external duties might include 'reasonable quantities of work for the Royal Colleges in the interest of the wider NHS', but the definition of reasonable is not developed and should, therefore, be a matter for local negotiation.[6] Taking into account the above national guidance, the College recommends that a physician undertaking such duties should agree, as part of the job plan review, that the supporting professional activities, other NHS responsibilities and external duties require significantly more than 2.5 PAs. The College has suggested the following guidelines:[7]

■ A physician undertaking the duties of College tutor – a role crucial to trusts for the education and support of senior house officers (SHOs) – might expect to agree one to two *additional* supporting PAs, depending on the size of the trust and numbers of SHOs, with an appropriate reduction in PAs for direct clinical care.

■ A physician undertaking the duties of regional adviser should expect to agree two *additional* supporting PAs (ie 4.5 PAs) and, depending on the model of working between deputy/CPD advisers, one to two additional supporting PAs might be appropriate.

The precise balance of PAs for direct clinical care and the supporting professional activities, other NHS responsibilities and external duties will need to be negotiated at the job plan review and will reflect local issues, including the size of the trust and the additional workload involved. Some duties, such as taking part in national working parties or committees, may be agreed on an ad hoc basis and special category leave may be appropriate for specific duties. However, it is essential that any formal position, such as College tutor, specialty adviser, regional adviser, work for the deanery and so on, is recognised and has a formal agreed sessional commitment.

Direct clinical care

The other notable change in the 2003 contract comes within the definition of direct clinical care, which incorporates work that might previously have been described separately under administration in a job description. It is clear that any activity that involves the care of individual patients should be included in PAs of direct clinical care. This includes a wide range of duties: clinic letters, reviewing and communicating results, providing advice to GPs and other healthcare practitioners, telephone consultations, seeing relatives, multidisciplinary team meetings, X-ray meetings, case conferences/presentations, prioritising referrals, organising investigations, supervising other members of the healthcare team, providing clinical reports and other clinical correspondence, addressing complaints or critical incidents and so on.

Many specialties identify substantial clinical activity for work relating to outpatients, including requesting additional information and organising investigations before seeing the patient, or reviewing results and providing a detailed management plan to GPs and other professional colleagues without seeing the patient. For direct clinical care there will be a minimum of 1.5, and often 2.5, PAs needed to cover these various duties, the balance reflecting the individual's specialty, work practice and local circumstances. This is reflected in the outline of clinical work of consultants in the various specialties in Part 2 of this document.

Predictable emergency work out of hours, and during normal working hours, must be scheduled in the PAs separately from other clinical duties. Emergency specialty work is reflected in the specialty statements in Part 2, but for those physicians practising acute medicine, the time and resources required to undertake this workload is set out in the following chapter.

Changing casemix, increasing complexity of cases and supervision of other members of the team

The specialty chapters also outline the time required to assess and advise new and follow-up patients in outpatient clinics, or for relevant specialty investigations and procedures. Many factors influence guidance on the number of patients that may be seen in one session. Time to offer guidance and supervision to trainee doctors in clinics has been highlighted in previous editions of this document. Current training reforms have led to the development of competency-based curricula and objective measures of assessment of progress. Such formal assessments may include direct observation (Mini Clinical Evaluation Exercise (mini-CEX)), Directly Observed Procedural Skills (DOPS) and 360-degree assessments of behaviour and interpersonal skills. The reduction in hours of work for trainees means that the programmes must be structured to utilise every training opportunity. Substantial additional time will be required for intensive training and for formal assessment of the clinical competencies of trainees to ensure career progression.

The changes in the delivery of healthcare outlined in the introduction, with many other healthcare professionals contributing to the clinical care of patients, impact on the workload of consultant physicians. The time needed for physicians to discuss the management of patients seen by clinical nurse specialists should be considered, and also the impact of the change in casemix. As GPs with a special interest (GPSIs) take on the care of more patients with chronic problems, and as the flexible workforce championed by the Modernisation Agency takes on new roles and responsibilities, so the complexity of patients seen by the consultant physician increases. Physicians' assistants (medical care practitioners) may prove hugely beneficial to the service for patients, and of substantial benefit to physicians themselves, but they, and other members of the healthcare workforce, will require supervision. In addition, involving patients directly in decisions about their management requires time to explain the nature of the clinical problem, and the choices, risks and benefits of the different investigations and treatments available, and to discuss practical ethical issues. These matters are time-consuming, and will directly reduce the numbers of consultations or procedures that can be undertaken in any session of PA.

5 Supporting staff and facilities

CONSULTANT'S OFFICE

In previous editions of this document, the College has made it clear that a private office is essential for the work, both clinical and managerial, of a consultant physician. We remain convinced that this is highly desirable. Privacy is necessary for confidential conversations with patients, relatives, trainees and many other professional colleagues. Telephone calls are often sensitive and confidential, as are clinical letters, papers and patient records. However, with the expansion in consultant numbers and greater emphasis on working in teams, it *may* be satisfactory to share an office with another colleague working in a complementary manner. New job descriptions may reflect innovative ways of working where consultants have responsibilities across multiple sites, including sessions in the community. In which case, sharing an office with a colleague, again, *may* be satisfactory provided there is ready access to a private room for sensitive interviews and phone calls. All consultants must have a personal computer with access to the Internet.

SECRETARIAL SUPPORT

Secretarial support of appropriate seniority and experience is essential for the work of any professional and the College has recommended that a full-time personal secretary supports a consultant physician. With the emphasis on working in teams, there may be occasions where a number of secretaries support a team, but the College believes that adequate, efficient secretarial support implies a ratio of at least one secretary per full-time consultant.

CLINICAL INFORMATION AND INFORMATION TECHNOLOGY

The safe care of patients requires ready access to existing medical records, to results of previous investigations and consultations, and to information regarding clinical care in other hospitals and in primary care. Such up-to-date information is often lacking. As a result, patients with complex medical histories and drug regimens may have to be managed as emergencies without adequate clinical records. This is dangerous. It is also inefficient as it may lead to unnecessary investigation and delay in diagnosis.

Information derived from clinical records is necessary to support activity analysis, performance review, service planning, health surveillance and all aspects of clinical governance including audit. Hospital episode statistics (HES), derived from paper medical records, are now being used to inform the appraisal of individual consultants. At present, the validity of the data is poor, largely because there is little clinical involvement in the process of data extraction and aggregation. The College is working to improve the quality of records, both paper and electronic, by developing evidence-based standards for their structure and content. It is also encouraging greater involvement of consultants in secondary data extraction, particularly for appraisal, in order to improve data validity. Major investment in the IT infrastructure in the health service creates good opportunities for physicians to influence the quality of records, data and information. Further details can be obtained from the Health Informatics Unit (HIU) website: **www.rcplondon.ac.uk/college/hiu**

STUDY LEAVE AND CONTINUED PROFESSIONAL DEVELOPMENT

Doctors are charged with personal lifelong learning and professional development. They must demonstrate this through the acquisition of educational credits, in order to meet the requirement of the revalidation process established by the GMC. The credit requirements are a minimum of 50 education credits per year, including 25 non-clinical credits over the five-year cycle. Credits, both clinical and non-clinical, can be derived from personal, internal or external activities but, in any one-year period, a minimum of 25 credits must be external. There must, therefore, be adequate time and funding for study leave supplementary to attending local hospital educational activities. The consultant is an employee of the NHS; the expenses of continuing medical education (CME) are a duty of the employer and funding for CME/continuing professional development (CPD) must be identified for each physician. Educational needs should be identified at the annual appraisal. The credits achieved should reflect the practice of the individual consultant, with appropriate time for general medicine/acute medicine as well as the specialty, to ensure practice is kept up to date and clinically safe. We strongly advocate the use of the College's online system, accessed through the website, for the collection of CPD records.

6 Acute medicine: quality of care

The College has produced a number of reports in recent years addressing the delivery of acute medical services and how the needs of patients might best be met. Specialisation in medicine has promoted advances in investigative and therapeutic techniques, which have resulted in improved outcomes. Patients expect specialists to be involved in their care, and higher medical training has evolved to meet the needs of both the specialist service and the requirement for specialty training. With increasing specialisation, however, many physicians feel less able to undertake acute, general medical work at a time when the emergency medical workload is rising. This tension between the benefits of increased specialisation and the need to retain high quality general medical skills is well recognised. It is compounded by the unprecedented and rapid changes in established working patterns, driven by the imperative to meet the European Working Time Directive (EWTD) and the changes in training set out in *Unfinished business* and *Modernising medical careers*.[8,9] Historically, there has been a failure to recognise the medical time and resources required to provide acute medical care.

In Part 2 of previous editions of this document, the specialties set out their recommendations for the resources and the time required to assess or treat specific numbers of patients, and the manpower required to deliver the service. Emergency work was fitted in around the elective commitments, but the rising emergency workload has threatened to compromise safe practice and to overwhelm those physicians trying to deliver the service.

These issues have now been comprehensively addressed in the recent College report, *Acute medicine: making it work for patients*.[10] The report builds on previous recommendations from *The interface of accident & emergency and acute medicine* and *The interface between acute general medicine and critical care*.[11,12] It defines the practice of acute medicine (the preferred term) as that part of general internal medicine (GIM) concerned with the immediate and early specialist management of adult patients with a wide range of medical conditions who present in hospitals as emergencies. It notes that over the next 10 years, the majority of acute medicine at consultant level will continue to be delivered by physicians practising acute medicine with another specialty interest. There will be increasing support from consultants in acute medicine, with the aim to have at least three consultants in acute medicine in every acute trust by 2008. All trainees in GIM will require appropriate training in acute medicine, but following the recognition of acute medicine for subspecialty training by the Joint Committee on Higher Medical Training (JCHMT) in July 2003, there will need to be a planned increase in specialist national training numbers (NTNs) for those wishing to acquire accreditation in the subspecialty.

The report sets out specimen job plans for both physicians with a special interest in practising acute medicine, and for consultant physicians in acute medicine. Both job plans include 2.5 PAs for supporting professional activities, as detailed earlier in this document. The precise balance will vary, depending on local models of care, but the physician with a specialist interest might devote four PAs to direct clinical care in acute medicine and 3.5 PAs to direct clinical care in the specialty interest. The consultant physician in acute medicine might have five direct clinical care PAs, one PA for acute medicine unit (AMU) service development and management and 1.5 PAs for other clinical activities, such as sessions in high dependency units, intensive care units or emergency clinics and specialist procedures.

At present, there are only around 100 physicians in acute medicine, and most emergency care is provided by about half of the 7,582 consultant physicians in the UK who participate in the acute take rota. Consultants who undertake medical emergency duties spend, on average, 12 hours a week on general medicine, compared with 20 hours in their specialty. With the 2002 Census suggesting that these physicians work an average of 64 hours per week it is crucial that adequate time in their job plans be identified to fulfil this commitment safely.

STANDARDS OF MEDICAL CARE

Many emergency patients are referred, or present, to hospital without a firm diagnosis. Many are elderly but, whatever their age, they require and expect effective specialist management of their acute illness. Any hospital that receives emergency patients must provide comprehensive investigative and treatment services 24 hours a day. There must be adequate numbers of appropriately trained staff to manage patients in an expert and timely manner and to enable assessment and development of a management plan for all patients within four hours of presenting to hospital as an acute medical emergency. A medical team should comprise enough doctors of sufficient experience to manage the clinical work for which the hospital has responsibility. Some units have a consultant physician based on AMUs, directly supervising the SHOs and SpRs, and it is envisaged that as numbers of physicians in acute medicine increase, so they will be increasingly present on AMUs.

The acute medicine report makes the following specific recommendations:

- The College recommends that a doctor with the appropriate skills in acute medicine should be based in the receiving unit at all times. This would usually be a SpR, or equivalent middle-grade doctor, who should have the MRCP(UK) qualification and two years' recent experience managing acutely ill patients. When on take they should have no other scheduled commitments.

- There must always be consultant cover to support the medical team on call.

- The College recommends that at house officer (HO) or SHO level, one hour should be allowed for each patient to assess, document, investigate and gather results, and to prescribe and initiate treatment.

- The SpR should be available 24 hours a day to review cases, deal with the critically ill and take referrals from other colleagues.

- A consultant physician should review all patients within 24 hours of admission. Fifteen minutes should be allowed to assess each new patient on the post-take ward round. Thus, a consultant physician can see 16 patients in one four-hour session of PA. This may require the cancellation of other commitments and will require a consultant-led ward round at least twice a day in all but the smallest trusts.

These recommendations will allow clinical directors to calculate the sessions required to cover the service and to identify time in job plans. It will be apparent that current practice in the UK often falls below these standards. The number of PAs required to meet this service will be considerable in busy trusts, and initial calculations may be met with incredulity. Yet from all perspectives, both from those organising and delivering healthcare and from the patients receiving it, one hour for a junior doctor to fully assess, investigate and treat an acutely ill patient is not excessively lengthy, nor is 15 minutes very long for a senior physician to review a new acutely ill patient and draw up a management plan. Such standards have improved care in outpatients and specialty care and have been long overdue in acute medicine. There will then be better understanding of the time and resources required to manage acutely ill patients.

In previous editions, the College has recommended that a team on call should comprise a consultant and at least three resident medical staff: a SpR, SHO and HO. Unfortunately, the requirement to reduce junior doctors' hours of work to meet the EWTD is resulting in almost all resident doctors working in shifts. This represents a major challenge to quality of care and patient safety, as continuity of care may be lost and the team structure may all but disappear. The responsibility for patient care has to be handed over from one team to another, and though adequate time for handover is essential it does not compensate for the difficulties in transferring care. The loss of opportunity to follow up patients who they have admitted and to learn from the natural history of disease, plus the difficulties in attending formal teaching sessions, have had a major adverse impact on the training of junior doctors.

The sense of personal responsibility for the continuing welfare of patients is eroded by shift work. This, and the loss of senior example and leadership in a close-knit team, is a major factor in the unease amongst the profession regarding quality of care and potentially falling medical professionalism. Nevertheless, it seems inevitable that almost all resident doctors will be working full shifts and, therefore, the College has undertaken robust surveys to provide data to the DH on staffing levels in acute hospitals and has drawn up advice on how best to deliver the cover. Additionally, the College has developed the following series of standards of good medical practice to improve continuity of care, all of which are amenable to external audit.[13]

STANDARDS TO IMPROVE CONTINUITY OF CARE FOR MEDICAL INPATIENTS

1   A patient should know the name of the medical team responsible for his or her care.

2   A medical team should know the name and location of every patient under its care.

3   Medical teams should not routinely have patients outlying from their home wards.

4   A single medical team should be responsible for a patient's care at any one time.

5   Doctors should have sufficient protected time for patient handover.

6   On transfer of care, a patient's new team should have immediate access to all necessary clinical information.

7   Out-of-hours (evenings, nights and weekends) doctors should be aware of the patients under their care who are particularly unwell.

8   All clinical actions and annotations in patient notes should be traceable to the doctor concerned.

9   A patient's resuscitation status must be stored sensitively but also be accessible immediately.

10 Doctors should know the outcome of their decisions.

11 When designing a junior doctors' medical rota the first priority should be daytime continuity of care on the wards.

12 A discharge letter, summary or report should leave the hospital within 24 hours of a patient's discharge.

DETAILS OF OUT-OF-HOURS COVER AND THE HOSPITAL AT NIGHT TEAM

The College advises that in order to devise a rota that will provide 24-hour cover, with adequate flexibility to allow prospective cover for annual and study leave and optimal time for continuity of care and specialist training, 10 junior doctors at each grade or competency level are required. Fewer than 10 for each grade of interchangeable staff results in extreme inflexibility for a 56-hour week. The College considers that a rota with less than eight doctors in each interchangeable cell results in a rota that is unacceptable in terms of both continuity of care for patients and opportunities for daytime training.

Hospitals with small numbers of trainee staff will be unable to construct rotas with 24-hour medical cover. Solutions may include service reconfiguration, or rationalisation and collaboration between neighbouring hospitals. Skillmix changes may release some junior doctor time when other members of the healthcare team undertake tasks previously carried out by doctors. Flexible cross-cover arrangements may allow a limited number of junior doctors to cover greater numbers of patients, provided that the safety and management of patients is not compromised and trainees are not required to work outside their competence. Cross cover in specialist areas provides opportunities but clinical safety is paramount. The Academy of Medical Royal Colleges has collaborated with the DH Hospital at Night project and has developed a model of out-of-hours cover by a generic out-of-hours medical team (OoHMT).

Whilst offering advice regarding potential models for cover, the College has continued to express grave concern regarding the quality of clinical care in many hospitals that are struggling to meet the EWTD, and maintains the position that it may not be possible in some trusts to meet the Directive in August 2004 and safeguard patient care. Much of this work is set out in a number of papers on the College website: **www.rcplondon.ac.uk/news/ewtd.asp**

7 Quality of healthcare

In addition to their direct clinical duties, consultant physicians undertake a wide range of other duties to maintain and improve the quality of healthcare. These professional responsibilities include local service development and management roles, and participation in local audit and clinical governance programmes. They may also take part in national audit programmes and many undertake advisory roles in the wider interest of the NHS, such as work for the DH, the Royal Colleges and specialty societies. Physicians have responsibilities for the education, training and assessment of medical students, junior doctors, and other members of the healthcare team, and a personal commitment to keeping their own knowledge and skills up to date. Many physicians will have academic and research commitments in addition to their health service duties.

PROFESSIONAL RESPONSIBILITIES IN EDUCATION, TRAINING AND ASSESSMENT, AND RESEARCH

Much undergraduate and postgraduate teaching is undertaken by NHS staff, both in teaching hospitals and in district general hospitals. Physicians act as educational supervisors for trainee medical staff and contribute to their education and training, both in formal, structured programmes and in the traditional context of the clinical management of patients. The development of competency-based training and assessment and the implementation of *Modernising medical careers* herald major changes in medical training.[9] Additionally, the reduction in working hours with the EWTD, and the inevitable move to full shifts, means that there is less time available for formal and experiential learning and a reduced service commitment from trainees. The competing pressures of service provision and training are well recognised, and are a major challenge for the future.

Conversely, much direct clinical care is delivered by physicians with academic university contracts, and they have competing pressures from their research and academic duties and their health service duties. The commitment to research differs from basic science to clinical research, and varies depending on the institutions in which physicians work, and the appointments they hold. Many physicians will not undertake fundamental scientific experiments, but all doctors have a duty to contribute where they are able in order to support long-term, continued progress in healthcare. Clinical academic physicians find particular difficulties when the pressures of clinical services impact on their academic activities.

With the development of extended and new roles for many of the healthcare workforce, physicians have additional responsibilities for teaching and training of nursing staff and allied health professionals in the multidisciplinary team. Trainers, however, must not only have the time to teach but must also be properly trained in the delivery of quality-assured training and in the assessment of competencies. The College offers a wide range of support through its 'Physicians as Educators' training programmes and a series of workshops in the Consultants Development Programme, which assist physicians in meeting these new challenges and support their personal CPD. The College supports CPD by offering a range of CME programmes, based both at the College and across the regions, by accrediting external events for CPD, and by maintaining a personal CPD record for Fellows and Members.

CONSULTANTS IN MANAGEMENT AND ADVISORY ROLES

All physicians will have a management role in the running of their own service, and will, through their commitment to improving the quality of their service, be continually engaged in service development. At different times in their careers they may undertake additional formal management duties, or be involved in major service changes and development bids. They may act as a leader of a clinical or multidisciplinary team, or as lead clinician of a specialist department, or they may undertake formal responsibilities as clinical or medical directors. Consultants play a key role in facilitating change, and trusts are dependant on their senior clinicians for providing professional advice on medical matters and the strategic direction of the trust. By virtue of their experience and seniority, consultants are ideally placed to advise on the best use of limited resources, and to ensure the safety of patients. All physicians hold this responsibility. The College supports consultants in their broader management roles through the Consultants Development Programme.

Clinical and medical directors have a range of additional responsibilities including risk management, the investigation of complaints and critical incidents, clinical governance and professional performance, plus their general management responsibilities which include the delivery of agreed activity, meeting national targets and remaining within budget. Clinical directors have responsibilities for annual appraisal and job plans of consultant colleagues and coordinate and monitor the workload, performance and training needs of other medical staff in the directorate. Medical directors have corporate responsibilities and provide professional medical advice to the trust board. These clinicians act as the bridge between the trust board and senior management team, and the body of clinicians without formal management roles. Time for these duties must be reflected in the job plan.

Many physicians undertake a wide range of activities outside their trusts, for the wider interest of the NHS. These contributions are vital to the future of the NHS. They include advisory roles in postgraduate education, specialty societies or charities, research funding bodies, service inspections, development of national guidelines or national service frameworks (NSFs), and a range of requests for expert advice from the DH or other national bodies. Additional College activities include curriculum development, examining and standard setting. Time must be allocated for these duties, and this is reflected in the recent advice from the DH.

STANDARDS OF CLINICAL PRACTICE

The principles contained in the GMC statements regarding the duties of a doctor outline the standards of care that patients should expect from medical practitioners.[5] The GMC stipulates that doctors should keep their knowledge and competence up to date, must be aware of changes in statutes and legislation, and must work with others to ensure quality of care.

The Federation of the Royal Colleges of the UK has built on the standards set out by the GMC in *Good medical practice*, producing *Good medical practice for physicians*.[14] This document defines standards for physicians in each of the areas identified by the GMC, along with evidence that should be collected to support them. Additionally, in 20 appendices published on the College website there is guidance on specialty standards and evidence for the main medical specialties (**www.rcplondon.ac.uk/college/pa/prof_gmpfp.htm**).

It follows that all doctors must partake in, and be seen to partake in, CPD activities. Doctors must be aware of recommended standards for practice emanating from national bodies such as the NSF and the National Institute for Clinical Excellence (NICE), or specialty societies, and must demonstrate to their colleagues and to the public that they continue to maintain high quality clinical care. This requires an audit process in which the structures, processes and outcomes of care are systematically evaluated both against absolute standards, as set out in the documents referred to above, and against a relative standard derived from the performance of peers. Audit is a demanding and time-consuming activity but essential for physicians to demonstrate that care is of an acceptable standard or to identify what needs to be changed to improve current practice. The results of assessments of the quality of care are as important as data collected on the amount of care delivered.

The annual appraisal process should ensure review of an individual's work and performance (quantity and quality), identify any personal or professional development needs and highlight resource issues that compromise or threaten high quality practice. The appraisal process and folder, including data from both CPD and audit (including patient surveys or questionnaires), provide the documentation to meet the requirements for professional revalidation. The Government has set up a system for assuring and monitoring the performance of the NHS, via national performance indicators and the Healthcare Commission.

The College has taken a lead in setting and promoting the highest standards of medical practice. Measuring the quality of practice demands the setting of standards (guideline production) and the development of measurement instruments that can assess whether performance meets the standards. The Clinical Effectiveness and Evaluation Unit (CEEu) leads these activities, with input from all the disciplines making up the clinical team and from patient organisations. College guideline work includes projects that are entirely in-house such as the *National clinical guidelines for stroke.*[15] The College also houses the National Collaborating Centre for Chronic Conditions, a collaborative multiprofessional centre commissioned by NICE to develop an average of three new clinical guidelines each year. These guidelines are produced according to systematic methods so that all appropriate evidence is retrieved, critically appraised and augmented by expert opinion from the multidisciplinary groups.

The CEEu also promotes a series of shorter guidance documents from specialty societies that cover more limited areas of medicine in a manner pertinent to the general physician. These are still evidence based but produced at a fraction of the cost and are appearing as a series in the College journal, *Clinical Medicine*. The standards are nationally relevant, but the benchmark is usually defined by reference to the performance of similar units treating similar types of patients.

Measurement of performance requires that, for each topic, an appropriate multidisciplinary group defines what data needs to be collected, how to facilitate collection and how to record and analyse results, in order to provide a reliable and robust report for clinicians and managers. A sufficient number of hospitals should take part so that the benchmarking process is seen to be of value. Once data are available the College can feed the data back to the clinicians and chief executive officer (CEO) in each hospital and subsequently send a subsidiary report to the StHA and others with responsibility for use of the data.

The CEEu has pioneered two successful approaches to national performance benchmarking. The first is typified by the National Sentinel Audit of Stroke Care, which collects a 'snapshot' of the organisation, process and outcome of care on 40 consecutive patients and compares the results to care across other participating units. The stroke audit is repeated every two years and has demonstrated that the results are robust and have facilitated changes that have led directly to better care. In the most recent iteration, all hospitals in England, Wales and Northern Ireland have taken part voluntarily, confirming local support for the process. Government bodies such as the NHS Clinical Governance Support Team (CGST) and the Healthcare Commission have also made use of the data and the NSF for Older People recommends that all hospitals take part.

The second type of data collection is the Myocardial Infarction National Audit Project (MINAP), which collects a limited number of data items selected to address key targets in the NSF for Coronary Heart Disease. The data are collected using a sophisticated database package, the Central Cardiac Audit Database (CCAD), which allows local teams to view full data on local patients but ensures that only anonymous data can be viewed by others, including the central analysis team. The system operates in real time, and allows full comparison of trusts across the country. Every three months a more detailed report is made available to the teams and to the CEO in each trust.

The success of these projects results from the ability to feed in robust, comparative data from many hospitals. Careful and accurate interpretation has gained the clinical confidence of professionals and credibility with managers. Both the MINAP and stroke projects have shown substantial changes in clinical practice that are linked to improved patient outcomes. Results are being shared with SHAs and with the Healthcare Commission where they feed into the performance assessments of hospitals. The CGST has used the stroke data to work with hospital managers to help them understand the clinical and financial implications of running a service.

Beyond specific in-house projects, the CEEu works closely with the specialty societies, through the Clinical Effectiveness Forum, to facilitate the development of guidelines and disseminate knowledge more widely. Funding and time constraints limit progress, but the College is committed to improving the quality of patient care through setting standards and auditing practice.

8 Consultant workforce

One of the key aims of the Medical Workforce Unit is to provide accurate and clinically relevant data on the numbers and working patterns of hospital consultants in order to inform workforce planning. The unit carries out the annual Census of physicians, recently extended to cover the whole of the UK on behalf of the Federation of Medical Royal Colleges. Findings from the Census are published by the Federation each year.

Census data are used to support the College in improving standards in clinical practice for the benefit of patients. Information about the workload of physicians identifies the large numbers of patients requiring care in acute medicine and the specialties. It is evident that the time available for patient care may be less than ideal. The time required for direct clinical care, in addition to management and administrative activities, keeping up to date, training and all of the other professional activities results in great pressure on individual consultants and the service as a whole. These difficulties should be identified in the job planning process for an individual physician within each trust. Data produced by the College demonstrate the size of the problem nationally. Figures from the College are used in planning the future consultant physician workforce in collaboration with the DH, and can be used to model the impact of the EWTD and the 2003 consultant contract. The information supplied by the Medical Workforce Unit is valued by the specialties for their own planning, and for use in developing national service frameworks.

The most recent Census of consultant physicians was carried out in September 2003.[16] The information resulting from this has highlighted a number of issues relevant to the work of the College in setting standards in medical practice and in improving the quality of care for patients. There were 7,854 consultant physicians (7,318 whole time equivalents (WTEs)) working in the NHS in the UK, representing an increase of 3.6% compared to 2002, although across England, Wales and Northern Ireland there has been an average increase of 6.2% per year over the past 10 years.

In general, consultants in acute specialties work nearly 60 hours per week but the average for all consultants is 50 hours per week. The EWTD restricts working hours to 48 per week, which equates to 12 PAs under the 2003 consultant contract. In order to meet the requirements of the Directive, 1,323 (16.8%) more consultants will be required if there is to be no reduction in clinical activity. Many more consultants will be required to maintain the clinical service if consultants remain under the old contract or work only 10 PAs per week under the new contract. For example, across the UK, it is calculated that there would need to be 3,808 additional consultants under the old consultant contract to meet the EWTD, and 2,911 additional consultants across the UK if physicians worked 10 PAs.

It is widely accepted that additional consultants are required. In the NHS Plan, the Government set a target of 7,500 more consultants by 2004.[3] For England, Wales and Northern Ireland, this would mean an additional 1,681 consultant physicians, giving a total of 7,284. By the end of September 2003, there was a deficit of 972 consultants against this target. The current expansion rate of the past 12 months (3.6%) will not achieve the target. There are insufficient numbers of trained individuals to take up consultant posts. If every post advertised last year had been filled, the expansion rate would have been of the order of 15%.

Pragmatic estimates of the workforce requirement to meet the clinical need for each specialty over the next few years are set out in the following tables. The figures may differ from the final targets identified by each specialty as desirable, and set out in the specialty sections in Part 2. Clearly, very large increases will not be possible in the immediate future, although the overall view of many specialties is that at least 100% more consultants are required.

Surveys have indicated that most women and some men in SpR posts might choose to work part-time in the future and this must be taken into account in planning. Of current numbers of SpRs, 42% are female and, although the overall proportion of women in consultant posts is increasing slowly (currently 21.7%), 42% of the consultant force aged 34 and younger are female. There is evidence that the increase in numbers of women graduating from medical school may mean that the number of women doctors will exceed male doctors by the year 2012.

In some specialties, for example clinical pharmacology and infectious diseases, a high proportion of consultants hold academic posts, thus the numbers required to deliver the clinical service to patients will be affected by the requirement to provide teaching and commitments to research. Changing clinical practice or arising unforeseen issues, such as potential bio-terrorism, can also have a sudden impact on workforce planning.

PATTERN OF CONSULTANT WORK

Direct patient care

Overall, 47% of consultants stated that they were on call for unselected emergency admissions. Over 80% of consultants on call are from diabetes and endocrinology, gastroenterology, respiratory medicine and geriatric medicine, and from numerically smaller specialties such as clinical pharmacology. Most physicians were on call for patients of all ages but 29% of geriatricians were on call only for patients over 75 years of age. The mean frequency of on-call duties was 1:10.8. There were 21% of consultants on call at more than one location and 6% of consultants were single-handed in their specialties.

In the acute medical specialties, an average of 59 patients were admitted on take – a significant increase compared to 2000 when it was reported that 49 patients were admitted on take.[17] Of physicians in acute specialties, 45% continued the care of these admissions, although an average of 19 patients per week were transferred to other specialties for particular problems requiring specialist care. In acute specialties, 81% of respondents followed up general medical problems in their clinic; an average of four each week. An average of nine patients were transferred to other specialties for outpatient follow up after discharge and 11 were discharged to the care of their GP for follow up.

Consultants in the acute specialties who undertake general medicine spent, on average, 12 hours per week on this, mostly on ward work, although a mean of four new outpatient referrals each week were general medical in nature.

Consultants spent an average of 21 hours per week in their main specialty (of which 11 were in outpatients, six on the wards and the remainder in other activities). Consultants in cardiology and gastroenterology spent about nine hours per week in special procedures. It was reported by 27% of consultants that they were on call for duties other than acute medical take. Two-thirds of these were on a specialty on-call rota to cover general tasks and 28% for specialty-specific tasks such as emergency gastrointestinal endoscopy and bronchoscopy.

Gastroenterologists make up 41% of the consultants in this group and they also make up the largest proportion of consultants on call for other duties apart from acute takes (14.2%).

Consultants have many other responsibilities in the NHS in addition to general medicine and their main specialty commitment; nearly 10% have an additional specialty. Furthermore, consultants spend a mean of 32 hours per week in other work, some of which is direct patient care. This includes communications (to GPs, other doctors, patients and their relatives), education and training, CPD, work for the postgraduate deaneries or as medical or clinical director for their trust, and academic research in support of the wider NHS.

RECOMMENDATIONS

Consultant workforce
There need to be sufficient consultants to provide a safe and high quality healthcare service in hospitals. The recommendations by the various specialties are set out in Part 2 of this document and the immediate needs in tables 1–6.

The workforce needs to be expanded to meet the current and future needs, and the changing agenda in education and working hours. However, the College also recommends that other ways of working should be explored. These include the development of physicians specialising in acute medicine, and enhancing and extending the role of nurses and other non-medical healthcare professionals. Additional administrative and secretarial support, to release consultants from unnecessary clerical duties, would impact favourably on the workload, allowing more time for direct clinical care.

The opportunities for flexible and part-time working at different stages in a consultant's career should be enhanced. There should also be more opportunities for working part-time after retirement.

Consultants in the medical specialties

WORKFORCE FIGURES

The following tables (pages 23–28) summarise the returns of the 2003 Census of consultant physicians. The tables also incorporate estimates of consultant requirements provided by the specialties for Part 2 of this document. These figures may need to be reviewed in the light of recommendations arising out of deliberations that have a bearing on the workforce, such as those on skillmix and national service frameworks, besides other developments in practice and service delivery.

Consultants in the medical specialties: numbers in post and estimates of numbers required for UK, England, Wales, Northern Ireland and Scotland.

Information provided by the medical specialties and from the Royal College of Physicians Consultant Census, September 2003.

Table 1: United Kingdom. Population 58,251,978.

| Specialty | Consultants required* | | | Additional consultants required | | |
	Per 250k population (WTEs)	Total (WTEs)	Consultants in post now (WTEs)	WTEs	Percentage increase	Annual % expansion needed over 10 years
Allergy	0.15	35	17	18	106	7
Audiological medicine	0.28	65	32	33	104	7
Cardiology	7.70	1,794	700	1,094	156	10
Clinical genetics	1.00	233	114	119	104	7
Clinical neurophysiology	0.75	175	69	106	153	10
Clinical pharmacology and therapeutics	1.00	233	64	169	264	14
Dermatology (no NCCG support)	4.50	1,049	447	602	135	9
Diabetes and endocrinology	5.00	1,165	579	586	101	7
Gastroenterology	6.95	1,619	711	908	128	9
Genitourinary medicine	3.00	699	267	432	162	10
Geriatric medicine	7.05	1,643	1,030	613	59	5
Haematology	3.70	862	589	273	46	4
Immunology	0.49	114	51	63	124	8
Infectious diseases and tropical medicine	0.83	193	71	122	172	11
Medical oncology	1.72	401	182	219	120	8
Neurology	3.90	909	403	506	125	8
Nuclear medicine	0.50	117	58	59	101	7
Palliative medicine	2.00	466	236	230	97	7
Rehabilitation medicine	1.00	233	125	108	86	6
Renal medicine	2.45	571	307	264	86	6
Respiratory medicine	6.00	1,398	614	784	128	9
Rheumatology	2.78	648	468	180	38	3

* Based on estimates submitted by specialties.
WTE = whole time equivalent.

Table 2: England. Population 48,630,500.

Specialty	Consultants required*			Additional consultants required		
	Per 250k population (WTEs)	Total (WTEs)	Consultants in post now (WTEs)	WTEs	Percentage increase	Annual % expansion needed over 10 years
Allergy	0.15	29	17	12	72	6
Audiological medicine	0.28	54	29	25	88	7
Cardiology	7.70	1,498	580	918	158	10
Clinical genetics	1.00	195	91	104	114	8
Clinical neurophysiology	0.75	146	62	84	135	9
Clinical pharmacology and therapeutics	1.00	195	47	148	314	15
Dermatology (no NCCG support)	4.50	875	372	503	135	9
Diabetes and endocrinology	5.00	973	471	502	106	8
Gastroenterology	6.95	1,352	595	757	127	9
Genitourinary medicine	3.00	584	242	342	141	9
Geriatric medicine	7.05	1,371	821	550	67	5
Haematology	3.70	720	472	248	52	4
Immunology	0.49	95	43	52	122	8
Infectious diseases and tropical medicine	0.83	161	49	112	229	13
Medical oncology	1.72	335	156	179	114	8
Neurology	3.90	759	343	416	121	8
Nuclear medicine	0.50	97	49	48	98	7
Palliative medicine	2.00	389	191	198	104	7
Rehabilitation medicine	1.00	195	100	95	95	7
Renal medicine	2.45	477	238	239	100	7
Respiratory medicine	6.00	1,167	518	649	125	8
Rheumatology	2.78	541	406	135	33	3

* Based on estimates submitted by specialties.
WTE = whole time equivalent.

Table 3: Northern Ireland. Population 1,685,267.

Specialty	Consultants required* Per 250k population (WTEs)	Consultants required* Total (WTEs)	Consultants in post (WTEs)	Additional consultants required WTEs
Allergy	0.15	1	0	1
Audiological medicine	0.28	2	1	1
Cardiology	7.70	52	22	30
Clinical genetics	1.00	7	2	5
Clinical neurophysiology	0.75	5	1	4
Clinical pharmacology and therapeutics	1.00	7	2	5
Dermatology (no NCCG support)	4.50	30	10	20
Diabetes and endocrinology	5.00	34	13	21
Gastroenterology	6.95	47	16	31
Genitourinary medicine	3.00	20	1	19
Geriatric medicine	7.05	48	29	19
Haematology	3.70	25	14	11
Immunology	0.49	3	1	2
Infectious diseases and tropical medicine	0.83	6	2	4
Medical oncology	1.72	12	3	9
Neurology	3.90	26	8	18
Nuclear medicine	0.50	3	0	3
Palliative medicine	2.00	13	4	9
Rehabilitation medicine	1.00	7	2	5
Renal medicine	2.45	17	12	5
Respiratory medicine	6.00	40	14	26
Rheumatology	2.78	19	9	10

* Based on estimates submitted by specialties.
WTE = whole time equivalent.

Table 4: Wales. Population 2,874,200.

| Specialty | Consultants required* | | Consultants in post | Additional consultants required |
	Per 250k population (WTEs)	Total (WTEs)	(WTEs)	WTEs
Allergy	0.15	2	0	2
Audiological medicine	0.28	3	1	2
Cardiology	7.70	89	33	56
Clinical genetics	1.00	11	6	5
Clinical neurophysiology	0.75	9	1	8
Clinical pharmacology and therapeutics	1.00	11	1	10
Dermatology (no NCCG support)	4.50	52	19	33
Diabetes and endocrinology	5.00	57	30	27
Gastroenterology	6.95	80	33	47
Genitourinary medicine	3.00	34	8	26
Geriatric medicine	7.05	81	46	35
Haematology	3.70	43	31	12
Immunology	0.49	6	1	5
Infectious diseases and tropical medicine	0.83	10	3	7
Medical oncology	1.72	20	4	16
Neurology	3.90	45	11	34
Nuclear medicine	0.50	6	0	6
Palliative medicine	2.00	23	9	14
Rehabilitation medicine	1.00	11	4	7
Renal medicine	2.45	28	13	15
Respiratory medicine	6.00	69	28	41
Rheumatology	2.78	32	19	13

* Based on estimates submitted by specialties.
WTE = whole time equivalent.

Table 5: Scotland. Population 5,062,011.

| Specialty | Consultants required* | | Consultants in post (WTEs) | Additional consultants required |
	Per 250k population (WTEs)	Total (WTEs)		WTEs
Allergy	0.15	3	0	3
Audiological medicine	0.28	6	1	5
Cardiology	7.70	156	65	91
Clinical genetics	1.00	20	15	5
Clinical neurophysiology	0.75	15	5	10
Clinical pharmacology and therapeutics	1.00	20	14	6
Dermatology (no NCCG support)	4.50	91	46	45
Diabetes and endocrinology	5.00	101	65	36
Gastroenterology	6.95	141	67	74
Genitourinary medicine	3.00	61	16	45
Geriatric medicine	7.05	143	134	9
Haematology	3.70	75	72	3
Immunology	0.49	10	6	4
Infectious diseases and tropical medicine	0.83	17	17	0
Medical oncology	1.72	35	19	16
Neurology	3.90	79	41	38
Nuclear medicine	0.50	10	9	1
Palliative medicine	2.00	40	32	10
Rehabilitation medicine	1.00	20	19	2
Renal medicine	2.45	50	45	5
Respiratory medicine	6.00	121	54	67
Rheumatology	2.78	56	34	22

* Based on estimates submitted by specialties.
WTE = whole time equivalent.

Additional WTE consultants needed to meet population requirements. United Kingdom.

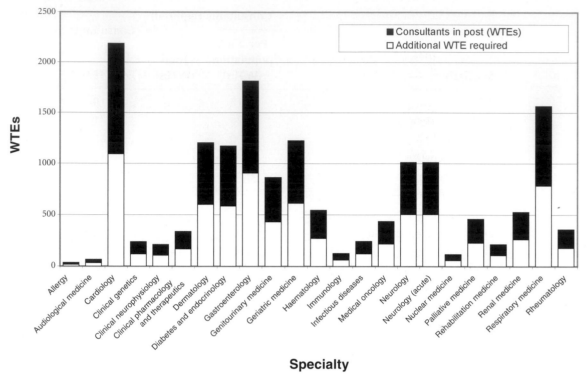

References

1. Royal College of Physicians. *Consultant physicians working for patients.* 1st edition. London: RCP, 1999.

2. Royal College of Physicians. *Consultant physicians working for patients.* 2nd edition. London: RCP, 2001.

3. Department of Health. *The NHS cancer plan: a plan for investment, a plan for reform.* London: DH, 2000.

4. Irvine, Sir D. *Patient centred professionalism – decision time.* The 2003 Duncan Memorial Lecture. www.kingsfund.org.uk/PDF/duncanmemorial.pdf

5. General Medical Council. *Good medical practice.* London: GMC, 2001.

6. Department of Health. *AL(MD) 3/2003 Introduction of the 2003 consultant contract (England).* London: DH, 2003.

7. Royal College of Physicians. *Guidance on the new consultant contract and its implications for job plans (programmed activities),* 2004. www.rcplondon.ac.uk/professional/consultantcontract/index.asp

8. Donaldson, Sir Liam. *Unfinished business: proposals for reform of the senior house officer grade.* London: NHS, 2002.

9. Department of Health, Scottish Executive and Welsh Assembly Government. *Modernising medical careers: the next steps.* London: DH, 2004.

10. Royal College of Physicians. *Acute medicine: making it work for patients.* Report of a working party. London: RCP, 2004.

11. Royal College of Physicians. *The interface of accident & emergency and acute medicine.* Report of a working party. London: RCP, 2002.

12. Royal College of Physicans. *The interface between acute general medicine and critical care.* Report of a working party. London: RCP, 2002.

13. Royal College of Physicians. *Continuity of care for medical inpatients: standards of good practice.* London: RCP, 2004.

14. Royal College of Physicians. *Good medical practice for physicians.* London: RCP, 2004.

15. Royal College of Physicians. *National clinical guidelines for stroke.* 2nd edition. Report of an intercollegiate working party. London: RCP, 2004.

16. The Federation of the Royal Colleges of Physicians of the United Kingdom. *Census of consultant physicians in the UK, 2003. Data and commentary.* London: The Federation of the Royal Colleges of Physicians of the United Kingdom, 2003.

17. The Federation of the Royal Colleges of Physicians of the United Kingdom. *Census of consultant physicians in the UK, 2000. Data and commentary.* London: The Federation of the Royal Colleges of Physicians of the United Kingdom, 2000.

PART 2

WORK IN THE SPECIALTIES

Introduction

Part 1 of *Consultant physicians working with patients* describes the duties and responsibilities of consultant physicians and the ways in which they work to maintain and improve the quality of patient care. It emphasises the importance of working with patients, and of clinical engagement in service development and commissioning of healthcare services. It sets out recommendations for resources, time, manpower and facilities required to allow physicians to practise high quality medicine.

Part 2 describes each of the medical specialties, the organisation of specialist services and the facilities and staff required to meet the clinical needs of patients. Through the work of our Medical Workforce Unit and our joint specialty committees we are able to give advice regarding workforce requirements and the content of consultant job plans.

SPECIALTY STATEMENTS

The joint specialty committees and specialist societies have drawn up statements within a common format, but outlining the characteristics of each specialty and the variations in organisation and practice. The styles and presentations necessarily vary, reflecting the differing approaches, but the information and key concerns are consistent.

Each section has been prepared through wide consultation within each specialty and therefore carries particular authority; they may be referred to as position statements for the specialties. They will inform and support clinicians and managers in identifying deficiencies and in planning the development, provision, organisation and delivery of services.

A further aim of the statements is to inform and guide the preparation of job plans and the annual appraisal. With the advent of the 2003 consultant contract, consultant duties are now expressed as 'programmed activities' (PAs) rather than the traditional notional half-day. All new job descriptions will be expressed in terms of PAs, and the job plans in the statements reflect this. We believe the specimen job plans will be useful to established consultants at annual appraisal, whether they elect to stay with their existing contract or elect to change. Many duties, including work to maintain and improve the clinical service, were previously recorded as 'administration' in flexible sessions. Any activity that involves the care of individual patients should now be included as direct clinical care. This includes clinic letters, reviewing and communicating results, providing advice to GPs and other healthcare practitioners, telephone consultations, seeing relatives, multidisciplinary team (MDT) meetings, X-ray meetings and case conferences/presentations, prioritising referrals, organising investigations, providing clinical reports and other clinical correspondence, addressing complaints or critical incidents and so on.

For many specialties there is substantial clinical activity for work relating to outpatient consultations or procedures. Some specialties have identified, for example, 0.5 PA to support each outpatient clinic, others have identified between 1.5 and often 2.5 PAs required to cover these various clinical duties, reflecting differing specialties and work practice.

Professional work to maintain and improve the quality of the clinical service, as well as service development, now needs to be included under the PAs for supporting professional duties. The supporting professional activities include research, education and training, management, clinical governance, audit, appraisal, continuing professional development (CPD) and revalidation. Where individual clinicians have an increased commitment to teaching, research, specific management roles or other additional duties, this needs to be formally recognised in the job plan by an appropriate increase in the number of PAs for supporting professional activities. Physicians may have rotating commitments with other colleagues and may agree an annualised job plan. Some may undertake external duties that are formally recognised within the job plan; others may agree ad hoc activities under special category leave.

The Clinical Academic Contract (England) 2003 allows clinical academic physicians to agree an integrated job plan with their NHS and university employers. Physicians with a significant academic commitment will have separate PAs identified for university and NHS work. Clinical academic contracts will vary but, in general, will be based on five PAs for the university and five involving work for the NHS.

Many existing consultants are working in excess of 10 PAs. New consultant posts should have a job description based on 10 PAs, although the successful candidate may agree additional sessions with the trust after appointment. The statements describe the different aspects of patient care and the duties and workload represented in one PA. The job plans illustrate a range of different activities, reflecting current clinical practice. The precise balance between PAs for direct clinical care, supporting professional activities, additional NHS responsibilities and external activities will be negotiated individually at the job plan review.

Broadly, each specialty statement describes:

- The specialty and clinical needs of patients.
- Organisation of the service at primary, secondary and tertiary levels, including clinical networks and community arrangements, patterns of referral and relationships with other services.
- Ways of working with patients to ensure a patient-centred service, outlining the importance of patient choice, involving patients in decisions about their treatment, and opportunities for education and promoting self-care as well as the role of carers. Details of patient support groups, expert patient programmes, other relevant information and discussion regarding support for patients with chronic conditions are included.
- The work of the MDT, and the interspecialty and interdisciplinary liaison required to deliver care, including reference to general practitioners with a specialist interest.
- The characteristics of a high quality service and the resources required for ensuring this, including clinical workforce and support staff and specialised facilities.
- Quality standards and measures of the quality of specialist services, including specialist society guidelines, national service frameworks (NSFs) and National Institute for Clinical Excellence (NICE) guidelines.
- Details of the work of consultants in the specialty, including contribution to acute medicine, direct clinical care, work to maintain and improve the quality of care, service development, education and training, appraisal and mentoring of other staff, continuing medical education (CME) and clinical governance, research, management and leadership, and regional and national work.
- The duties, responsibilities and areas of work of academic physicians, with particular reference to the clinical contribution to NHS work.
- Workforce requirements for the specialty.
- Specimen job plan.

Allergy

i Description of the specialty and clinical needs of patients

Allergic disorders are wide-ranging and cross organ-based disciplines. Allergists require expertise specific to allergy and knowledge of diseases managed by a number of other specialties, particularly respiratory medicine, dermatology, ear nose and throat (ENT) medicine and paediatrics.

Allergic disease varies from mild to life-threatening. There has been a doubling in prevalence of the more common allergic disorders – asthma, eczema and rhinitis – in the last two to three decades. One-third of the population suffer from allergic disease and impaired quality of life, resulting in considerable direct cost to the health service.[1] Allergy is one of the most common chronic disorders. It has been suggested that part of the increase in prevalence may be related to a westernised lifestyle and lack of infection in childhood.

In addition, there has been a rapid rise in serious and multisystem allergic disease and the emergence of new disorders. Severe anaphylaxis originating outside hospitals occurred in one in 3,500 of the UK population in 1994, and the incidence is rising.[2,3] Hospital admissions increased seven-fold over 10 years and doubled over four years.[4] Anaphylaxis occurs in 1.2–16.8% of the US population, depending on aetiology.[5] The incidence of peanut allergy – the commonest food cause of fatal and near-fatal reactions – has trebled over four years. Peanut allergy now affects 1.6% of children.[6,7,8] Up to 8% of healthcare workers have latex allergy, yet only the second case of latex allergy was described in 1979.[9,10] Others are affected by drug allergy/intolerance, which accounts for 5% of hospital admissions, and by other food allergies. Much of this serious disease occurs in patients who also have allergic asthma, rhinitis and eczema.

Traditionally, much of allergy care has been provided by organ-based specialists. More recently, immunologists and paediatricians with a special interest in allergy have provided a part-time service in allergy as an add-on to their main specialty, usually in limited areas or in general practice. There are a small number of specialist allergy services run by consultant allergists, mainly in academic centres.

The rise in severe and life-threatening allergic disease and multisystem allergic disease – the allergy epidemic – has created a new and substantial demand for the expertise of a consultant allergist. Further, management of the newly emerged disorders (nut allergy, latex allergy and drug allergies) requires knowledge gained from dealing with large numbers of patients. For many patients, this need is unmet. It is not appropriate for severe or non-organ-based disorders to be dealt with by non-specialists. The lack of access to specialist care for many patients and long waiting lists are unacceptable in a modern health service. This system of healthcare delivery does not manage disease optimally and leads to unnecessary cost to the NHS.

A Royal College of Physicians expert working party has made proposals to improve patient care.[11] Key to development of services is the creation of at least one major allergy centre in each region (or population of about five million), staffed by sufficient adult and paediatric allergists. This requires an increase in the number of consultants and a substantial expansion in allergy trainees. Such an investment would provide the infrastructure and expertise to begin to develop services throughout the region. The proposed programme for change would provide care in the first instance for the more serious disorders, and would be the focus for education in primary and secondary care. The proposals are a rational approach to the construction of a new pattern of allergy services within the NHS in response to the developing epidemic.

A House of Commons Health Committee enquiry into the provision of allergy services in 2004 endorsed the College report. It identified that there is a problem and that the appropriate response is to develop a national allergy service. The Committee went further, making recommendations for implementing change within manpower (see later) and comissioning, and for a major allergy centre in each area of the country. [12]

Allergy is a small specialty with its own training programme and certificate of completion of specialist training (CCST).

ii Organisation of the service and patterns of referral

Allergy is a specialty recognised for specialist commissioning. Disorders which should be seen in tertiary centres are listed in the Department of Health (DH) definition of specialist allergy services (definition no. 17).[13]

Currently, allergy services are extremely poor and fail to meet the clinical need.[14,15] Services have developed ad hoc in academic units and there is no tradition of NHS investment. Of 101 allergy services, six are run by consultant allergists providing a full-time service; nine by consultant allergists providing part-time services; and the remaining 86 clinics are part-time and run by consultants in other specialties who offer a limited spectrum of diagnostic and treatment facilities.[16] There is a shortage of consultant allergists; large parts of England have none. Full-time services led by consultant allergists are mainly in London and the south-east.

GPs, who deal with the brunt of allergic disease, have little or no training and little access to specialist advice. Patients have difficulty accessing allergy services, either because they do not exist or because of waiting lists or restricted access in some trusts. The British Society for Allergy and Clinical Immunology (BSACI) and the National Allergy Strategy Group (NASG) held discussions with the DH to highlight the need to improve services. Current services and proposals for allergy care have been outlined most recently in the College report *Allergy: the unmet need. A blueprint for better patient care.*[11,15]

In a model of allergy care there would be three tiers, as follows:[11,15]

1) Simpler allergic diseases would be dealt with in primary care.

2a) Consultant allergists in smaller centres in teaching hospitals and in district general hospitals (DGHs) would provide secondary care.

2b) Until the shortage of allergists can be corrected, organ-based and other specialists with an interest in allergy (dermatologists, respiratory physicians, ENT specialists, paediatricians, immunologists) would contribute to secondary care.

3) Regional allergy centres would deal with the more specialised tertiary problems, and provide secondary care for their locality. Currently, because of the lack of provision described at 2a above, regional centres provide secondary care for a larger area.

The College proposed that the immediate aim should be to develop regional allergy centres to provide expertise, improve geographical equality of care and to act as an educational resource and training centre for each region. These specialist centres should be drivers for change, while giving access for the most serious allergy cases. The College proposals are designed to move the service towards a clinically rational and patient-sensitive pattern of provision.

Special patterns of referral

Because of the lack of allergists, major centres receive both secondary and tertiary referrals from within and outside their area. Systems must be in place to ensure that urgent referrals (anaphylaxis, life-threatening angioedema) are seen quickly. Anaesthetists need rapid access to their regional centre for diagnosis of anaphylaxis during anaesthesia, and should establish referral systems.

iii Working with patients: patient-centred care

Opportunities for education and promoting self-care

Good allergy care requires accurate diagnosis and, importantly, identification of triggers which may then be avoided. Avoiding allergic triggers, for example foods or drugs, completely ameliorates symptoms, and reduces acute attacks (anaphylaxis, urticaria or angioedema) and chronic illness (asthma, rhinitis or eczema). Early whole-system effective intervention prevents chronic illness developing.[17]

Patients can contribute to self-care. Drugs are provided in management plans for self-treatment of acute attacks in case of mistaken exposure to the allergic trigger or in idiopathic reactions, for example in food-induced reactions, anaphylaxis to insect stings or glottal oedema. There is evidence that this reduces the burden of disease (see *Clinical work* below). Where avoidance is not possible, symptomatic relief can be obtained with the correct medicine. Informing and involving the patient is a crucial aspect of effective allergy care and nurse specialists contribute to this.

Access to information and patient support groups

The patient support groups – Allergy UK and the Anaphylaxis Campaign – are members of the NASG and support the College proposals. The most common reason for calls to their helplines is difficulty in being referred to an allergy clinic, or finding one able to deal with their specific problem.

iv Interspecialty and interdisciplinary liaison

Working with other specialists

Regional centres should have a minimum of two consultants and, ideally, two paediatric allergists. Allergists should work as part of a larger clinical team, including allergy specialist registrars (SpRs) and specialist nurses, to provide an efficient service and because of the clinical risks involved in certain procedures and treatments (eg challenge testing and immunotherapy). Links with adult and paediatric dietitians ensure that patients avoiding foods long term have nutritionally adequate diets.

Allergists liaise with other specialists including respiratory physicians, dermatologists, immunologists, ENT consultants and paediatricians. These consultants may refer patients to allergy or be involved in the care of allergy patients. Allergists in regional centres have a key role in educating GPs and other consultants who deal with allergy patients in their region. A clinical immunology laboratory service run by a consultant immunologist must be available.

Community paediatric teams are needed to provide support for children at risk of anaphylaxis in schools.[18] A community paediatrician should provide support in his/her area and liaise closely with colleagues in other health authorities and the allergy team. Agreed protocols for school visits must be in place. Community paediatric nurses carry out school and nursery visits to train staff in avoidance of allergen (eg nuts), and recognition and management of reactions. They should have access to the allergy consultant for queries.

Occupational health physicians refer staff who have latex allergies, other occupational allergies or adverse reactions to vaccination. Allergy and occupational health consultants should lead in the development, implementation and review of the trust latex policy.

Anaesthetists from a wide geographic area liaise with allergists in regional centres. Established systems for referral of patients with suspected anaphylaxis during anaesthesia should be in place. The majority of these patients need to be treated in major allergy centres that have appropriate expertise and receive a sufficient volume of patients.

Multidisciplinary team working

Allergy specialist nurses   Nurses with appropriate training are key members of the team. They carry out skin prick testing; provide advice on allergen avoidance; train patients to use self-treatments (adrenaline autoinjectors and inhalers); monitor patients undergoing immunotherapy and challenge tests; support doctors in treatment of acute reactions including anaphylaxis; at times, use questionnaires to support history taking in defined disorders; and may support follow up of certain disorders.

Dietitians (adult and paediatric) trained in allergy   Dietitians assess the nutritional adequacy of diet, advise on diagnostic exclusion and long-term diets. This is an important role in paediatric allergy.

Pharmacy and drug information service   This service will search for ingredients of drugs, provide capsules for drugs for challenge tests, drugs for skin testing and challenge tests, and information on adverse reactions.

v   Delivering a high quality service

Characteristics of a high quality service: requirements for consultant allergists

Consultant allergists should have completed an accredited training programme and be on the specialist register of the General Medical Council (GMC). Applicants from outside the UK will be expected to demonstrate comparable quality of training, as assessed by the Joint Council for Higher Medical Training (JCHMT) of the College. Allergists should not work in isolation; they must have appropriate support staff including specialist allergy nurses.

The concept of a quality driven service, with standards of care clearly defined in contracts, provides a framework in which the allergy care for a community can be improved.

Resources required for a high quality service

The table below gives an overview of standards and resources required in any specialist allergy centre. This is what is currently proposed for the regional allergy centres – the change drivers which will establish the service and enable a more rational and patient-sensitive model to emerge. Workforce requirements are described in the main text. The requirements should be linked to the 2003 consultant contract, with explicit standards for service quality.

The service standard	Specialised facilities and resources required
Referral ▪ all referrals letters prioritised by the allergist ▪ explicit standards set for time from referral to first appointment for urgent and routine cases ▪ 24-hour advice available from an allergist ▪ dedicated administrative support staff.	*Referral* ▪ time for consultant to triage and review referral letters ▪ standards (determined locally) for time to first appointment for urgent and routine cases (due to the shortage of allergists this is not always a reasonable time, but urgent cases should be seen preferentially) ▪ sufficient consultant staff to provide 24-hour cover and allergy advice for existing allergy outpatients, inpatients, A&E, admissions unit and GPs ▪ dedicated secretarial and clerical support staff.
Outpatients ▪ ability to diagnose and manage all types of allergic disease ▪ adequate time for complex cases ▪ appropriate investigations available, eg skin test extracts, common foods for skin prick testing, and a system for asking patients to bring unusual foods for skin testing ▪ allergy specialist nurses ▪ appropriate interpretation of skin prick tests ▪ appropriate interpretation of intradermal tests ▪ support from adult and paediatric dietitians with knowledge of allergy ▪ defined number of patients per clinic* ▪ established links with community paediatric teams ▪ patient literature to consolidate verbal information (see below).	*Outpatients* ▪ a dedicated allergy team of trained consultant allergists and adequate numbers of medical staff ▪ dedicated clinic space, defined consulting rooms and facilities for day cases (see below) ▪ integrated facilities with outpatient and day cases seen in the same setting to improve efficiency and use of expertise ▪ allergy specialist nurses, with space to work ▪ skin testing rooms ▪ couches for safe management of at least 20 patients in one immunotherapy session, in case of anaphylaxis, and space for recuscitation around each couch ▪ immediate access to treatment for anaphylaxis (by allergist) ▪ inhalers, nebulisers, oxygen, peak flow meters, spirometry, all drugs, IV lines and fluids, tilting couches, cardiac arrest box (adult and paediatric), latex free equipment ▪ pharmacy service (with a locked refrigerator and drug storage) to supply drugs for skin testing or challenge ▪ drug information service ▪ dedicated dietitian service (adult and paediatric) with standard methods of referral to establish if a diet is nutritionally adequate and provide advice on exclusion diets ▪ easy access to, and close liaison with, lung function laboratory ▪ full investigations including immunology and imaging

continued

*Allergy patients are usually complex, and detailed history taking is essential. New patients commonly require 45 minutes and follow-up patients, 20–25 minutes. Four new and two old patients per clinic is the maximum, but will depend on case complexity and support staff.

The service standard	Specialised facilities and resources required
Outpatients	*Outpatients* ▪ child-orientated clinic with play facilities in paediatric waiting area, play assistants where possible, and appropriate paediatric dress for nurses and doctors ▪ community paediatric team with dedicated time for support of children at risk of anaphylaxis in schools ▪ liaison with community paediatrician: agreed management plan, systems for implementation in schools (local area and distant) and proforma letters, eg requesting teacher training at schools with a child at risk of anaphylaxis ▪ literature on various disorders (see below) ▪ dedicated secretarial support staff trained in allergy terminology and policies, especially to handle telephone enquiries from existing and prospective patients, GPs, nurses and other hospital specialists.
Day case management ▪ an agreed definition of a day case and recognition of the time required to perform the various investigations, procedures or treatments ▪ protocols and agreed systems for approach to diagnosis ▪ sufficient caseload of each category of day case to ensure expertise ▪ ability to investigate, exclude or confirm drug allergy ▪ expertise and ability to carry out inhaled and oral challenges ▪ ability to interpret results of investigation and challenge, and to provide a clear and high quality report, eg for anaphylaxis during anaesthesia ▪ 24-hour advice available after discharge of day cases. *Immunotherapy clinic* ▪ immunotherapy performed by trained medical and nursing staff (an allergy team) with a patient load large enough to ensure continuing standards of care ▪ defined number of patients per session, eg 20–25 patients per two doctors, according to risk assessment (ideally, two doctors per clinic for safety reasons) ▪ expertise in carrying out immunotherapy safely and facilities for resuscitation	*Day case management* ▪ adequate numbers of medical and nursing staff trained and experienced in allergy day case investigation ▪ adequate numbers of medical and nursing staff trained and experienced in immunotherapy ▪ appointment system ▪ facilities where day case patients undergoing challenge tests can remain for a session or all day with supervision by trained nursing staff (this may be in outpatients) ▪ trained medical staff to supervise high-risk procedures such as challenge tests and immunotherapy ▪ consent forms and information sheets for the above ▪ defined procedures and protocols, including monitoring for immunotherapy ▪ accurate record keeping, especially of adverse reactions ▪ allergy specialist nurses and continuous nursing cover ▪ couches for safe management of at least 20 patients in one immunotherapy session in case of anaphylaxis and space for recuscitation around each couch ▪ immediate access to drugs and equipment for treatment for anaphylaxis and other acute allergic reactions (See *Outpatients* above) ▪ locked refrigerator and standard systems for use and storage of controlled drugs

continued

The service standard	Specialised facilities and resources required
Day case management ▮ quality standards for care of patients, decision making and monitoring for adverse reactions ▮ competence to treat anaphylaxis, acute asthma and other allergic reactions ▮ regular advanced life support training (adult and paediatric) of medical and nursing staff.	***Day case management*** ▮ facilities to make up dilutions of drugs for skin testing in day case clinic ▮ pharmacy service to supply drugs for skin testing and drugs/placebos for blinded challenge testing ▮ drug information service ▮ procedures for advance ordering of drugs for testing or challenge ▮ systems to provide regular advanced life support training.
Inpatients ▮ access to inpatient beds with junior staff cover.	***Inpatients*** ▮ agreed access to inpatient beds with junior staff cover (often shared with respiratory medicine but to be determined locally).
Literature for patients ▮ specialist literature and verbal information: treatment plans for acute allergic reactions (anaphylaxis or glottal oedema); adrenaline autoinjector instructions; diet sheets, (how to avoid foods); diagnostic exclusion diets; symptom calendars; allergen avoidance measures; proforma 'to whom it may concern' letters to highlight drug allergies (for anaphylaxis during anaesthesia, hereditary angioedema); medic alert application forms.	***Literature for patients*** ▮ medical, nursing and secretarial staff to produce, explain and distribute literature ▮ high quality websites for patients to access information.
Patient support ▮ information available and literature displayed.	***Patient support*** ▮ information available and literature displayed ▮ nursing and secretarial staff ▮ contact with patient support groups.
Records ▮ hospital notes with IT access as determined locally by the trust.	***Records*** ▮ trained administrative and appointment staff ▮ secretarial support ▮ outpatient records storage ▮ IT systems for access to appointment system and laboratories.
Communications with primary care ▮ letters sent to primary care outlining patients' diagnoses and proposed management.	***Communications with primary care*** ▮ secretarial staff ▮ full-time allergy service ▮ agreed protocols and proformas ▮ Locally determined IT systems.
Office and equipment ▮ office facilities for all members of the allergy team.	***Office and equipment*** ▮ offices for consultants (close to clinic, ideally), specialist nurses, trainees and secretaries ▮ space for clinic administrator and adequate record storage ▮ IT facilities.

Continued

The service standard	Specialised facilities and resources required
Data collection: workload ▪ coding of allergy workload ▪ data collection for monthly and annual numbers of outpatients, day cases, inpatients, and the source (primary care trust) of patients ▪ data on casemix ▪ audit of allergy work.	***Data collection: workload*** ▪ IT support systems within the trust to collect allergy data ▪ consultant/specialist nurse time to monitor demand, workload and casemix seen ▪ time for audit.
Teaching and training ▪ teaching and training of SpRs, students and nursing staff in clinic ▪ clinical meetings to discuss cases and ensure standards are maintained.	***Teaching and training*** ▪ adequate space and time in clinic for teaching (adjusted number of patients seen) ▪ weekly clinical meetings attended by medical and nursing staff.

Workforce requirements: clinical and support staff

▪ A minimum of two consultants allergist are required; they should not work alone.

▪ As the paediatric allergy service develops, consultants should be supported by two paediatric allergists.

▪ There should be at least two allergy SpRs in major centres to provide cover and to enhance training.

▪ Other medical staff, including associate specialists and GPs with a special interest (GPSIs), should be encouraged.

This is a high volume specialty with complex patients so it is essential to have adequate cover at all times and continuity of service. A team approach is crucial to provide for a high quality efficient service.

vi   Quality standards and measures of the quality of specialist services

Standards of care need to be defined and developed. There is a lack of validation of procedures for investigation of certain disorders. The BSACI is developing guidelines for investigation of specific disorders and updating guidelines on immunotherapy.[19] Consultants in major allergy centres conduct clinical research to produce evidence in support of the development of guidelines and to provide advice on best practice.

Clinical governance

Many of the requirements are listed under *Characteristics of a high quality service* above.

Measures of quality

▪ protocols for monitoring immunotherapy, accurate data collection (including adverse reactions), systems to check dose and safe administration

▪ challenge testing protocols, information sheets, consent forms, use of appropriate investigations, diagnostic outcome, apppropriate management of reactions

- training of the entire allergy team, including nursing, secretarial and other support staff
- outcome data, for example the incidence of further reactions in nut allergy, effective control of disease, identification of causes of anaphylaxis
- effectiveness of systems for allocating appropriate appointments, for example to a specialist clinic or day case clinic
- quality and appropriateness of the support literature for patients, for all disorders seen
- levels of paediatric facilites and staff expertise with children and families in clinics where adult physicians see children
- regularity of advanced life support training (adult and paediatric) for medical and nursing staff
- documentation of patient throughput (outpatients and day cases) and the nature of casemix to demonstrate that adequate numbers of specific disorders are seen in a tertiary service
- patient satisfaction data
- GP feedback (including rate of referral).

CLINICAL WORK OF CONSULTANTS IN ALLERGY

Most of the work in allergy is outpatient or day case based, with only a minimal inpatient component. Most NHS consultants have five clinics a week, some in general allergy and some in specialised clinics or day case sessions according to the consultant's interest, such as immunotherapy, day case challenge tests, anaphylaxis or venom allergy. As allergic disease becomes more severe, diagnostic challenge tests and immunotherapy are increasingly important. In the future, novel therapies to replace conventional immunotherapy are likely to increase workload.

Providing advice by telephone or letter without seeing the patient is becoming more common. The shortage of allergists, and lack of knowledge of allergy in primary care, means that consultants often provide GPs with information and act as an educational resource. There is also considerable out-of-clinic work related directly to patient care in major centres.

Contributions made to acute medicine

Allergists do not participate in the on-call rota for general medicine. However, consultants in allergy provide:

- a consultation service for urgent problems (anaphylaxis, asthma, angioedema)
- a consultation service for drug allergy including skin testing for penicillin allergy
- a consultation service for anaesthetic problems, pre-operative or post-reaction
- management of latex allergic patients on elective or emergency admission (in conjunction with the trust latex allergy policy), and a major contribution to the formulation of the trust latex policy
- consultation in A&E (eg anaphylaxis)
- urgent training in use of adrenaline autoinjector before discharge from ward or A&E.

Direct patient care

Outpatient work

General allergy clinics   The ratio of new to follow-up patients varies with the complexity of referrals and type of service but averages 1:1. A clinic might include four new plus two review patients per doctor. Extra time must be allocated for teaching and to review patients.

Immunotherapy clinic   Approximately 20 patients can be seen per clinic. Ideally, this should be staffed by two doctors plus specialist nurses, because of the risk of anaphylaxis,.

Day case challenge session   Typically, two patients can be seen in one sesssion but this depends on the number of doctors and nurses, facilities and local arrangements.

Special clinics within allergy (optional depending on specialist interests and type of centre):

- immunotherapy clinic
- challenge sessions, eg drug or food challenge
- paediatric allergy clinic (the lack of paediatric allergists means the majority of children are currently seen by adult allergists but facilities and staff should be child orientated)
- anaphylaxis clinic, including nut allergy
- drug and general anaesthetic allergy clinics
- venom allergy clinic.

Specialised investigative and therapeutic procedures

- skin prick testing and intradermal skin testing
- immunotherapy
- challenge testing: oral, parenteral and bronchial challenge tests
- occupational allergy testing.

Immunotherapy

Immunotherapy patients are seen as day cases. Management protocols and specialist nurses are essential. Systems must be in place for monitoring the patient's pulse, blood pressure and peak flow pre-injection and at 30 and 60 minutes post-injection. Symptoms should be monitored throughout to enable early detection and treatment of allergic side effects including anaphylaxis. Staff must be trained in the treatment of acute severe allergic reactions. Drugs, oxygen and a nebuliser must be immediately available. A patient having two injections will typically be in the clinic for over two hours if treatment is uneventful, and substantially longer if there is an adverse reaction.

Challenge/complex investigation sessions

These sessions are mainly for the investigation of drug allergy, food allergy or occupational allergy. They may involve skin prick tests, intradermal tests and/or challenge. As some of these investigations are not validated, major allergy centres have to deal with larger numbers of patients so that approaches to diagnosis can be evaluated and national standards set. Patients with antibiotic allergy, local anaesthetic allergy, general anaesthetic allergy, aspirin and non-steroidal anti-inflammatory drug (NSAID) sensitivity, other drug allergies and some food allergies are seen in this setting. All clinics require adequate support staff including specialist nurses. The number of patients seen depends on the complexity of the procedure.

Work to support clinics

A typical job plan for a consultant in a major centre should allow about two hours per clinic for work relating to outpatients, and time for other clinical work. This includes:

■ reviewing referral letters and allocating these to the appropriate clinic

■ advising GPs by telephone or letter without seeing the patient

■ requesting information before patients are seen (for example, anaesthetic and drug charts in case of an anaphylaxis during a general anaesthetic, or details of drugs given and reactions caused in multiple antibiotic allergy) in order that the patient can proceed directly to a complex investigation or challenge test, and to avoid wasted consultations

■ requesting additional information after the patient is seen (for example, ingredients of foods or other products to identify possible causes of anaphylaxis) and planning/preparing substances for challenge testing

■ dealing with requests relating to existing patients not currently being seen (for example, those having further allergic reactions), liaising with schools in the case of children at risk of anaphylaxis, dealing with patients with new acute allergies, updating treatment plans, investigating and identifying ingredients of meals to determine causes of anaphylaxis

■ literature searches for complex or rare cases.

In addition, writing letters is a more complex and time-consuming task than in other specialties, and requires absolute accuacy because of the severity of the reactions and high risk. For example a child with nut induced anaphylaxis requires:

■ a letter to their GP

■ a written treatment plan outlining (parent) treatment of acute reactions

■ a letter to the community paediatric team (in or out of area) requesting school visits to train teachers

■ a letter to the head of school informing them of the allergy, the management and the proposed school visit

■ literature for parents on nut avoidance and how to use an adrenaline autoinjector.

A patient with anaphylaxis during anaesthesia requires:

■ a letter to the referring anaesthetist, copied to the GP

■ a 'to whom it may concern' letter (copied to anaesthetist and GP) outlining the cause, drug(s) to be avoided and drugs likely to be safe for use in future general anaesthesia

■ an application for a medic alert bracelet (the allergist should provide the wording for the inscription)

■ an entry in the drug allergy/risk section of hospital notes

■ a report to the Medicines Control Agency (MCA).

Inpatient work

Requests for an allergy opinion are common. Ward referrals are seen on the wards or in outpatient clinics. There are occasional inpatients. Rush immunotherapy requires the presence of a doctor at all times during treatment. Challenge testing, either as a day case or inpatient, requires a high level of doctor input and immediate access to treatment for reactions. If a reaction is protracted patients may need to be admitted after day case challenge.

Specialist on call

Allergists are on call for advice in emergencies and for other specialties in the case of anaesthetic allergy, drug allergy and latex allergy etc. The allergist should be available to patients for advice by telephone during the night following day case procedures such as immunotherapy and challenge testing.

Clinically related administration

See *Work to support clinics* above. Administration includes writing letters at point of referral (eg advice to GP or refusing to see patient), prioritising letters, arranging day case procedures, writing clinic protocols and guidelines, and literature searches.

Work to maintain and improve quality of care

This work encompasses duties in clinical governance, professional self-regulation, continuing professional development (CPD), and education and training of others. For many consultants at various times in their careers it may include research, serving in management and providing specialist advice at local, regional and national levels.

Service developments that deliver improved patient care

- Referring patients with nut allergy to specialist allergy clinics reduces morbidity and mortality by limiting the frequency and severity of further reactions, and by providing effective self-treatment should a reaction occur, thereby reducing A&E attendance and hospital admission, and improving quality of life.[20,21]
- Children with glue ear and rhinitis can be managed by allergists. Allergic rhinitis is an important cause and treating this can avoid ENT surgery.[22,23]
- Immunotherapy avoids the complications of medical therapy, reduces chronic disease, reduces long-term drug use and improves quality of life.[24,25,26,27]
- A single consultation with a specialist allergist is more effective than multiple referrals to a series of organ-based specialists in dermatology, ENT and respiratory medicine. Allergists consider the whole patient and identify allergic triggers, often enabling avoidance of allergens, better control of disease and reduced need for drugs and further consultations.
- Challenge testing enables diagnosis or exclusion of drug allergy and improves diagnosis of food allergy/intolerance.
- The use of specialist nurses reduces waiting lists.
- Liaison with community paediatricians improves care for children at risk of anaphylaxis.[18]

ACADEMIC MEDICINE

There is a strong tradition of academic allergy in the UK. Most of the major allergy centres have been developed with academic funding and are headed by academics. Thus, clinical expertise and service delivery rely heavily on academics, and the NHS input into allergy is small. The NHS workload of academic allergists depends on their academic responsibilities and individual job descriptions, but they make an important contribution to the work of the NHS department and often set up tertiary services (specialised clinics). Evidence-based guidelines on diagnosis and management are needed in many areas of allergy, and academic allergists make a major contribution to clinical research and towards the development of guidelines. They also have a role in training allergy SpRs.

WORKFORCE REQUIREMENTS FOR ALLERGY

At present there are 26.5 whole time equivalent (WTE) consultant allergists in England (DH workforce data 2003) and none in Wales, Scotland or Northern Ireland. The College and the Scottish Executive have made recommendations for an increase in allergy SpR and consultants posts.[11,28]

In total, over 100 allergy clinics exist within the UK.[16] High patient demand means that most are run by doctors with an interest in allergy, but without specialist training or expertise, as an add-on service to their main specialty.[15] Whilst these consultants make a valuable contribution to patient care, clinics which are an offshoot from the provision of another service are only a partial response to patient need. Allergy service provision by other specialists as an add-on to their main specialty is no longer adequate. A substantial expansion in the number of trained full-time allergists providing a dedicated allergy service is needed. For an effective national system of allergy patient care, these consultants and clinics need to be networked with allergy specialist centres. Unfortunately, within the UK only six such centres and nine part-time centres offer allergy services run by specialist allergists (five of which are in London or the south-east).

The current situation fails to deliver basic standards of care to allergy patients, fails to comply with clinical governance, and is completely inadequate for the increasing number of patients with severe, multisystem or non-organ based allergic disease. Substantial expansion is required to provide patients with a first class service to match that available elsewhere in the developed world. Improvement is required across the board, in primary, secondary and tertiary care, to achieve more equal access to appropriate allergy services throughout the country, and to gear the training of doctors and nurses to achieve these ends.

Both now and in the immediate future, demand will outstrip service supply by a very large measure. A vision of how a mature allergy service might be configured, and a change programme addressing how to get there, are required. This section addresses the workforce aspects of both.

Immediate proposals: the change programme

The College working party report on allergy services (supported by the BSACI and the NASG) and the House of Commons Health Committee report proposes that a key step is the creation of a network of regional specialist allergy centres.[11,12,15] These services in adult and paediatric allergy would provide expertise for more complex diseases, and training, research and leadership within the nascent national allergy service. They would also improve geographical distribution of allergy services. In the mature service these would become regional tertiary centres. A core of experts is essential to set standards and support developments in primary care, where the bulk of allergy care will eventually be delivered. Thereafter, other developments can follow. There are two immediate needs:

1. *To create or adequately staff regional allergy centres (a minimum of one per region).*
   This requires a minimum of two additional consultant allergists and two paediatric allergists per region, more in less densely populated areas (to cope with demand and waiting times in established centres and to set up services in regions where none exist).[11,12] Appreciation of factors relating to workforce planning has matured since the College report. Department of Health workforce data show that two additional allergy national training numbers (NTNs) are required to maintain the present allergy consultant numbers. The House of Commons report recommended that an additional 20 adult and 20 paediatric consultants are required (phase one of development).

2. *To substantially increase the number of centrally funded SpR posts.*
   A large increase is needed to feed the consultant expansion recommended, and even to maintain the present consultant workforce, as DH data predicts negative growth. The DH Workforce Review Team and the House of Commons Health Committee recommended an increase of 20 centrally funded NTNs in allergy. The Health Committee recommended a parallel increase of 20 trainees in paediatric allergy.

Long-term aim: a mature specialist allergy service (secondary and tertiary)

The aim is to create consultants in other teaching hospitals and in DGHs. Following the start up, the service would be extended to provide allergist-led services in most major teaching hospitals. Later, a service might be developed in selected DGHs. Current provision is so inadequate that even a moderate improvement would require an enormous expansion of consultant numbers.

Calculations

Assumptions of population/patient need

It is estimated that 50,000 people per million need to see a specialist consultant allergist (5% of the UK population), that is about 300,000 in the UK, and that 5,000 people per million need to see a consultant allergist in any year (workload spread over 10 years). This estimate is derived as follows:

- *Epidemiological data*   At least one third of the population and 40% of children have allergic disease.[1,11]

- *Clinical estimates*   Assume about 85% of these will be dealt with in general practice or in allergy clinics run by consultants in other specialties, or may not need to see a doctor. Therefore, assume 15% of those with allergic diseases (about 5% of the population) need to see a consultant allergist. This figure is based on the prevalence of life-threatening, severe or multisystem allergic disease, drug, food, latex and venom allergy and the need for complex investigation, challenge testing and immunotherapy.

- *Immunotherapy and diagnostic challenge tests*   Need is currently difficult to estimate but worldwide use of both is growing. Minimum estimates are that >60 cases per million require immunotherapy for venom and severe pollen allergy (with 50 attendances required per patient) and >150 adults per two million population per annum require more complex investigation/challenge testing (eg for drug allergy). Immunotherapy and challenge testing both have specific safety requirements.

It should be noted that for many disorders prevalence data is not known, but referrals to major allergy centres suggest that anaphylaxis and severe allergic reactions (eg glottal oedema and severe angioedema) are increasing in frequency; that there are many new allergies, particularly to drugs and foods; and that there is more multisystem disease.

Assumptions to calculate consultant manpower to see these patients

Patient throughput

- The workload to provide for the 5% of the population who need to see an allergist will be spread over a 10-year period. Thus, 0.5% (5,000 patients per million population) will need to be seen each year as new patients.

- There is a high rate of discharge after a single outpatient consultation (this is current practice but a proportion are discharged earlier than clinically indicated because of considerable service pressures). This is becoming less realistic as the proportion of patients with more complex disease increases.

Other assumptions in calculating caseload

- A consultant works 42 weeks per year (allowing for annual leave, study/professional leave and bank holidays).

- A programmed activity (PA) is four hours under the 2003 contract in England.

- A consultant has four to five clinics per week.

Consultants needed per million population

The nature of clinic work will vary according to the degree of specialisation in the centre. In a regional allergy centre, three to four clincs might be outpatients, one immunotherapy and one challenge/complex investigation session. In a teaching hospital or DGH with a smaller allergy unit, there might be five outpatient clinics and no challenge or immunotherapy sessions. The number and nature of patients seen will vary. As services develop, the most complex cases, immunotherapy and challenge testing will largely be catered for in the regional centres.

The following calculations are based on specialist work in a major full-time allergy centre offering a tertiary and secondary service.

> Patients with allergy requiring referral to a specialist allergist in any year: 0.5% of 1 million = 5,000
>
> *Outpatient clinics*   Four new and two old patients are seen per clinic, if adequately supported by specialist nurses. This makes 504 new and 252 old patients per annum per consultant.
>
> *Immunotherapy session*   20 patients can be seen per two doctors, which equates to 10 patients per doctor per week. This makes 420 patient attendances per annum (12–21 visits are required per patient per annum).
>
> *Challenge/complex investigation session*   Two patients attend per doctor per week, which equates to 84 patients per annum.
>
> One consultant will see approximately 500 new, 250 review and 500 day cases (immunotherapy and challenges) per annum. 10 consultants will see approximately 5,000 new patients per annum.
>
> Thus, 10 consultants are required per million population (assuming that the at-risk population is seen over 10 years). This equates to 2.5 consultants per 250,000 population. Therefore, 520 consultants are needed for 52 million population (England and Wales).
>
> Present number   27
>
> Additional number for regional centres (phase 1)   20 adult + 20 paediatric consultants = 40
>
> Therefore, number required for other centres (phase 2)   453

Thus, a total of 493 additional allergy consultants are required, a considerable proportion of whom would be in paediatric allergy. The requirement for allergists could be reduced by, say, 20% as organ-based physicians, immunologists and general paediatricians with an interest in allergy continue to contribute to allergy care, for example in allergy affecting only one organ, isolated asthma or eczema.

CONSULTANT SPECIMEN JOB PLAN (IN A TERTIARY CENTRE)

The following is an outline of the work of a NHS consultant allergist in a tertiary centre, as in a regional allergy centre in phase one of development of the service. It should be recognised that the job plan of an academic allergist in a major centre will differ. This job plan should not be seen as prescriptive, particularly as the service is developing.

Activity	Workload	Programmed activities (PAs)
Direct clinical care		
Clinical sessions (outpatients, day cases, ward work)		**4–5**
Work related to clinics and clinical advice		**2–2.5**
Other clinical work and clinical administration		**0.5–1**
On call		**0.25**
Total number of direct clinical care PAs		**7.5 on average**
Supporting professional activities (SPA)		
Work to maintain and improve the quality of healthcare	Education and training, appraisal, departmental management and service development, audit and clinical governance, CPD and revalidation, research	**2.5 on average**
Other NHS responsibilities	eg medical director/clinical director/lead consultant in specialty/clinical tutor	**Local agreement with trust**
External duties	eg work for deaneries/Royal Colleges/specialist societies/Department of Health or other government bodies etc	**Local agreement with trust**

Calculation of clinical programmed activities required for a population of 250,000
Approximately 11 PAs are required to deliver five clinics.
So, 2.5 × 11 = 27.5 PAs (= 2.75 WTE consultants) required for a population of 250,000.

Trainee manpower

There are few trainees at present. There is an immediate need to substantially increase numbers, otherwise even a minimal consultant expansion is unachievable. A further 20 NTNs are required to feed the first phase of development and to begin to grow the specialty. Because allergy is one of only two specialties predicted to have negative growth (minus 6% by 2012, and minus 3% after one new NTN is appointed), two additional NTNs are required to maintain the present consultant workforce. There is training capacity in the major allergy centres, most of whom can accommodate three trainees, and other developing allergist-run centres.

Summary of workforce needs

▪ An estimated 5,000 people per million population have allergic disease of sufficient severity/complexity to see a specialist allergist in any one year.

▪ 2.5 consultant allergists (or 27 PAs) are needed to provide services for 250,000 population.

▪ This workload requires 520 allergists to cover adult and paediatric services (England and Wales).

▪ The assumptions used mean these figures are minimum estimates. New caseload is now seen over a period of 10 years.

▪ Development of an adequate allergy services is proposed in two phases:

Initial expansion The start-up programme to grow the service requires an immediate expansion of 20 consultant allergists and 20 additional SpRs in adult allergy. Concomitant development in paediatric allergy is required, with 20 additional paediatric allergists and expansion of training in paediatric allergy. This would establish one major allergy centre providing adult and paediatric tertiary level services for a population of about five million, and local secondary services, thus providing a core of expertise across the country.

Long-term plans Phase two of development, providing adequate secondary and tertiary services, requires up to 520 allergists (for adult and paediatric services).

Note: In 2001 there was insufficient information available to allow a more precise estimate of the workforce requirements in this specialty. This recent estimate provides a firmer basis for workforce planning but this, too, will need to be reviewed in the light of developments in practice and service delivery.

References

1. The UCB Institute of Allergy. *European Allergy White Paper. Allergic diseases as a public health problem*. Belgium: The UCB Institute of Allergy, 1997.

2. Stewart AG, Ewan PW. The incidence, aetiology and management of anaphylaxis presenting to an accident and emergency department. *Q J Med* 1996;**89**:859–64.

3. Sheikh A, Alves B. Hospital admissions for acute anaphylaxis: time trend study. *BMJ* 2000;**320**:1441.

4. Gupta R, Sheikh A, Strachan DP, Andersen HR. The burden of allergic disease in the UK. *Clin Exp Allergy* 2004;**34**(4):520–6.

5. Neugut A, Ghatak AT, Miller RL. Anaphylaxis in the United States: an investigation into its epidemiogy. *Arch Intern Med* 2001:**161**:15–21.

6. Tariq SM, Stevens M, Matthews S, Ridout S *et al*. Cohort study of peanut and tree nut sensitisation by the age of 4 years. *Br Med J* 1996;**313**:514–17.

7. Grundy J, Matthews S, Bateman B, Dean T, Arshad SH. Rising prevalence of peanut allergy in children: data from 2 sequential cohorts. *J Allergy Clin Immunol* 2002;**110**: 784-9

8. Chiu L, Sampson HA, Sicherer SH. Estimation of the sensitisation rate to peanut by skin prick test in the general population: results from the National Health and Nutrition Examination Survey 1988–94 (NHANES III). *J Allergy Clin Immunol* 2001;**107**:S192 (abstract).

9. Leung R, Chan HJ, Choy D, Lai CKW. Prevalence of latex allergy in hospital staff in Hong Kong. *Clin Exp Allergy* 1997;**27**:167–74.

10. Liss GM, Sussman GL, Deal K *et al.* Latex allergy: epidemiological study of 1351 hospital workers. *Occup Environ Med* 1997;**54**:335–42.

11. Royal College of Physicians. *Allergy: the unmet need. A blueprint for better patient care.* A report of the Royal College of Physicians working party on the provision of allergy services in the UK. London: RCP, 2003, pp 1–93.

12. House of Commons Health Committee. *The provision of allergy services.* London: The Stationery Office, 2003.

13. Department of Health. *National specialised services definitions set. Specialist services for allergy –* definiton no. 17 (all ages), December 2002. www.dh.gov.uk/assetRoot/04/01/96/05/04019605.pdf

14. Ewan PW. Provision of allergy care for optimal outcome in the UK. *Br Med Bull* 2000;**56**:1087–1101 (Ed. Kay AB).

15. Ewan PW, Durham SR (for British Society for Allergy and Clinical immunology). NHS Allergy Services within the United Kingdom: proposals to improve allergy care. *Clin Med* 2002;**2**:122-7.

16. British Society for Allergy and Clinical Immunology. *National Health Service allergy clinics.* 3rd edition. London: BSACI, 2001.

17. Warner JO for the ETAC study group. A double blind randomised placebo-controlled trial of cetirizine in preventing the onset of asthma in children with atopic dermatitis: 18 months treatment and 18 months post-treatment follow-up. *J Allergy Clin Immunol* 2001;**108**:929–37.

18. Vickers DW, Maynard L, Ewan PW. Management of children with potential anaphylactic reactions in the community: a training package and proposal for good practice. *Clin Exp Allergy* 1997;**27**:898–903.

19. British Society for Allergy and Clinical Immunology. Position paper on allergen immunotherapy. Report of a BSACI working party. *Clin Exp Allergy* 1993;23 (Suppl 3):1–44.

20. Ewan PW, Clark AT. Long-term prospective observational study of patients with peanut and nut allergy after participation in a management plan. *Lancet* 2001;**351**:111–15.

21. Ewan PW, Clark AT. Efficacy of a management plan based on severity assessment in longitudinal and case controlled studies of 747 children with nut allergy: proposals for good practice. *BMJ* 2004 (submitted).

22. Alles R, Parikh A, Hawk L *et al.* The prevalence of atopic disorders in children with chronic otitis media with effusion. *Pediatr Allergy Immunol* 2001;**12**:102–6.

23. Parikh A, Alles R, Hawk L *et al.* Treatment of allergic rhinitis and its impact in children with chronic otitis media with effusion. *J Audiol Med* 2000;**9**:104–117.

24. Varney VA, Gaga M, Frew AJ *et al.* Usefulness of immunotherapy in patients with severe summer hayfever uncontrolled by anti-allergic drugs. *BMJ* 1991;**302**;265–9.

25. Durham SR, Walker SM, Varga E-M *et al.* Long term clinical efficacy of grass-pollen immunotherapy. *N Engl J Med* 1999;**341**:468–75.

26. Nasser SMS, Ewan PW. Depot corticosteroid treatment for hay fever causing avascular necrosis of both hips. *BMJ* 2001;**322**:1589–91.

27. Varga EM, Durham SR. Allergen injection immunotherapy. *Clin Allergy Immunol* 2002;**16**:533–49.

28. Scottish Medical and Scientific Advisory Committee. *Immunology and allergy services in Scotland.* Edinburgh: Scottish Executive, 2000.

Audiological medicine

i Description of the specialty and clinical needs of patients

Audiological medicine is the medical specialty concerned with the investigation, diagnosis and management of adults and children with disorders of balance, hearing, tinnitus and auditory communication, including speech and language disorders in children. An audiological physician provides clinical leadership to a multidisciplinary team (MDT), and specialist medical opinion within the integrated care pathway. Non-medical members of the team undertake the majority of the assessment procedures and rehabilitative and follow-up care. Audiological medicine is best described as audiovestibular medicine.

Approximately 20% of the UK population have significant hearing loss as judged by the Medical Research Council (MRC) National Study of Hearing,[1] 5% suffer troublesome tinnitus, and one-third of the population experience symptoms of dizziness/imbalance by the age of 60. Multifactorial imbalance and falls are a major problem for those over 60 years. In children, 1.1 in 1000 are born deaf, 0.9 in 1000 develop or acquire deafness, 25% will have temporary conductive hearing loss in the pre-school period and 10% will experience delay in speech acquisition. 20% of deaf children have additional handicaps. The provision of neuro-otological services for patients with dizziness/vertigo, imbalance or falls is a priority for all departments of audiovestibular medicine. Deafness, tinnitus and vertigo are often chronic, and patients require an explanation of their disorder based upon accurate diagnosis, treatment where possible, and effective rehabilitation to empower them to manage their own healthcare.

Single-handed consultants cover the whole spectrum of service provision in audiovestibular medicine, but those working in teaching hospitals with other audiological physicians may subspecialise.

Inpatient consultation provides an opinion on auditory and vestibular disorders. Most inpatients are seen in the outpatient department where appropriate test facilities are available.

Outpatient services, equally split between adults and children, are the primary medical workload. Emphasis is on evaluating audiovestibular function in the context of the overall medical condition for diagnosis and treatment, and to initiate rehabilitation delivered by a MDT. Separate outpatient clinics are organised for adult neuro-otology, adult tinnitus, adult learning disability and mental health, paediatric audiovestibular medicine, paediatric vestibular disorders, and speech and language disorders. More than 50% of paediatric consultations take place in a community setting.

Screening and surveillance programmes for detection of congenital or early-onset hearing loss are overseen by a consultant community paediatrician (audiology) who also leads follow-up diagnostic services. This workload will increase with the full implementation of universal newborn hearing screening by 2005.

ii   Organisation of the service and patterns of referral

Primary, secondary and tertiary levels

Audiovestibular medicine is an activity which involves the MDT working alongside managers to set mutually agreed targets and goals.[2]

There is no formal provision of service at primary care level, although this may change if primary care trusts (PCTs) lead newborn hearing screening. A significant proportion of paediatric audiological services are provided as secondary care in the community, most commonly led by a consultant community paediatrician (audiology). Targeted neonatal and school hearing screening and surveillance are organised as part of the community programme.[3] This is supervised and supported by a tertiary centre in the hospital or community, and led by an audiological physician, consultant community paediatrician, consultant otologist or consultant scientist. Some secondary services for adults are now provided in a primary care setting by general practitioners with a special interest (GPSIs) in otology. Tertiary adult services and most tertiary children's services are hospital based and include sophisticated neuro-otological test facilities, access to cochlear implant programmes, bone-anchored hearing aid programmes and specialised services such as cleft palate clinics. Integrated multidisciplinary care is a key feature of these services.

Most departments accept referrals directly from primary care, from second-tier community clinics and at the tertiary level from consultant colleagues (see section iv).

Clinical networks and community arrangements

A 'hub-and-spoke' network exists in thinly spread services. In the adult sector, there are no structured audiovestibular services in primary care. There are some community centres in which adults with hearing impairment may be assessed and provided with auditory amplification. Direct access hearing aid services for patients over 60 years are run by audiologists who work to strict guidelines for referral to an appropriate consultant audiological physician or otolaryngologist.

Relationship with other services/agencies

Multiagency working is fundamental to audiovestibular medicine, in common with other specialties with an emphasis on chronic conditions. Education services share the care of deaf children. Social services are important in terms of both employment and appropriate domestic support. Voluntary bodies, including the Royal National Institute for the Deaf (RNID) and the National Deaf Children's Society (NDCS), play a vital role in ensuring appropriate facilities are available for the hearing impaired and laying down criteria for good practice.

Complementary services

Conjoined services include nurses in tertiary centres and health visitors in the community, together with teams of volunteers helping new hearing aid users, particularly the housebound.

iii   Working with patients: patient-centred care

Patient choice and involving patients in decisions about their treatment

Rehabilitation of those with auditory and vestibular disorders depends upon deciding strategy and setting goals in partnership with the patient. Decisions to refer for surgery are part of the treatment plan agreed with the patient. Parent and patient choice determine the management strategy as it cannot succeed without their support. Community attitudes to deafness differ across different ethnic and cultural groups in relation to resistance to surgery, desire for genetic testing, disquiet in the deaf community about the role of cochlear implantation, or the debate of when and whether to introduce British Sign Language (BSL), for example. Parents have to decide, on the basis of unbiased information, which approach will be in their child's best long-term interest. This can be very difficult for parents of newly diagnosed deaf children with no previous experience of deafness or the emotive nature of the issues involved. The audiological physician has to be especially sensitive to the concerns and anxieties of the families of deaf children.

Opportunities for education and promoting self-care

Audiovestibular medicine is fortunate in working alongside voluntary organisations that provide excellent information and education for patients and carers alike. Although education services promote a child's independence in hearing care, the same has not always been true of hospital services for adults. There is frequently insufficient time to train patients adequately in the care and use of hearing aids. This may be addressed to some extent in the Modernising Hearing Aid Services (MHAS) programme.

Patients with chronic conditions

The majority of patients with hearing and balance disorders have chronic or relapsing conditions. Patient empowerment is crucial to their care.

The role of the carer

Parents and carers are crucial to the successful adaptation of children and those with learning disability. Adults with auditory and vestibular disorders depend upon the support of 'significant others' for their rehabilitation.

Access to information, patient support groups and the role of expert patients

Information is available from websites, special libraries, and written material produced by educational, health and patient support groups. It is part of the statutory duty of the doctor at diagnosis to give patients information on relevant support groups. Patient support groups are an essential part of the team and the following list is not exclusive: RNID, Hearing Concern, Meniere's Society, the British Tinnitus Association (BTA), the British Deaf Association (BDA), the Royal Association for the Deaf (RAD), Sign (the National Society for Mental Health and Deafness), the Council for the Advancement of Communication with Deaf People (CACDP), Usher's Society, Sense, NDCS, AFASIC, etc. Some services already use adult role models, local self-help groups or patient volunteers as expert patients. This will expand as resources allow.

Availability of clinical records and results

Paediatric services already give parents copies of any reports. This will be implemented, in line with government recommendations, for those adults who desire this information as soon as resources allow.

iv Interspecialty and interdisciplinary liaison

Multidisciplinary team working

Both adult and paediatric audiovestibular medicine services are delivered by MDTs of health professionals together with those from other services. Teams include audiologists, speech and language therapists, hearing therapists, psychologists, behavioural therapists, educational audiologists and physiotherapists.

Working with other specialists

The key specialty in this respect is mental health. There are a small number of psychiatrists specifically for the deaf, but all mental health services for both adults and children have a crucial role to play in the shared care of many patients. Other closely linked specialties include genetics, radiology, nephrology, infectious diseases, neurology and neurosurgery, paediatrics and neonatology, plastic surgery and maxillofacial surgery, and otolaryngology.

Working with GP specialists

Some GPSIs in otolaryngology are concerned with aural care and audiovestibular disorders in adults and this area could be expanded usefully.

v Delivering a high quality service

Characteristics of a high quality service

- All patients presenting with dizziness, imbalance, falls and ataxia, and many of those with severe/profound hearing loss, with or without other handicaps, should have access to comprehensive diagnostic and multidisciplinary rehabilitative facilities. These facilities are specialist and best provided for a population of 500,000 rather than 250,000.
- A high quality service depends upon the integration of audiovestibular medicine into the national provision of neurosciences.
- Services should be patient centred with best practice unrestricted by resources.
- Patients, their families and carers expect, and should receive, clear, unbiased, up-to-date information in an accessible form.
- There should be adequate time and expertise for the counselling that is required in chronic disorders and disability.
- First language interpretation, including BSL, should be available whenever needed, and there should be prompt access to other paramedical and medical disciplines when needed for effective care.
- National guidelines on waiting times should be met and all aspects of the service should be audited.
- In paediatric practice, all hearing-impaired children should be identified before four months of age and have access to appropriate amplification, specialist speech and language therapy, educational support and aetiological investigation.

- Specialist psychiatric services should be accessible to all who need them.
- Children should be given sufficient time in a child-friendly and family friendly environment.
- Care must be integrated across health, education and social services, with seamless transition from paediatric to adult care.
- In adult practice, all patients with auditory and vestibular symptoms should have rapid access to diagnostic and rehabilitation facilities. Dizziness, imbalance and vertigo in particular require accurate diagnosis and appropriate medical treatment as a basis for rehabilitation.
- Tinnitus services should be rehabilitative as well as diagnostic.
- All hearing aids should be provided on a 'right-first-time' basis and a full range of hearing aids should be available using MHAS protocols, which should be universally implemented by 2006.

Resources required for a high quality service

Specialised facilities

Suitable space is required for the provision of auditory and vestibular testing. As this function is highly specialised it is best designed for a population of 500,000 spread across several sites. Some of the facilities will be available on all sites and some in the central facility only. Audiometric booths must meet international standards and all rooms must meet health and safety requirements and be suitable for infection control. All facilities should have pushchair and wheelchair access.

Specialised facilities required by an audiovestibular medicine service for a population of 500,000

Hearing testing:

Paediatric
>   3 large paediatric sound-proof test booths with viewing areas
>   1 standard booth with viewing area for children
>   1 child-friendly hearing aid fitting room
>   1 acoustically-treated child-friendly hearing aid prescription room
>   1 parent counselling room

Adult
>   4 standard audiometric sound-proof test booths
>   1 evoked-response booth
>   2 acoustically-treated hearing aid prescription rooms
>   3 hearing aid fitting rooms
>   2 comfortable rooms for hearing therapy
>   1 large room for group relaxation classes
>   1 seminar room
>   1 waiting room
>   5 offices for two people each

Vestibular testing:

Paediatric
>   A child-friendly, purpose-designed, dark vestibular test room with play area

Adult
>   2 large, dark vestibular laboratories with sink and clean mains water
>   1 large room for group relaxation and balance retraining
>   1 counselling and cognitive therapy room.

Specialised facilities required include a full range of sophisticated audiological test equipment (audiometers, visual-reinforced audiometry, impedance bridge, otoacoustic emission equipment, speech audiometry, electrophysiological equipment and central auditory test facilities) together with appropriate resources and facilities for calibration of equipment and prescription of hearing aids.

Specialised vestibular equipment includes facilities for caloric testing, eye movement recording (including electro-oculography and/or video-nystagmography), rotational testing and posturography in the main centre with video-nystagmography and a couch for positional testing in each location.

Access to tertiary radiology (with provision for magnetic resonance imaging (MRI) or computed tomography (CT) with anaesthesia), genetics, neurology, otology, ophthalmology and paediatric facilities are essential for diagnosis. Access to psychology, physiotherapy and speech and language therapy is essential for rehabilitation.

Details of the up-to-date equipment (less than five years old) required for a population of 500,000 is described in *Audiological medicine in a modern NHS*.[4]

Workforce requirements: clinical and support staff

Audiovestibular medicine depends upon a MDT and the workforce requirements for clinical and support staff are therefore crucial to the service.

Audiological medicine in a modern NHS contains recommendations for the staff required to serve a population of 500,000.[4] This covers vestibular and hearing services combined (paediatric and adult) in community and hospital sites, with universal neonatal hearing screening and digital hearing aid provision, and ensuring that each professional has a peer. It refers also to the staff required for a team based at a main unit working across several sites and providing support for ear, nose and throat (ENT) clinics.

Table 1. Non-medical staffing requirement for the service provided by an audiological centre

Professional		Child		Adult	Total (500,000)	Total (250,000)
Audiological scientists	Grade C	1	or	1	1	1
	Grade B	1	or	1	1	1
	Grade A	1	or	1	1	1
Audiologist	MTO5	1		(1)	1–2	1
	MTO4	2		2	4	2
	MTO3	1		1	2	1
	MTO2	1		1	2	1
	MTO1	0		2	2	1
	ATO	2		2	4	2
SALT for hearing impaired		2		1	3	1–2
Educational audiologists/ATHI		2		0	2	1
Deaf role model/sign language teacher		1		0	1	0.5
Social worker/counsellor		1		1	2	1
Hearing therapist		0		2	2	1
Physiotherapist		1		1	2	1
Psychologist		1		1	2	1
Nurse/healthcare assistant		1		3	4	2
Medical secretary		2		2	4	2
Receptionists		2		2	4	2
A and C records staff		2		2	4	2

MTO = Medical technical officer
ATO = Assistant technical officer
SALT = Speech and language therapists
ATHI = Advisory teachers for the hearing impaired

vi Quality standards and measures of the quality of specialist services

Specialist society guidelines

Audiological medicine in a modern NHS was published in 2001 by the British Association of Audiological Physicians (www.baap.org.uk) and sets out the standards to be expected in a high quality service.[4] The NDCS and the RNID have published quality standards documents on a variety of topics including paediatric audiology and bone-anchored hearing aids.

National Institute for Clinical Excellence (NICE) guidelines

NICE guidelines have been superseded by the MHAS and the Modernising Children's Hearing Aid Services (MCHAS) programmes of the Modernisation Agency. The RNID has set down the criteria for modernising hearing services for adults and children.

Clinical governance

This is delivered at national and local level by regular clinical and medical audit against published guidelines and quality standards of the professional and voluntary organisations.[4]

Children's hearing impairment services working groups established by the NDCS, with user participation, have a regulatory role.

CLINICAL WORK AND/OR LABORATORY WORK OF CONSULTANTS IN AUDIOLOGICAL MEDICINE

Direct clinical care

A population of 250,000 generates approximately 1,000 new medical referrals a year and 1,000 follow-up medical appointments. The follow-up rate is kept low, despite the fact that the specialty is largely concerned with chronic disease, because much of the work is undertaken by non-medical members of the team. Non-medical audiologists provide a direct access service for hearing impaired adults and almost all the rehabilitation service. This consists of approximately 400 new referrals and 4,000 follow-up appointments for a population of 250,000. A 'red flag' system operates whereby selected patients are referred on to audiological medicine or otology.

Inpatient work (consultation only)

Consultants and specialist registrars (SpRs) in audiological medicine do not participate in the on-call rota for acute general medicine. They do, however, manage two acute presentations: sudden hearing loss and acute intractable vertigo. Both conditions require urgent admission, investigation and management in collaboration with otology. In an average district general hospital (DGH), approximately four patients per week are likely to be referred from other specialties.

Outpatient work

A consultant audiological physician working alone in an outpatient clinic may see four to six new patients or 6–12 follow-up patients per programmed activity (PA) (children generally need longer than adults). The number will depend on the consultant's experience, the complexity of the problem and the availability of support staff. Whenever possible, audiovestibular investigations should be carried out at the same attendance. Specialist registrars are largely confined to teaching hospitals, so in the average DGH the consultant is likely to work unsupported. Where SpRs are available the increased number of patients seen is offset by the time required for training and the number of PAs required will be similar.

Specialised investigative and therapeutic procedure clinics

Specialised clinics within audiological medicine vary considerably from trust to trust, depending on the nature of the hospital, the allocation of resources, the workload of the individual consultant and the availability of support from other medical disciplines. The aim of all clinics should be to provide a 'one-stop' service, often with joint consultations and time for team discussions of complex cases. These clinics include those for vertigo and imbalance in adults or children, and those for tinnitus. A consultant is likely to undertake one such clinic per week, seeing four new patients.

Specialist on call

There is no formal on-call requirement.

Other specialist activity including activities beyond the local services

Many audiological physicians undertake clinics in more than one hospital, or in outreach clinics in DGHs, community clinics, primary care groups and schools for the deaf or learning disabled. The scope of this work and the way in which the clinics are conducted varies widely.

For those unable to attend hospital clinics for the provision of hearing aids and appropriate auditory rehabilitation, domiciliary visits or visits to old people's homes are undertaken, usually by non-medical members of the team.

Clinically related administration

As so much of the work involves multiagency working, the clinics generate a considerable communication burden for doctor and secretary alike. The audiological physician provides input into the statement for special educational needs, and receives requests from patient agencies and others for information and documentation to support entitlements such as the disability living allowance.

Work to maintain and improve the quality of care

This work encompasses duties in clinical governance, professional self-regulation, continuing professional development and education and training of others. For many consultants at various times in their careers it may include research, serving in management and providing specialist advice at local, regional and national levels.

Leadership role and development of the service

The role of clinical lead in a MDT will be one of leading clinical governance and working with managers and other clinical staff to put service developments into a clinical context.

Service developments that deliver improved patient care

Time allocated to consultants for this work includes: one PA for continuing medical education (CME); one PA for teaching junior and allied staff; one PA for administration and management; and one PA for clinical research – making a total of four PAs per week. Senior consultants will also have national committee or editorial work of 0.5–1 PA per week.

Current proposals and developments to improve the provision of audiological care include:

■ *Universal neonatal screening*   This is a recent initiative with pilot sites currently evaluating the efficacy and feasibility in the UK using otoacoustic emissions. A critical review has clearly demonstrated that universal neonatal hearing screening is the most cost-effective and highest-yield method of defining congenital bilateral hearing impairment.[5]

■ *Genetics*   Recent advances in the Genome Project and the identification of genes associated with deafness are encouraging aetiological investigation of deafness at all ages.

■ *One-stop vestibular clinics*   These are required for the dizzy patient to limit the occupational and social morbidity caused by disorders of balance.

Education and training

Consultants will be involved in training for undergraduate and postgraduate medical junior staff and other clinical staff, lecturing and examining for MSc and BSc courses, and working with the Hearing Aid Council and other professional bodies. Those consultants attached to undergraduate teaching hospitals will be involved in selection and examination procedures.

Mentoring and appraisal of medical staff and other professional staff

As a senior member of the team these aspects may be a significant responsibility for the consultant.

Continuing medical education

As the specialty is small and fragmented much CME takes place nationally and internationally.

Clinical governance

The consultant will be expected to take a lead in clinical governance.

Research – clinical studies and basic science

As medical education becomes more self-directed and trainee audiologists develop a portfolio of skills and knowledge, research across all disciplines should expand.

Local management duties

As specialty lead the consultant will work closely with management both strategically and on a daily basis.

Regional and national work

In a small specialty, work for the Royal College of Physicians, the Department of Health (DH), specialist societies, patient groups, deaneries and other national bodies is a greater burden than in large specialties where the majority of consultants may not need to get involved if they are not so inclined.

ACADEMIC MEDICINE

Clinical contribution to NHS

Audiological medicine is a developing specialty with three professors and academic trainees. They are responsible for taking the lead in promoting evidence-based medicine. Each academic department runs a tertiary clinical service: paediatric audiological medicine (Manchester), adult auditory rehabilitation (Cardiff), and vestibular medicine (London).

Teaching

An MSc programme in audiological medicine in London provides part of the higher specialist training programme in this specialty.

Research

Academic staff have taken a lead in training, research, and piloting and validating new rehabilitation and management strategies.

Other academic activities

Academic staff act as external examiners in related academic courses.

WORKFORCE REQUIREMENTS FOR AUDOLOGICAL MEDICINE

Current workforce numbers

- Consultant audiological physicians: 39 (includes three professors and one senior lecturer), this equates to 29 whole time equivalent (WTE) consultants in post.
- Consultant community paediatricians in audiology: 20
- SpRs: 17 (5 flexible)
- Registrar retainers: 2
- Senior house officers: 2, combined with ENT (1) and paediatrics (1)
- Associate specialist: 1
- There are no non-consultant career grade doctors (NCCG) or GPSIs.

Consultant programmed activities required to provide a specialist service to a population of 250,000

The tertiary and technologically advanced nature of the specialty determines that it is best organised for a population of 500,000. The calculations in *Audiological medicine in a modern NHS* were based upon a sample of three DGHs, which had at least one consultant audiological physician, two of which had an establishment for one SpR. The total population covered by the three hospitals was 900,000.[4]

A minimum of three WTE consultant audiological physicians, one consultant community paediatrician (audiology) and one WTE consultant audiological scientist (state registered) was recommended for a population of 500,000. On the basis of these recommendations, the long-term aim may be that a DGH serving 250,000 population requires 20 consultant audiological physician PAs, to include eight outpatient PAs for the hospital, four PAs for the community service and eight PAs for supporting activities. However, an initial increase of 104% across the UK is thought to be an appropriate target over the next few years, equivalent to 0.28 WTE consultants per 250,000 population. The aim must be to provide the best service for patients using an appropriate balance of audiological physicians, community paediatricians and audiological scientists working closely with their ENT surgical colleagues.

CONSULTANT WORK PROGRAMME/SPECIMEN JOB PLAN

Activity	Workload	Programmed activities (PAs)
Direct clinical care		
Inpatient work	4–8 patients	0.5–1.0
Outpatient clinics		4–6
Adult and paediatric[1]	New patients: 4–8 adults per clinic; up to 6 children Follow-up patients: 8–12 adults per clinic; up to 6 children Outpatient review of inpatients: 4–12 adults per clinic; up to 6 children	
Specialist clinics	2–4 patients/clinic Adult vestibular service Adult tinnitus clinics Paediatric vestibular Adult learning disability hearing clinic Neonatal hearing service	 0–1 0–1 0–1 1 0.5
Work outside the base hospital	Special schools	0–1
On-call for specialist advice and emergencies	Depends on available resources Depends on the centre	} 0.1–1
Clinically-related administration		1.5–2
Acute medicine	Very rare	0.1
On-take	None	
Academic medicine	Clinical care Teaching and research	3 6
Total number of direct clinical care PAs		**7.5 on average**
Supporting professional activities (SPA)		
Work to maintain and improve the quality of healthcare	Education and training, appraisal, departmental management and service development, audit and clinical governance, CPD and revalidation, research	**2.5 on average**
Other NHS responsibilities	eg medical director/clinical director/lead consultant in specialty/clinical tutor	**Local agreement with trust**
External duties	eg work for deaneries/Royal Colleges/specialty societies/Department of Health or other government bodies etc	**Local agreement with trust**

A 50:50 split between paediatric and adult outpatient clinics is assumed for the purposes of the above table, although the distribution of work varies widely for individual jobs and individual trusts.

Full audiological and vestibular testing facilities are required to support inpatient and outpatient work.

References

1.   Davis, AC. *Hearing in adults.* London: Whurr, 1995.

2.   Dixon J, Lewis R, Finlayson B, Gray D. Can the NHS learn from US managed care organizations? *BMJ* 2004;**328**: 220–22.

3.   Bamford J, Davis A. Neonatal hearing screening: a step towards better services for children and families. *Br J Audiol* 1998;**32**:1–6.

4.   British Association of Audiological Physicians. *Audiological medicine in a modern NHS.* London: BAAP, 2001.

5.   National Deaf Children's Society. *Quality standards in paediatric audiology.* London: NDCS, Vol. 1, 1994; Vol. 2, 1996.

Cardiology/cardiovascular medicine

i Description of the specialty and clinical needs of patients

The subject of cardiology focuses on the wide range of disorders that can affect the structure and function of the heart itself. The term *cardiovascular medicine* is also frequently used, recognising the functional inter-relationship between the heart, systemic arterial and venous systems, and the vascular supply to the lungs. The process of atherosclerosis and the extremely important risk factor of diabetes mellitus commonly have significant adverse effects on organs and systems other than the heart. The concept of cardiovascular medicine, therefore, reflects the broad overall training and clinical attitudes that are required of a cardiologist.

Recent developments have emphasised the importance of subspecialties within cardiology:

- Percutaneous coronary intervention (PCI) is a developing method of restoring an adequate arterial blood supply to ischaemia myocardium without recourse to coronary artery surgery.
- In the field of electrophysiology, the advent of implantable defibrillators, together with advances in invasive techniques for ablating atrial and ventricular arrhythmias, have led to therapeutic advances for patients with rhythm disorders.
- The selection of appropriate treatment for patients with heart failure has expanded considerably over the past five years. The National Institute for Clinical Excellence (NICE) has clarified the appropriate drug therapy for such patients and developments in pacing offer the possibility of improving the quality of life of patients with cardiac failure.
- The increasingly specialist needs of adult patients with congenital heart disease are now well recognised in cardiological circles. Units for providing both lifestyle and specialist cardiac advice to this group of patients are being established across the UK.
- Developments in non-invasive imaging continue to influence the way in which cardiac patients are investigated. Magnetic resonance imaging (MRI), echocardiography (ECHG) and radionuclide scanning are key components of the management of patients with cardiovascular disorders.

General cardiology involves the care of many patients admitted on acute medical take with a broad range of disorders. Increasingly, patients require appropriate referral to cardiologists who have a subspecialty interest.

ii Organisation of the service and patterns of referral

Primary, secondary and tertiary levels

Primary care　Many cardiovascular disorders can be managed effectively with good cooperation between primary and secondary care. Recent development of rapid-access chest pain clinics and heart failure clinics provide examples of improvement in the management of patients who may be presenting with the first symptom of coronary heart disease, or in whom the diagnosis and treatment of heart failure needs to be established. Both primary and secondary prevention of coronary disease are important responsibilities in primary care. Symptoms of relatively minor disorders of cardiac rhythm, often presenting as palpitations, are a frequent reason for consultations in general practice. In some primary care trusts (PCTs) there are no specific arrangements for appropriate management of the many patients who present with atrial fibrillation.

Increasingly, primary care will follow up patients who have been seen and treated in secondary and tertiary care. The appropriate clinical management of patients with prosthetic heart valves and implanted electrophysiological devices will need to be communicated to the primary care setting. Training programmes for general practitioners with a special interest (GPSIs) in cardiology are likely to make a useful contribution to the primary/secondary care interface.

Secondary care   In recent years there has been striking success in ever more sophisticated cardiac diagnosis and therapy in district general hospitals (DGHs). This trend has been facilitated by a greater number of consultant cardiologists working in DGHs and by improved access to non-invasive investigations such as exercise tests, radionuclide scans, ECHG and non-invasive electrophysiological testing. The biggest change diagnostically lies in the increased numbers of cardiac catheterisation laboratories which are now located in DGHs. This not only saves patients from travelling to tertiary centres for coronary angiography (now a routine but invasive investigation), but also facilitates timely diagnosis for the large number of patients admitted to hospital with chest pain syndromes.

Routine permanent pacing procedures are increasingly carried out in a DGH. This is an obvious benefit to elderly patients and will reduce the number of temporary pacing procedures that need to be performed. Future developments are likely to occur in the fields of PCI and electrophysiology. It seems likely that more interventional procedures will be performed in DGHs without on-site surgical cover. Similarly, patients who require an implantable defibrillator are likely to be managed in the DGH rather than a tertiary centre.

Tertiary care   After appropriate triage, many patients require and benefit from the subspecialty services available in tertiary centres. These include:

  ▪ PCI with on-site surgical cover
  ▪ coronary artery and valve surgery after appropriate liaison with cardiac surgeons
  ▪ adult congenital heart disease centres with appropriate support from specialists in cardiac imaging
  ▪ cardiac surgery
  ▪ invasive electrophysiology
  ▪ non-invasive imaging including cardiac MRI and sophisticated ECHG and radionuclide techniques.

Most tertiary centres make significant contributions to research and development in both clinical and basic science disciplines.

Clinical networks and community arrangements

Cardiac networks are now established in most parts of the UK and play a vital role in coordination of primary, secondary and tertiary care. Networks typically serve a number of PCTs, secondary care trusts and one or two tertiary providers. Longer-term strategic decisions (for example concerning revascularisation or imaging strategies) should be developed within the structure of the network.

Taking into account patients' views from a number of sources, cardiac networks should ensure the success of the entire patient journey, focusing particularly on areas of interface between primary, secondary and tertiary care. Networks will also be involved in regular audit activity against national service framework (NSF) standards and will promote equity of access to healthcare within their sectors. Cardiac networks usually work closely with the coronary heart disease (CHD) collaborative to support innovation and sharing of practice and experience.

Relationship with other services/agencies

The changes in the pattern of delivery of cardiological care indicated above will, in an era of consultant appraisal and revalidation, inevitably affect the configuration of consultant cardiology posts. In particular, the relationship with general internal medicine (GIM) is likely to change.

The professional demands on both interventional cardiologists and invasive electrophysiologists will be substantial in terms of maintaining clinical competencies (performing procedures) and keeping up to date with new developments in these highly technical specialties. Professionally, it is not possible for such consultants to maintain competency across the breadth of GIM.

In the past, these competing competencies have not caused planning difficulties since the majority of such specialised cardiology posts have been located in tertiary care. In future, with the increased availability of cardiac catheterisation laboratories in secondary care (DGHs), pressure may come for interventional cardiologists to undertake general medical duties. In general, such pressures should be resisted. Cardiologists will have a close interest in acute medicine where the triage and treatment of acutely ill medical patients fall within the natural competency of a fully trained cardiologist. Furthermore, the appropriate management of patients with acute coronary syndromes, including acute myocardial infarction (MI), will increasingly fall exclusively within the remit of cardiologists in hospitals, particularly where there are on-site cardiac catheterisation facilities.

The focus of cardiology input into acute medicine will tend to change from a general unselected on-call structure towards managing the large number of acute cardiology patients on the coronary care unit (CCU) or acute medical wards. These patients should be seen on a daily basis by a cardiologist. In such circumstances, responsibility for both acute medicine and interventional cardiology may be possible, but the much broader range of competencies required for the ongoing care of patients with general medical problems will not be compatible with maintaining competency in coronary intervention or invasive electrophysiology.

By contrast, cardiologists with special training in heart failure, non-invasive imaging or adult congenital heart disease are likely to continue to make a substantial contribution to a general cardiology on-call service in addition to a subspecialty on-call commitment.

iii Working with patients: patient-centred care

Patient choice and involving patients in decisions about their treatment

The majority of patients in clinical cardiovascular medicine do have symptoms but some have no active symptoms and require prophylactic drug or procedural therapy. In either case, following appropriate investigations patients will be advised by their consultant cardiologist about the options for treatment.

All drug therapy including preventative therapy for coronary disease – antiplatelet agents, lipid-lowering drugs, antihypertensive agents, and anti-arrhythmic drug therapy or long-term treatment with anticoagulants – should always be discussed in detail with the patient. Indications for drug therapy, including benefits and possible adverse reactions, should be understood by each patient. The rationale for invasive investigations, treatment with devices or cardiac surgery should always be discussed as part of the procedure for obtaining informed consent. In a minority of instances, the cardiologist will give a clear recommendation, which will be expected to substantially improve longevity or avoid a major risk of sudden death. In the majority of cases two or more options for therapy will usually be presented to the patient.

The involvement of close relatives or carers facilitates discussion with the patient. Such discussions may involve relatively complex technical concepts. Booklets are available from both the British Heart Foundation (BHF) and the British Cardiac Society (BCS) to facilitate patient understanding.

Ethnic and religious considerations should be addressed, for example when guidance on fasting might interfere with life-saving drug administration or when the administration of blood products is of relevance to invasive or surgical procedures.

Opportunities for education and promoting self-care

Effective, structured patient education is the key to long-term compliance with therapy. Education about cardiovascular disease is essential since patients with cardiac disorders may have healthcare beliefs that do not accurately relate to their individual cardiovascular pathology. Cardiac education should always be a central component of cardiac rehabilitation programmes. The most effective education programmes involve collaboration between cardiologists, nurses and other healthcare professions such as dietitians and physiotherapists. Lifestyle issues, with regard to primary and secondary prevention of coronary disease and the inter-relation between diabetes and vascular disease, are a key focus of patient education programmes.

Patients with chronic conditions

Patients with heart failure, hypertension or a pacemaker benefit from the continuity of care delivered by specialist clinics where cardiologists work in partnership with specifically trained nursing or technical staff. Arrangements for monitoring long-term treatment with anticoagulants such as warfarin can be successfully devolved to primary care.

The role of the carer

The carer for a patient with a cardiovascular disorder has a vital role. Carers provide emotional and intellectual support when patients are confronted with life-threatening decisions, support lifestyle changes and ensure the safe administration of long-term drug therapy. Most cardiovascular consultations are facilitated by the presence of a carer.

Access to information, patient support groups and the role of the expert patient

The most common source of information for patients is the Internet. Cardiologists should be accustomed to discussing developments in clinical care and research findings with patients who have accessed such material on the web.

Both the BCS and the BHF have a series of patient-focused leaflets which provide information about cardiac investigations and treatment.

Patient support groups, generally organised locally, have been a feature of cardiology for many years. The BCS has set up Heart Health Partnership UK (HHPUK), a national affiliation between local groups, and has links with the British Cardiac Patients Association. The BCS is currently collecting a database of patients who will advise them as expert patients.

Availability of clinical records/results

The availability of the results of clinical investigations is central to the effective management of patients with cardiac disorders. Liaison with primary care in a timely and accurate way enables effective preventative measures to be delivered. The timely availability of results for cardiac surgeons or other cardiological subspecialists is essential for a high quality clinical service.

The availability of image servers to handle digitally the large amount of information contained in coronary angiograms has largely overcome the problems associated with storage and retrieval of film and CD angiographic images.

iv   Interspecialty and interdisciplinary liaison

Multidisciplinary team working

For many years cardiology has relied on multidisciplinary working with cardiac nurses, cardiac technicians and radiographers on an everyday basis. Pharmacists, physiotherapists and dietitians also contribute to the management of patients with cardiac disorders.

Working with other specialists

Cardiologists work closely not only with subspecialists within their own field but also with cardiac surgeons, general and acute physicians. The ability to work effectively with other specialists is an essential attribute for consultant cardiologists.

Working with GP specialists

The College and the BCS welcome the opportunity of developing the concept of GPSIs in cardiology. Such practitioners could make a very useful and effective contribution to meeting the demands of high quality cardiovascular care. This exciting new development will only be successful if it is linked to an effective training programme with a national curriculum and standard of assessment, and to a programme of continuing professional development (CPD) for the GP specialist.

v   Delivering a high quality service

Characteristics of a high quality service

■ accurate transfer of information, especially given the nature of many cardiac disorders

■ patient access to both general cardiology and specialist cardiology in a timely manner, and before irreversible adverse outcomes such as myocardial infarction or sudden death occurs

■ high quality IT and excellent secretarial services, particularly IT developments such as the electronic patient record

■ efficient access and referral for cardiac surgery

■ appropriate coordination of care for children and adults with both simple and complex congenital heart disease.

Resources required for a high quality service

Specialised facilities

■ PCI for both acute and chronic presentations of coronary artery disease

■ non-invasive imaging techniques such as ECHG, cardiac MR, isotope scanning and spiral CT scanning

■ resynchronisation therapy and transplantation for management of patients with advanced heart failure

■ interventional electrophysiology and implantation of cardiac defibrillators.

Provision of resources for the above needs to balance ease of geographical access for patients with high quality subspecialised investigation and treatment. Both human and technological resources need to be used in a cost-effective manner.

vi   Quality standards and measures of the quality of specialist services

Specialist society guidelines

The specialty advisory committee (SAC) in cardiology has developed a competency-based curriculum and is involved in the project to develop new methods of clinical assessment. The SAC and affiliated groups: the British Cardiovascular Intervention Society (BCIS), the British Pacing Electrophysiology Group (BPEG), the British Paediatric Cardiac Association (BPCA) and the British Society for Echocardiography (BSE), are all working to develop competency-based standards and measures of quality. The SAC and the education department of the College will be assisting these groups in developing methods based on modern standards.

National Institute for Clinical Excellence (NICE) guidelines

The College and the BCS have worked with NICE to develop a number of policies relevant to cardiology. Existing and imminent guidance covers:

■ IIb IIIa inhibitors

■ use of intracoronary stents

■ drug-eluting stents

■ treatment of heart failure

■ use of clopidogrel in patients with acute coronary syndromes

■ interventions in cardiology other than PCI, for example alcohol ablation for septal hypertrophy and valvuloplasty

■ myocardial perfusion scintigraphy for the diagnosis and management of angina and MI

■ smoking cessation

■ MI early thrombolysis

■ dual-chamber pacing

■ clopiodgrel and dipyridamole in the prevention of occlusive vascular events

■ implantable cardioverter defibrillators for the treatment of arrhythmias.

Current NICE guideline documents will all be reviewed, and the College and BCS will contribute to those reviews. In addition, an ongoing programme is considering new areas of cardiology that will require a report from NICE (**www.NICE.org.uk**).

Clinical governance

Cardiology has been the vanguard of developing clinical governance at both national and local levels. The central cardiac audit database collects sufficient patient information to permit adjusted comparisons of clinical care. To obtain full benefit from the national programme requires quality IT to be installed in all cardiac centres. The Clinical Effectiveness and Evaluation Unit (CEEu) of the College has worked with the BCS in developing the Myocardial Infarction National Audit Project (MINAP), which is generally perceived to have improved the timing and quality of drug prescribing for patients with acute MI.

CLINICAL WORK AND/OR LABORATORY WORK OF CONSULTANTS IN CARDIOLOGY

Contributions made to acute medicine

Cardiology welcomes the advent of the concept of acute medicine. Currently, most cardiologists will be involved either in a general medicine acute take rota or will be part of a cardiology on-take service. Based in a DGH, the cardiologist's role usually focuses on patients within the CCU and its associated 'step down' clinical care area. Growing evidence in the literature documents the benefits of PCI as optimal treatment for patients with ST segment-elevation MI and early revascularisation for non-ST segment-elevation MI or unstable angina. The direction for cardiology will undoubtedly be to focus attention in the A&E department and medical acute admissions unit. In this context, the cardiology service will become an integral part of the overall pattern of delivering acute medical care.

Direct clinical care

Three patterns of direct patient care are recognised within cardiology:

■ *Consultants based entirely in a DGH* This may be with or without access to on-site invasive cardiology (cardiac catheter lab). Consultants will often, though not necessarily, be involved in acute general medical takes. They will deliver a cardiological consultation service to the hospital and provide advice to general physicians, surgeons and obstetricians will form a considerable part of their workload. Consultant attendance on CCU ward rounds will be the norm with each consultant leading, on average, two CCU ward rounds per week.

■ *Consultants based both in a DGH and in a tertiary centre* These consultants are less likely than those in the first category to be involved in general medical takes. The development of acute medicine is welcomed by cardiology because of the high incidence of patients with acute coronary syndromes in A&E and on medical admission units. Cardiologists with a particular interest in PCI will wish to work with the acute medical team. Other cardiologists will bring their expertise in electrophysiology, adult congenital heart disease, non-invasive imaging or management of heart failure to patients whose care is delivered in the tertiary care setting.

■ *Consultants located geographically entirely within tertiary centres* A relatively small number of cardiologists are in this category. Work is focused on the subspecialty interest outlined above.

Other specialist activity including activities beyond the local services

Besides a role in general cardiology and acute medicine, most cardiologists will be expected to develop an area of special interest. These areas of interest have been outlined in the introduction to this paper. Consultants would be expected to provide evidence of the quality of such special interests, for example through the appraisal process, continuing medical education (CME) attendance, membership and contribution to the affiliated groups of the BCS. Attendance at regional, national and international meetings would be expected.

Clinically related administration

Contributing to local networks, patient pathways, and working in a multidisciplinary environment to develop healthcare delivery, all form part of the clinical duties of a cardiologist. Active liaison with cardiac surgeons, general and acute physicians, primary care and cardiological subspecialists is necessary for the delivery of the highest quality care to individual patients.

Work to maintain and improve the quality of care

This work encompasses duties in clinical governance, professional self-regulation, CPD and education and training of others. For many consultants at various times in their careers it may include research, serving in management and providing specialist advice at local, regional and national levels.

Leadership role and the introduction of service developments

Service developments within cardiology invariably require multidisciplinary working, for example with cardiac technicians, specialist cardiac nurses or clinical managers. Cardiologists continue to have a leadership role within the field of service development and consequently need to maintain their team-working and leadership skills. Cardiologists work with local management to develop integrated care pathways and to implement NICE guidelines in routine clinical care. The entire patient journey from GP referral to completion of cardiac care, and equity of access for patients are key objectives within cardiovascular medicine.

Education and training

Because cardiovascular disease is the most common cause of death and highly prevalent in the population, education and training are essential at all levels, from patients to undergraduates, house officers, senior house officers (SHOs) and specialist registrars (SpRs). The SpR training programme is curriculum driven and competency based. There has been a substantial increase in the number of SpRs in cardiology and most consultant cardiologists will be involved in training SpRs, as organised by specialty training committees in the relevant deaneries. Formal training programmes are organised by the BCS where one day a year is given specifically to SpR training issues, plus locally organised training days.

Mentoring and appraisal of medical staff and other professional staff

Appraisal and assessment of SpRs is an increasing responsibility for the consultant cardiologist. Mentoring for professionals allied to medicine (PAMs) will help to develop a highly skilled clinically competent group of healthcare workers who will contribute to the delivery of high quality cardiovascular care.

Continuing medical education

Cardiologists' CME is regulated by the Federation of the Royal Colleges of Physicians. The BCS, through its annual scientific meeting and the *Education in Heart* series, provide CME, now accredited by the European Board for Accreditation in Cardiology (EBAC).

Research – clinical studies and basic science

The British Society for Cardiovascular Research (BSCR) and the British Atherosclerosis Society are affiliated groups of the BCS and both recognise the importance of basic science. Nationally, research is supported by the BHF at clinical and basic science levels through project and programme grants, chairs, senior fellows, intermediate fellows and junior fellows. The medical director of the BHF is a member of the BCS council. Consultant cardiologists are encouraged, either individually or in collaboration with their full-time academic colleagues, to conduct high quality cardiovascular research.

Regional and national work

All deaneries have specialist training committees in cardiology comprising consultant cardiologists, educational supervisors and SpR representatives. The BCS encourages the involvement of all consultant cardiologists and a new system of regional representatives has been set up. The society is run on a day-to-day basis by the president, president elect, secretary, assistant secretary, treasurer and chair of the programme committee. Affiliated groups address the subspecialist areas of ECHG, heart failure, intervention, nuclear medicine, pacing/electrophysiology, primary care, rehabilitation, technology (cardiac technicians), training and nursing.

The College has a system of regional representatives in place who will also act as regional representatives for the BCS. The SAC deals with all issues with regard to SpR training and the curriculum. The joint specialty committee provides the link between the College and the BCS.

There are a number of Department of Health (DH) working parties advising on manpower, PCI for acute infarction and academic medicine.

Current workforce numbers are:

- approximately 700 WTE consultant cardiologists
- 411 SpRs in cardiology.

The BCS cardiac workforce working group has made detailed recommendations for future service provision.[1]

ACADEMIC MEDICINE

The duties, responsibilities and areas of work of academic physicians

The duties and responsibilities of academic cardiologists are diverse. They range from a substantial focus on basic science research in the areas of atherosclerosis, heart failure, cardiomyopathy and electrophysiology, to clinical science, leading clinical trials relating to risk assessment and treatment for patients with conditions as varied as acute coronary syndromes or heart failure.

Clinical contribution to NHS

Clinically based academic cardiologists make important contributions to the NHS in terms of the organisation and delivery of both healthcare and training programmes.

Teaching

The commitment of any individual academic will depend on his or her research interest; both undergraduate and postgraduate teaching are growing areas of responsibility for academic cardiologists. In general, these responsibilities are shared with NHS consultant colleagues.

Research

The BHF provides major financial support in terms of endowed chairs and project and programme grants. The system of junior BHF fellowship provides a valuable link between NHS training programmes and academic cardiology.

WORKFORCE REQUIREMENTS FOR CARDIOLOGY

Current workforce numbers

There are currently approximately 700 WTE consultant cardiologists in the UK.

Number of consultants required to provide a specialist service to a population of 250,000

The fifth joint report on the provision of services for patients with cardiac disorders by the BCS and the College recommended that there should be one cardiologist per 50,000 head of population and therefore five cardiologists for a population of 250,000.[2]

National consultant workforce requirements

A target of at least 1,500 cardiologists is the figure recommended by the 2002 joint report. This estimate includes work in acute medicine but does not include a desirable increase in the number of academic cardiology units, or take into account the development of emergency angioplasty in the future. This target of 1,500 cardiologists is achievable and would equate to 7.7 WTE consultant cardiologists per 250,000 population. The BCS workforce planning group has estimated the number of cardiologists required and the number of subspecialists. The report is available at **www.bcs.com/download/221/BCS-Cardiac-Workforce-2004.pdf**[1] The increases projected in the recommendations are clearly not achievable in the short term.

CONSULTANT WORK PROGRAMME/SPECIMEN JOB PLAN

Consultant cardiologists work in a variety of different clinical settings and possess a wide range of clinical skills. The following job plan can be regarded as general advice.

Some cardiologists work predominantly in outpatients; some have general responsibilities for inpatients and some are procedure based, for example interventionalists or electrophysiologists.

Activity	Workload	Programmed activities (PAs)
Direct clinical care	Within the team of cardiologists, any individual would expect to devote 7.5 PAs on average to a selection of these activities.	
CCU ward rounds		**0.5–1**
Inpatient care plus referrals		**1–2**
Outpatient work		**2–3**
Specialised investigative or therapeutic clinical duties		**2–6**
Clinical administration (eg liaison with referring sources and on-ward referral for intervention or cardiac surgery; administration of waiting lists; working with nurse practitioners; writing reports/case summaries)		**1**
Total number of direct clinical care PAs		**7.5 on average**
Supporting professional activities (SPA) Work to maintain and improve the quality of healthcare	Education and training, appraisal, departmental management and service development, audit and clinical governance, CPD and revalidation, research	**2.5 on average**
Other NHS responsibilities	eg medical director/clinical director/lead consultant in specialty/clinical tutor	**Local agreement with trust**
External duties	eg work for deaneries/Royal Colleges/specialist societies/Department of Health or other government bodies etc	**Local agreement with trust**

A team of cardiologists will need to address the issues of:

▌ lead clinician

▌ audit

▌ delivery of higher specialist training

▌ general management

▌ clinical governance and risk management

▌ regional and national work:

    a)   postgraduate deanery with the specialty training committees

    b)   BCS and affiliated groups – intervention electrophysiology, heart failure etc (see Clinical work and/or laboratory work of consultants in cardiology)

    c)   manpower, education, clinical practice, programme committee for annual scientific conference and council committees

    d)   Royal College of Physicians – SAC, joint specialty committee, CME

▌ membership of national subspecialty groups promoting quality issues in clinical care

▌ IT for collecting reliable data in relation to clinical activities

▌ cardiac networks.

References

1. British Cardiac Society. *Cardiac workforce requirements in the UK*, April 2004. www.bcs.com/download/221/BCS-Cardiac-Workforce-2004.pdf

2. Fifth report on the provision of services for patients with heart disease. *Heart* 2002;**88**(Suppl 3):iii1–56.

Clinical genetics

i Description of the specialty and clinical needs of patients

Clinical genetics is a medical specialty that receives referrals of all ages from all branches of medicine and surgery. Clinical geneticists are physicians who have undergone higher specialty training in genetics after general professional training, usually in medicine or paediatrics (sometimes in other specialties such as psychiatry, obstetrics and gynaecology, ophthalmology and general practice). Higher specialty training covers a broad range of subspecialties including the genetics of adult and paediatric disorders, cancer, dysmorphology and neuropsychiatry. It also covers basic theoretical genetics, communication skills, laboratory experience and research skills. Specific clinical activities involve the diagnosis of genetic disorders and human malformations, genetic risk estimation, and support and management of families and individuals with genetic disorders. This includes discussion of the availability, implications and interpretation of genetic testing. The specialty has an increasingly important role in areas such as education of other professionals and the public, drawing up clinical pathways to reflect best practice, providing expert advice, and research and development.

The objectives of a clinical genetics service may be summarised as follows.[1]

- to diagnose persons referred to the service and provide relevant information to guide preventative and therapeutic care
- to explain the genetic basis of a disease or syndrome
- to support the identification and surveillance of relatives who are at risk for genetic disorders, to guide preventative and therapeutic actions if required
- to provide support to family members, both those affected and those who are not
- to educate the health community on genetic matters
- to contribute to genetic research that will benefit the population.

ii Organisation of the service and patterns of referral

Clinical networks and community arrangements

Clinical geneticists work within regional genetic centres and, together with genetic counsellors and laboratory scientists, provide genetic services to the population of a defined geographical region. These services are delivered through a network of central, joint and district clinics. In each region there are strong links with genetic laboratories, oncology and fetal medicine centres, and with community and primary care teams. The referrals to most genetic centres come from GPs and hospital specialties.

The regional genetic centres have formed a national network to provide information and diagnosis for individuals and families requiring specialist genetic expertise. Clinical genetic services are organised on a 'hub-and-spoke' model.[2] The regional genetic centre is the hub for the service incorporating a range of core services. Locally based clinics and support staff (secretarial and genetic counsellors) are closely linked with the regional centre.

Clinical genetics is mainly an outpatient specialty. Most genetic centres have a team approach to genetic referrals: the clinical genetics team discuss each referral and decide on an appropriate clinical management pathway. Many referrals concern genetic disorders and complex malformation syndromes that call for precise clinical diagnosis and calculation of risk. Where the diagnosis is known and where medical examination is not required, referrals may be seen by the genetic counsellor within the multiprofessional team without having direct contact with the consultant. The training of such genetic counsellors has been developed with the establishment of a registration scheme.[3]

Relationship with other services/agencies

Genetic services have close links with other specialties, particularly cancer services. Some regions use a system whereby patients complete a family history questionnaire to assess risk of inherited cancer. Families identified as being at moderate risk of having a genetic cause for a particular cancer are seen by a local clinician if surveillance is indicated. Families at high risk are seen in the genetics clinic for assessment and DNA predictive tests where these are available.

Clinical genetics centres undertake multidisciplinary clinics with other specialties and may hold disease-specific clinics to advise on surveillance for complications in specific disorders.

Genetic centres keep family-based records using a dedicated computer system. They administer their own appointments system and request medical records with consent from other hospitals to confirm diagnoses. Summary letters are sent to patients and referring clinicians following clinic appointments. Administrative and secretarial staff are, therefore, integral members of the genetic team.

iii   Working with patients: patient-centred care

Patient choice and involving patients in decisions about their treatment

The multiprofessional team approach in clinical genetics provides a patient- and family-centred approach. Individual and family diagnostic detail is ascertained and accurate, up-to-date information about risks and availability of testing is given. Information giving is non-directive and the individual or family is helped to make their own decisions about further diagnostic investigation or genetic testing. Ethical and religious considerations are paramount. The principles of privacy, consent, confidentiality and non-discrimination on the basis of genetic characteristics are upheld. Clinical geneticists liaise with patient support groups to ensure the provision of clear and accurate information.[4]

The Clinical Genetics Society (CGS) has delineated the core responsibilities of a consultant clinical geneticist to improve patient care.[5] They are as follows:

▪ diagnosis of genetic disorders affecting all ages and body systems, birth defects and developmental disorders
▪ investigation and genetic risk assessment
▪ information giving
▪ predictive testing for late-onset disorders using agreed protocols
▪ where appropriate, follow-up, support and coordination of health surveillance for specific genetic conditions

■ where appropriate, the offer of genetic services to extended families

■ where appropriate and where sufficient resources exist, maintenance of genetic family register services

■ liaison with genetic laboratories

■ participation in national genetic networks

■ education and training of genetic professionals and other healthcare professionals

■ acting as a resource of expertise and information to other specialists, GPs and other health professionals

■ research – clinical, biomedical, psychosocial and service related.

In this rapidly developing specialty the work of a clinical geneticist should be responsive to developments and changes in service need.

iv Interspecialty and interdisciplinary liaison

Genetic counsellors

Genetic counsellors have a background in nursing or science with specialist clinical genetic training. They may hold their own clinics with support and advice from consultants, for which consultant time should be allocated.

Laboratory genetic services

The clinical team works closely with molecular genetic and cytogenetic laboratory staff, especially concerning the indications for, and interpretation of, extremely specialised genetic tests, which may need to be tailored specifically to a particular family's clinical problem. Joint clinical and laboratory meetings are held to review case management.

Other specialists

Many genetic units hold multidisciplinary clinics and meetings with other specialties such as radiology, fetal medicine, oncology, neurology, nephrology, paediatric specialties, ophthalmology and cardiology.

v Delivering a high quality service

A high quality clinical genetics service should be part of a regional genetics centre, with full access to specialised genetic testing laboratories and a university department of medical genetics. The facilities required for clinical genetics services have been set out in a report from the College, and are summarised below:[2]

Facilities required to deliver a high quality clinical genetics service

Clinical facilities

■ appropriate and sympathetic outpatient area suitable for families and for adult and paediatric patients

■ access to full range of outpatient investigations

■ access to inpatient facilities for investigations (specific beds not required).

Office facilities

- adequate office space for consultant, other medical, co-worker and administrative/clerical staff
- secretarial support for clinic and other activities
- facilities for family record storage and retrieval
- library area for books, journals, database searching.

Information and IT requirements

- computer facilities for genetic registers (dedicated)
- desktop computer facilities and links to allow searches of internet-based and other databases
- software for malformation and other diagnostic databases
- regularly used journals and books .

General

- facilities for communicating between 'hub' and 'spoke' parts of the service
- support for travel of medical/counselling staff for peripheral clinics and home visits
- adequate study leave for national meetings and inter-regional audit.

vi Quality standards and measures of the quality of specialist services

Quality standards for clinical genetics services are discussed in a document from the College, and reviewed by the British Society of Human Genetics (BSHG) and the CGS.[1] Quality standards have also been created for the purposes of commissioning through the Genetics Commissioning Group (GenCAG), a subgroup of the National Specialist Commissioning Advisory Group (NSCAG). Not all centres are able to operate in the same manner. This principally reflects historical differences in staffing levels, the geographical locations of centres and the size and distribution of the populations served. The chief factor influencing access to service appears to be the availability of clinical genetics professionals.

Most centres provide:

- pre-consultation assessment
- clinical consultation
- post-consultation follow up
- inpatient consultations
- long-term contact and review of high risk individuals by genetic registers
- an urgent referral service for cases involving prenatal diagnosis.

Centres undertake regular audit activity and clinical governance to ensure adherence to quality standards.

CLINICAL WORK OF CONSULTANTS IN CLINICAL GENETICS

Clinical geneticists do not participate in the on-call rota for acute general medicine. They do, however, provide a consultation service for urgent problems (see below).

Direct clinical care

New patient clinics

The length of a consultation depends on the complexity of the case and whether or not genetic counsellors have been involved beforehand, but normally takes 45 minutes, occasionally one hour. A consultant working alone is usually able to see three or four new families in one session.

Specialist clinics

The number of patients seen depends on whether pedigree information is available beforehand, whether investigative procedures are carried out and whether the consultant works alone or with other specialists. The arrangements should be agreed locally.

Follow-up clinics

Follow up is often required to discuss the results of genetic tests and their implications. Each consultation might take 30 minutes. Without genetic counsellors more consultant clinics may be needed. In a new service most patients are first referrals, with few follow-up patients.

Review and recall

Many units have active review and recall systems supported by genetic registers and dedicated staff. The purpose of this form of anticipatory care is to inform individuals and families about technical advances and new information for health interventions, reproductive decisions and life-planning. Other units provide such a service within their routine working. Sessions for this work should be agreed locally.

Travel

District clinics allow equitable access to the service. Some are distant from the centre and require allowance for travelling time.

Junior medical staff

The work that can be undertaken by junior medical staff depends on their experience; most new entrants have no experience in the specialty. A consultant must set aside time to supervise their work. Overall, the contribution of a junior doctor might increase the amount of work that can be done in the clinic by 50%.

Supporting genetic counsellors

Part of the work of consultant clinical geneticists is to give training, support and advice to genetic counsellors and to encourage good team working and liaison.

Clinical discussion and laboratory liaison meetings

Attending regional and national clinical meetings (for example to discuss rare cases of dysmorphic syndromes) is necessary to ensure quality of clinical opinion. Joint clinical and laboratory meetings to discuss case management are an integral part of a consultant's work and should be recognised as a (fixed) commitment. Clinical geneticists attend multidisciplinary team (MDT) meetings relevant to their individual practice and specialist expertise.

On call for occasional urgent referral

Sessions must be allocated for emergency diagnostic work in early pregnancy. Inpatient ward referrals are undertaken as requested by other consultants. Some units also provide an emergency dysmorphology service to paediatricians and fetal pathology.

Work to maintain and improve the quality of care

This work encompasses duties in clinical governance, professional self-regulation, continuing professional development (CPD) and education and training of others. For many consultants at various times in their careers it may include research, serving in management and providing specialist advice at local, regional and national levels.

Leadership role and development of the service

Research and development of new diagnostic protocols and tests have arisen out of collaboration between clinicians and laboratory staff with the aim of improving care for patients with rare genetic disorders. Clinical geneticists take a leading role in the rational introduction of these improved service developments. A consultant may be the clinical director or hold other leadership or management roles within the service or NHS trust.

Teaching, training and education

The work of a clinical geneticist includes a large commitment to education, involving professional and non-professional groups.[6] It may be appropriate for a consultant in the regional genetic centre to have dedicated sessions to coordinate and organise teaching and training activities.[7] Increasing the educational provision for other health service professionals has been identified as an urgent national need to enable adequate provision of services to families.[8]

Mentoring and appraisal of medical staff and other professional staff

A clinical geneticist will appraise junior doctors, associate specialists and genetic counsellors working in the team.

Continuing professional development

The rapidly developing nature of clinical genetics requires that a clinical geneticist undertakes sufficient CPD, both external and internal, recognised by the College. This often requires attendance at international specialist meetings.

Clinical governance

Clinical genetics services have developed multidisciplinary clinical governance of patient care reflecting the integrated involvement of clinicians, genetic counsellors and laboratory staff.

Research

In a rapidly developing specialty where there are far more questions than answers, research forms an inherent part of the clinical geneticist's role. There is unanimity amongst practitioners that participation in research is essential to good clinical practice and that research activity should be broadly defined and not restricted to grant-funded or laboratory projects.[5] Legitimate research activities include clinical delineation and study of natural history, biomedicine, psychosocial aspects, service delivery etc and can all be performed either individually or in collaboration. It is important that consultant contracts and work plans reflect and acknowledge research demands.

Regional and national work

Clinical geneticists undertake College duties related to training, workforce planning and CPD. They advise the Department of Health and devolved governments on issues related to the provision of genetic services, genetic testing and the ethical implications of genetic advances. The CGS and the BSHG have widespread membership from clinical geneticists and take the lead in developments in clinical care.

ACADEMIC MEDICINE

The NHS workload of academic clinical geneticists depends on their academic responsibilities and individual job descriptions. Most academic clinical geneticists make a strong contribution to the routine work of the NHS department and undergraduate and postgraduate teaching, in addition to providing tertiary services. They supervise clinical research attachments leading to higher degrees. Major advances in clinical research have come from the close collaboration between clinical geneticists, laboratory scientists and the patients who attend genetics clinics.

WORKFORCE REQUIREMENTS FOR CLINICAL GENETICS

Clinical genetics services involve close team working between medical staff and genetic counsellors. Counsellors may be clinical nurse specialists or genetic counsellors with specific training in clinical genetics. The role and manpower requirements for such staff were set out in a College report.[7] The report recommended a minimum staffing level of two whole time equivalent (WTE) consultants and four genetic counsellors per million population for a general genetic service. Figures from the South West of Britain Audit and Training Group based on actual referral rates per million population support this. This does not include the rapid development of cancer genetics services. The requirement for a cancer genetics service has been identified as a minimum of one consultant per million population.[9]

The government white paper, *Our inheritance, our future*, published in 2003, highlights the fundamental role of regional genetic services to undertake programmes of genetic education.[8] There will be an increased workload engendered by the national antenatal and neonatal screening programmes and the mainstreaming of genetics in general medicine (for example cardiovascular genetics). This will require additional manpower.

The most recent annual Census of consultant physicians carried out by the College in September 2003 reported 114 WTE consultant clinical geneticists.[10] There is a need for continued planned expansion, coordinated with specialist registrar (SpR) posts. An initial expansion of 104% (to 233 WTE) should be the aim over the next few years. There is an increased demand to work less than full-time in clinical genetics. This is due to academic/research or personal commitments.

CONSULTANT WORK PROGRAMME/SPECIMEN JOB PLAN

Activity	Workload	Programmed activities (PAs)
Direct clinical care		
Outpatient new referrals	4 families	1
Cancer new referrals	6 families	1
Clinic preparation		2
Specialist clinics		
Follow up		
Ward referrals	2 families (variable)	1
Prenatals		
Telephone enquiries		
Team working with co-workers		
Multidisciplinary meetings		
Laboratory liaison	variable	2.5
Travel to peripheral clinic		
Total number of direct clinical care PAs		**7.5 on average**
Supporting Professional Activities (SPA)		
Work to maintain and improve the quality of healthcare	Education and training, appraisal, departmental management and service development, audit and clinical governance, CPD and revalidation, research	**2.5 on average**
Other NHS responsibilities	eg medical director/clinical director/lead consultant in specialty/clinical tutor	**Local agreement with trust**
External duties	eg work for deaneries/Royal Colleges/specialist societies/Department of Health or other government bodies etc	**Local agreement with trust**

A population of 250,000 requires one WTE clinical genetics consultant cover to run a clinical genetics service.

References

1. Royal College of Physicians. *Clinical genetic services. Activity, outcome, effectiveness and quality.* London: RCP, 1998.

2. Royal College of Physicians. *Commissioning clinical genetic services.* London: RCP, 1998.

3. Skirton H, Barnes C, Guilbert P, Kershaw A. Recommendations for education and training of genetic nurses and counsellors in the United Kingdom. *J Med Genet.* 1998;35(5):410–2. www.agnc.co.uk/training.htm

4. Genetic Interest Group. *Guidelines for genetic services.* London: Genetic Interest Group, 1998.

5. Clinical Genetics Society. *Role of the clinical geneticist,* March 2000. www.bshg.org.uk/Official%20Docs/ clingenrole.htm

6. Zimmern R, Cook C. The Nuffield Trust. *Genetics and health: policy issues for genetic science and their implications for health and health services.* London: The Stationery Office, 2000.

7. Royal College of Physicians. *Clinical genetics services into the 21st century.* London: RCP, 1996.

8. Department of Health. *Our inheritance, our future. Realising the potential of genetics in the NHS.* London: DH, 2003.

9. Department of Health. *Genetics and cancer services.* Report of a working group of the Chief Medical Officer. London: DH, 1996.

10. The Federation of the Royal Colleges of Physicians of the United Kingdom. *Census of consultant physicians in the UK, 2003: Data and commentary.* London: The Federation of the Royal Colleges of Physicians of the United Kingdom, 2003.

Clinical neurophysiology

i   Description of the specialty and clinical needs of patients

Clinical neurophysiologists undertake a variety of recordings and measurements of the electrical activity of the central and peripheral nervous systems. This information can be used to aid the diagnosis and management of a wide range of neurological conditions in all age groups. Activity is usually divided into four areas:

Electroencephalopathy (EEG)

The electrical activity of the brain (the EEG) can be recorded using either scalp (surface) or, in special circumstances, intracranial electrodes. The majority of studies are undertaken on an outpatient basis using scalp electrodes. Recordings may last from a half to several hours, particularly if a period of sleep is included. The principal indication for EEG is in the investigation of epilepsy and other disorders of consciousness. Since it is rare for brief recordings to capture a clinical attack, these EEGs are usually referred to as interictal recordings. Interictal EEG is used to classify the type of epilepsy or seizure disorder and to provide evidence to support a diagnosis of epilepsy.

EEG activity now includes more specialist studies such as ambulatory EEG and video telemetry monitoring. These studies monitor EEG for several days in an attempt to capture a clinical attack and characterise the associated EEG. Some patients, particularly those being considered for surgical treatment of intractable epilepsy, may require intracranial electrodes (depth or sub-dural electrodes) as part of video telemetry EEG studies.

EEG is also used in the diagnosis and management of other conditions such as encephalitis, Creuztfelt Jacob disease, coma, developmental and neurodegenerative disorders, including dementia. EEG studies may be undertaken during neurosurgical procedures to monitor cerebral activity, identify particular areas of cortical function and assist in the placement of deep-brain stimulators with intractable movement disorders.

Nerve conduction studies (NCS) and electromyography (EMG)

NCS recordings are made using electrical stimulation of the peripheral nerves. EMG activity measures the spontaneous and voluntary electrical activity produced in skeletal muscle. Many general medical disorders, as well as neurological disorders and trauma, can cause damage to the peripheral nervous system. EMG and NCS identify and characterise the site and nature of the pathological processes affecting the peripheral nervous system.

Evoked potential (EP) studies

These studies are used to monitor the response of the peripheral or, more commonly, central nervous system to a variety of sensory or cognitive stimuli.

Intraoperative monitoring (IOM)

Monitoring EPs, and in some cases EEG and NCS/EMG, can protect various neurological structures and systems during neurosurgery or orthopaedic surgery. Monitoring during functional neurosurgery for disorders such as Parkinson's disease and pain relief surgery can identify the correct neural structures for stimulation and lesioning.

ii   Organisation of the service and patterns of referral

Clinical neurophysiology is largely a consultant-provided service. The majority of neuro-physiological investigations are undertaken by consultant clinical neurophysiologists supported by trained neurophysiology technicians. In general, NCS/EMG and intraoperative monitoring (IOM) procedures are undertaken by medical staff. EEG and EP examinations are performed by technical staff and the results reviewed and reported on by consultant clinical staff. Some senior technical staff also perform NCS tests under consultant supervision. There are currently 31 specialist registrar (SpR) posts in the UK for the training of future consultant clinical neurophysiologists, but no junior staff at senior house officer (SHO) level.

Most consultant clinical neurophysiologists are based in neuroscience centres or larger district general hospitals (DGHs) with neurological services. Many consultants also cover local DGHs from their bases in the tertiary referral centres on a 'hub-and-spoke' model. A few consultants are based in larger DGHs with academic or teaching links to their local neuroscience centre. Clinical networks spanning strategic health authorities tend to be informal with some consultants taking the lead in highly specialised areas, usually as part of a multidisciplinary team (MDT).

Neurophysiological testing requires appropriate recording equipment, an appropriate environment and trained technical personnel. Therefore, neurophysiological services are usually only available in tertiary referral centres or larger DGHs.

The majority of investigations are carried out on an outpatient basis. However, some patients with severe neurological or medical/surgical conditions may require treatment and investigation as inpatients. Studies may be undertaken in intensive care units or special care baby units.

Special patterns of referral

Most patients are referred for investigation from other hospital consultants, principally neurologists, general physicians, rheumatologists, paediatricians and orthopaedic surgeons. Some neurophysiology departments provide access for GP referrals but this is usually limited to specific conditions or indications, except where GPs are specialists, for example in orthopaedics.

iii   Working with patients: patient-centred care

A neurophysiological opinion usually forms only part of the management of a patient as the majority of referrals come from consultants in the frontline specialties. Where referrals are accepted directly from primary care the patient needs to receive understandable information from the neurophysiology service to aid appropriate consent and any subsequent discussion of the management of their problem. The British Society for Clinical Neurophysiology (BSCN) has produced national guidelines on consent for neurophysiological procedures.

iv Interspecialty and interdisciplinary liaison

Multidisciplinary working is the foundation of investigation using EEG and EP; the consultant is totally reliant on the skills of the technician performing these tests.

There must be regular meetings and reviews between users of neurophysiological services and the medical and technical staff who carry out the neurophysiological studies. In centres undertaking complex surgical treatment for patients with epilepsy this may involve MDT meetings between neurologists, neurosurgeons, neuroradiologists, neuropsychologists and neurophysiology staff. Similarly, departments undertaking NCS and EMG testing may require MDT meetings between neurologists, paediatricians, and muscle and nerve histopathologists. In smaller centres or DGHs, which do not require MDT meetings, there should still be regular audit and review of activity between the referring clinicians and the neurophysiology department

v Delivering a high quality service

Resources required for a high quality service

An adequate neurophysiology service requires appropriate accommodation, testing equipment, and technical and other support personnel.

Specialised facilities

Accommodation

▪ The modern neurophysiology department should be a self-contained unit with a patient reception, clinical investigation rooms and office space. Scattered rooms located on wards or corridors do not provide an adequate or safe environment for a quality neurophysiology service.

▪ Clinical rooms should be of sufficient size to accommodate the testing equipment, examination chairs or couches, patients, medical and technical personnel together with the patient's carers and/or relatives.

▪ There must be suitable access for disabled patients or inpatients transferred on ambulance trolleys or beds.

▪ The department should contain suitable, separate office space for consultant and technical staff and for secretarial and administrative support staff.

▪ Neurophysiology departments should be sited for ease of access for outpatients who form the bulk of the patient workload.

▪ Testing equipment should be located well away from heavy electrical switchgear, which might preclude satisfactory recording.

▪ Departments undertaking video telemetry monitoring should be within easy reach of the monitoring suite.

Equipment It is essential that all departments have sufficient neurophysiology equipment to undertake the required EEG/EP or EMG activity. Equipment must be tested regularly for safety and accuracy. Many departments have now converted to digital EEG recording with significant advantages for storage retrieval and transmission of data. This is particularly important for smaller departments where there may not be a consultant neurophysiologist present on every working day.

Workforce requirements

Medical staffing The consultant clinical neurophysiologist should not work in isolation. Larger departments may contain two or more consultant neurophysiologists. Smaller DGH units, which may support only a single consultant, should have close links with a nearby larger clinical neurophysiology department. Each department should be led by a consultant clinical neurophysiologist with support from a senior member of the technical staff. The number of technical staff required will depend upon the workload of the department. For reasons of continuity of patient care and safety no department should be staffed with less than two whole time equivalent (WTE) technicians. Larger departments will require three or more trained technical staff and should be able to support a programme of technician training.

As this is a specialty that supports regional neurological centres, calculations based on 250,000 population are less relevant. However, based on national needs, it is estimated that 0.75 WTE consultants per 250,000 population are required. This would mean an additional 106 WTE consultants across the UK, representing an increase of 153% over the next few years.

Technical staffing The provision of suitably trained and qualified technical staff is essential for the safe and efficient operation of a neurophysiology department. There is a national shortage of suitably trained technicians and the numbers of technicians entering basic grade training has fallen in recent years. Larger departments, especially those in regional neuroscience centres, must develop basic-grade training programmes and attract suitably qualified and motivated applicants to these training places. Larger departments should also provide continuing post-basic training, particularly in more advanced areas such as video telemetry and IOM.

Administrative and secretarial staffing Neurophysiology departments should be equipped with adequate IT to support an appointment and reporting system. The system should provide statistical information regarding activity and waiting lists. There should be adequate secretarial and administrative support for the consultant neurophysiologists and technical staff undertaking the various studies: one WTE secretary per seven consultant programmed activities (PAs) in direct clinical care. Departments should set standards for waiting times for investigation and processing times for generation of reports and dispatch. The department should provide a system for prioritising requests, usually divided into urgent, soon or routine. Further subdivision may be helpful, for example in carpal tunnel screening clinics.

vi   Quality standards and measures of the quality of specialist services

Specialist society guidelines

Waiting time standards are outlined by the Association of British Clinical Neurophysiologists (ABCN). To provide a quality service for patients it is essential to set standards for waiting and reporting times. The following guidelines would provide an acceptable minimum standard of service for most departments:

- For routine investigations, waiting times should be less than four weeks for EEG and EP studies, and less than six weeks for NCS/EMG.
- More urgent cases should be seen within two days for EEG and one week for EMG.
- Urgent inpatient cases for both EEG and EMG should be seen within 24 hours.

CLINICAL WORK AND/OR LABORATORY WORK OF CONSULTANTS IN CLINICAL NEUROPHYSIOLOGY

Contributions made to acute medicine

Neurophysiologists are rarely directly involved in the delivery of care in general internal medicine (GIM).

Direct clinical care

Inpatient work

The volume of EEG, EMG and other investigations requested in support of acute medical care can be highly variable. In larger departments it may be possible to programme inpatient clinic slots for EEG and EMG with little wastage. Providing an inpatient service on sites away from the main base can be challenging and so may be limited to patients for whom transfer is not practical, for example critical care units and secure psychiatric facilities.

Outpatient work

The number of patients seen per EMG/NCS clinic will depend upon the complexity of the investigations required. Usually, between four and six patient appointments would be expected per four-hour PA of direct clinical care. This number should be reduced if the consultant is required to supervise concomitant carpal tunnel or peripheral nerve testing clinics undertaken by suitably trained technicians, or if supervising SpRs undertaking their own NCS/EMG clinic. The ABCN guideline is that least one hour of an NCS/EMG PA in direct clinical care should be for the generation of reports on patients seen in the clinic.

A consultant undertaking an EEG reporting session might be expected to report between 15 and 25 routine outpatient interictal EEGs per four-hour PA. This would include paediatric EEG studies and short-term sleep studies. The number of the EEGs reviewed per session should be adjusted downward if there is a significant teaching element for SpRs and technicians attending the reporting session.

The number of long-term ambulatory or video telemetry studies that could be reported in a session will depend on the degree of data analysis carried out by the recording technician. If there has been significant editing and data selection then four to six studies could be assessed per session. If the consultant does all the data analysis, only one or two studies could be assessed per session. It is good practice to involve the recording technicians in all consultant EEG reporting sessions.

Specialist investigative and therapeutic procedures

Larger departments in neuroscience centres are increasingly involved in IOM, which is highly labour intensive. The consultant may perform the studies, such as corticography or deep brain stimulation, or supervise technical staff in monitoring neurological structures, such as in scoliosis surgery.

Specialist on call

Few centres have enough staff to enable full consultant and technician on-call rotas for a reliable out-of-hours service for EEG – this being the test required most often. Various ad hoc arrangements tend to be in place.

Other specialist activity

Multidisciplinary team meetings must be fully recognised, formalised and auditable (the meeting must follow an agenda and the minutes be recorded etc).

Patient-related administration

This includes communication with and about patients with whom the consultant has had direct involvement or responsibility (phone calls, letters, emails, reading referrals). This would include consent issues, direct meetings and report writing. Work relating to complaints is part of the consultant's clinical governance responsibilities and so constitutes supporting professional activities (SPA).

Work to maintain and improve the quality of care

This work encompasses duties in clinical governance, professional self-regulation, continuing professional development (CPD) and education and training of others. For many consultants at various times in their careers it may include research, serving in management and providing specialist advice at local, regional and national levels.

This work falls within SPA and a consultant would devote 10 hours per week (2.5 PAs) to this on average. For many consultants the amount of time spent on research, serving in local management and leading in other activities such as audit will vary during their career. Other NHS responsibilities need to be agreed with the employer and included in the job plan.

ACADEMIC MEDICINE

The NHS workload of academic neurophysiologists depends on their academic responsibilities and individual job descriptions but, in general, academic neurophysiologists are a central component of a complex and technological discipline. Advances in the understanding of neurophysiological function of the nervous system are crucial to developing practice, and academic appointments make a strong contribution to the work of NHS departments.

In general, most academic neurophysiologists will need to devote at least two to four PA sessions to academic work rather than NHS service activity. Academic appointments should not include any significant sessional commitment outside the regional or academic centre. It is important that academic departments have sufficient technical and support staff, possibly including engineers and IT specialists to support clinical academic research.

CONSULTANT WORK PROGRAMME/SPECIMEN JOB PLAN

The range of activities in average mixed practice is reflected below. In some neurosciences centres a consultant may only work in one field viz. EEG, EMG or EP.

Travelling between multiple sites may have a significant impact on direct clinical care. This can be accommodated by reducing the length of the clinic/reporting session or taking the travelling time as extra direct clinical time in addition to the four-hour PA.

At least one hour in each four hour NCS/EMG clinic should be allowed for the generation of clinical reports.

EEGs are the main out-of-hours requirement, limited by the availability of technicians. Some neurosciences centres have a formal rota but most operate an ad hoc arrangement.

Activity	Workload (cases/patients)	Programmed activities (PAs)
Direct clinical care		
Routine outpatient EMG/NCS clinics	4–6	**2–5**
Inpatient EMG (department)	3–4	**0–1**
Inpatient EMG (portable multisite)	1–2	**0–1**
Reporting routine EEG and EPs/Technician NCS	15–25	**1–3**
Reporting (± performing) specialist tests, eg telemetry or visual electrophysiology	1–5	**0–1**
Intraoperative monitoring	1	**0–2**
Multidisciplinary clinics eg epilepsy or neuromuscular disease		**0–2**
Patient-related administration		**0–1**
Total number of direct clinical care PAs		**7.5 on average**
Supporting professional activities (SPA) Work to maintain and improve the quality of healthcare	Education and training, appraisal, departmental management and service development, audit and clinical governance, CPD and revalidation, research.	**2.5 on average**
Other NHS responsibilities	eg medical director/clinical director/lead consultant in specialty/clinical tutor	**Local agreement with trust**
External duties	eg work for deaneries/Royal Colleges/specialist societies/Department of Health or other government bodies etc	**Local agreement with trust**

Clinical pharmacology and therapeutics

i   Description of the specialty and clinical needs of patients

Clinical pharmacologists employed within the NHS usually combine their specialty with work as a general physician. About half of their time involves the supervision of acute medical admissions, managing medical inpatients and running outpatient clinics. These individuals will normally have another clinical specialty interest (for example cardiovascular risk management, toxicology) and will take a particular interest in prescribing issues on behalf of their employing NHS body.

The mission of the specialty is to improve the care of patients by promoting safe and effective use of medicines and to evaluate and introduce new therapies.[1] Therefore, clinical pharmacologists will often make wider contributions to the NHS clinical service. At a local level this may involve leading the drug and therapeutics committee, developing and maintaining a drug formulary, assessing new products, creating prescribing guidelines, reviewing medication incidents and promoting evidence-based therapeutics.

Some consultants may play a leading role in a medicines information service for local prescribers, usually with the support of a clinical pharmacist. At a national level, consultants in clinical pharmacology and therapeutics occupy many positions within key bodies such as the National Institute for Clinical Excellence (NICE), the Medicines Control Agency (MCA), the Committee on Safety of Medicines (CSM), the Joint Formulary Committee overseeing publication of the British National Formulary, the Medicines Commission, and adverse drug reaction monitoring (pharmaco-vigilance) schemes. The National Poisons Information Service (NPIS) is run almost exclusively by NHS clinical pharmacologists.

The work programme of a consultant in clinical pharmacology and therapeutics varies greatly, depending on the job setting. At the time of the last College Census, approximately two-thirds of consultants in clinical pharmacology and therapeutics held academic appointments within universities.[2] While having a service commitment, many of these individuals will have a strong research emphasis in their work that will contribute to knowledge about drug actions and their clinical usage. They will also play an important role in the planning and delivery of undergraduate teaching in therapeutics.

Other clinical pharmacologists at consultant level are employed by the pharmaceutical industry and are involved in the development of new drugs and early clinical trials in patients. Some also hold joint appointments with academic units or trusts, a trend that may grow in the future.

ii   Organisation of the service and patterns of referral

Primary, secondary and tertiary levels

Clinical pharmacologists are active in promoting safe and effective use of medicines at all levels. At the primary care level they develop and maintain formularies; at the secondary level they may lead the drug and therapeutics committee or run a drug information service; at a tertiary level they may be involved in organisations such as the CSM adverse drug reaction monitoring system, the NPIS and health technology assessment.

Clinical networks and community arrangements

The viability of local clinical networks is restricted by the small number of consultants. However, clinical pharmacologists often come together at national level in the setting of the CSM adverse drug reaction monitoring system, the NPIS and health technology assessment.

Relationship with other services/agencies

Clinical pharmacologists will usually have a close relationship with one or more of the following:

▪ clinical pharmacy service
▪ chief pharmacist
▪ medicines information unit
▪ medical director
▪ finance director
▪ clinical risk management committee
▪ primary care prescribing adviser
▪ director of public health
▪ regional adverse drug reaction monitoring centre
▪ local health authority.

Complementary services

The work of clinical pharmacologists in promoting safe and effective use of medicines is complemented by a clinical pharmacy service. Pharmacists often play an important role in supporting the work of professional committees, providing information about medicines, preventing and reporting medication incidents, and reporting adverse drug reactions. Some consultants will require an efficient laboratory service to support therapeutic drug monitoring or the assessment of poisoned patients. In some circumstances, the work of a clinical pharmacologist may involve close collaboration with a department of public health.

iii   Working with patients: patient-centred care

Patient choice, opportunities for education and promoting self-care

Clinical pharmacologists will not only be practitioners of patient-centred care within their own clinical area but, as part of their mission to deliver rational therapeutics, will also promote improved understanding of drug therapy issues and support concordance about prescribing decisions between local prescribers and their patients. These objectives may be achieved through education of doctors (at undergraduate and postgraduate levels) with emphasis on patient involvement in therapeutic choices, informed consent, and promotion of self-care, and through education of patients by disseminating relevant patient information. Clinical pharmacologists will also endeavour to improve the efficacy and safety of medicines through promotion of evidence-based medicine, development of guidelines and shared care protocols. They will, wherever possible, liaise with patient groups and lay representatives when developing prescribing policies.

iv Interspecialty and interdisciplinary liaison

The nature of medicines management activities means that clinical pharmacologists often have important relationships with many other specialist groups and primary care colleagues. Clinical pharmacologists often have medical subspecialties, particularly in cardiovascular medicine, where liaison with other clinical groupings such as cardiology and stroke medicine will be important. It is also likely that they will work as part of a multidisciplinary team (MDT) involving pharmacists and nurses in the pursuit of medicines management and when carrying out clinical trials.

v Delivering a high quality service

Characteristics of a high quality service

- a well-organised and efficiently run drug and therapeutics committee drawing on relevant local expertise
- an agreed local formulary
- development and regular review of local prescribing policies that support safe, evidence-based and cost-effective prescribing
- contribution to clinical risk management through regular review of medication incidents
- appropriate levels of adverse drug reaction reporting by local prescribers
- regular high quality education in rational prescribing for undergraduates and postgraduates
- early review of, and advice concerning, poisoned patients.

Resources required for a high quality service in clinical pharmacology

- inpatient medical beds (approximately 15–20) to support acute medical services with appropriate levels of nursing support
- junior staff support, including a specialist registrar (SpR), for the admission of unselected acute general medical cases
- outpatient facilities with access to clinical laboratory services and space for teaching
- clinical laboratory facilities, which may include access to special investigations such as drug assays, sometimes necessitating collaboration with other specialists (eg clinical biochemists)
- research facilities, which may include protected beds for clinical research together with appropriately trained nursing staff, laboratory facilities with technical support, or computer hardware for data management
- secretarial support for inpatient and outpatient activities, and other managerial responsibilities
- private office space, including appropriate IT facilities and space for filing
- library facilities
- teaching facilities for undergraduates and postgraduates, including image projection
- facilities to support the training of SpRs, including research facilities and computer and word-processing support
- an adequately staffed clinical pharmacy service including the facility to provide a medicines information service
- study leave and support for continuing professional development (CPD).

vi   Quality standards and measures of the quality of specialist services

Quality and standards in clinical pharmacology are largely expressed by local prescribers in the primary and secondary care sector in relation to the approach to medicines usage, rather than by clinical pharmacologists alone. The measurement of quality and standards in relation to the provision of a clinical pharmacology service is, therefore, problematic. However, potential means to ensure and measure quality include adherence to widely applicable national guidelines, dissemination of relevant prescribing information, implementation of cost-effective prescribing patterns and audit of prescribing practices.

CLINICAL WORK AND/OR LABORATORY WORK OF CONSULTANTS IN CLINICAL PHARMACOLOGY

Clinical pharmacologists have very varied patterns of working but most NHS and academic consultants are accredited in both clinical pharmacology and therapeutics and in general internal medicine (GIM) as their second specialty. However, the skills of clinical pharmacology and therapeutics are generic and fully applicable to other medical specialties. There are a small number of consultants who also practise in geriatric medicine, paediatrics, oncology, respiratory medicine or cardiology, and it is likely that the number of such consultants will increase as more varied training schemes are established.

Contributions made to acute medicine

Clinical pharmacologists have traditionally taken a particularly active role as general non-organ-based physicians in the on-call rota for the supervision of receiving and triaging acute emergency admissions. These duties should be undertaken with the support of an appropriate number of junior doctors including a SpR. Acute general medical admissions should, ideally, be admitted to a medical admissions unit with appropriate staffing levels and access to emergency investigations.[3] The on-call rota should not normally be more onerous than one in five. Each period of acute admitting must include a post-take ward round with the junior staff who were involved in the admission process. In some services two ward rounds may be required in a 24-hour period. Consultants who are responsible for the review of poisoned patients have more frequent post-receiving ward rounds.

Direct clinical care

Inpatient work

Activities will normally be devoted to supervising the management of general medical patients and the specialist work of the individual consultant. This work typically requires two ward rounds per week at fixed times.[4] The number of inpatients for which the consultant team is responsible should not normally exceed 20. Part of this time will be dedicated to inpatient referrals for patients with pharmacological or toxicological problems. Consultants expect to work in an adequately staffed ward with the appropriate facilities and ancillary services to care for a typical casemix of general medical patients. They should have the support of at least one junior doctor who has completed general professional training.

Outpatient work

Time will be allocated for seeing new patient referrals, including emergency referrals, and follow-up after discharge from A&E or a hospital ward. Consultants normally provide this service with the support of junior staff and must allow time for their supervision. It is reasonable to expect that assessment of a new patient will take approximately 30 minutes and follow-up patients approximately 15 minutes. Trainees require more time and should not work in isolation. A typical clinic might include four to six new patients and 10–15 follow-up patients. These sessions should include time for dictating clinic letters and administrative matters relating to the outpatient service. Some clinical pharmacologists also provide specialist clinics, for example in cardiovascular risk management or epilepsy. Patients are sometimes referred with specific therapeutic, toxicological or other drug-related problems.

Specialist investigative or therapeutic procedures

Clinical pharmacologists will not normally undertake specialist procedures other than those that arise from other specialty activities.

Specialist on call

The most likely on-call commitment to arise from a clinical pharmacology service is to provide emergency advice about the management of poisoned patients. This activity will usually be supported by a poisons information service and clinical pharmacologists may offer advice on a regional basis. Some academic specialists may have ongoing out-of-hours commitments to subjects involved in clinical trials.

Clinically related administration

Clinical pharmacologists will have administrative duties in keeping with their clinical workload. They may also be called upon to write specialist reports related to medication issues.

Work to maintain and improve the quality of care

This work encompasses duties in clinical governance, professional self-regulation, CPD and education and training of others. For many consultants at various times in their careers it may include research, serving in management and providing specialist advice at local, regional and national levels.

While supervision and management of general medical patients is a major direct contribution to the NHS service, most consultants in clinical pharmacology and therapeutics take on other roles that contribute indirectly to achieving local NHS service objectives and standards. These activities usually focus on the management of medicines in primary and secondary care, for example:

- leading or playing an important role in the activities of the drug and therapeutics committee and overseeing the use of drugs in both hospital and primary care
- managing a local drug formulary, which may be jointly agreed with a local GP
- editing and facilitating the production of local prescribing guidelines for common medical problems
- taking a lead role in reporting adverse reactions and reviewing local medication incidents

- undertaking health technology assessment, which might involve reviewing new and established drugs for clinical- and cost-effectiveness
- auditing and reviewing patterns of local drug use with the aim of maximising effective and safe use of medicines in the NHS.

All of these activities make an important contribution to achieving local objectives in clinical effectiveness, clinical risk management and clinical governance. Clinical pharmacologists are likely to play a major role in auditing and investigating local drug-related incidents.

Some consultants may provide a drug information service, often with the support of a clinical pharmacist. This may include a therapeutic drug monitoring service to advise on the management and prevention of medication errors, and an advice service on drug overdoses and management of adverse effects. Some consultants have a specialist interest in forensic pharmacology and provide expert advice in coroner's, criminal and civil cases. There should be adequate provision for all of these important public health and additional service commitments within a job plan.

ACADEMIC MEDICINE

Approximately two-thirds of consultants in clinical pharmacology and therapeutics hold academic posts, which accounts for the particularly diverse contributions that the specialty makes to the delivery of healthcare. Consultants in major teaching centres play a key role in the design and delivery of teaching in therapeutics to medical students.[5] For new medical graduates, prescribing drugs is a major activity and one that is associated with significant clinical risk. For these reasons therapeutics remains an important theme within any medical curriculum and requires appropriate support from clinical teachers. Clinical pharmacologists are also involved in the delivery of postgraduate training in therapeutics to other health professionals within the NHS, including GPs, nurses and pharmacists.

Research is a fundamental part of the work of many clinical pharmacologists. It may involve clinical research in patients and healthy volunteers, and some individuals lead teams of laboratory-based researchers. Drug-related research activities make an important contribution to the local and national NHS research and development strategy, providing important long-term benefits for patient care. The success of these activities will depend on the availability of suitable clinical and laboratory areas, recognition of the need for protected research sessions, and the support of appropriately trained clinical and technical staff. Clinical pharmacologists often have an important role on (or chair) local and multicentre research ethics committees because of their expertise in drug-related research.

WORKFORCE REQUIREMENTS FOR CLINICAL PHARMACOLOGY AND THERAPEUTICS

The 2001 consultant Census reported that there were 60 WTE consultants in clinical pharmacology and therapeutics in England and Wales, equivalent to one per 870,000 of the population.[6] The following calculation reflects the number of consultants needed to ensure that there are sufficient clinical pharmacologists to contribute to national bodies, and to provide a high quality local service with particular emphasis on medicines management, toxicology and academic activities such as teaching and research. The workforce will also contribute to the care of unselected acute general medical admissions. The calculation takes into account several important trends:

■ Drugs account for an increasing proportion of NHS expenditure (currently 15% of the total) and there are pressures to prescribe newer, more expensive medicines.

■ There is a requirement to contain costs by adopting agreed formularies, and making rigorous assessments of clinical- and cost-effectiveness of new drugs.

■ New medical schools are opening and there has been a significant expansion in medical student numbers to around 6,000 annually.

■ Acute general medical admissions are increasing year on year.

■ The increasing burden on physicians running a specialty service (eg gastroenterology, cardiology) is creating difficulties in providing acute medical cover.

■ Junior doctors' hours of work are decreasing.

■ Working time directives will have an impact.

Clinical pharmacology is one of the few specialties with decreasing numbers at present. Sufficient consultants are required to deliver the academic programme, including teaching. There is a strong case to be made for having one WTE clinical pharmacologist in every large district general hospital (DGH) for acute medicine and to address the specialty needs of the trust and the local primary care trust (PCT).

It is estimated, therefore, that the workforce requirement for consultants in clinical pharmacology and therapeutics is approximately 200 WTE. This number of consultants is based on providing:

■ one WTE consultant per DGH serving a population of 250,000 (with an expected annual drug expenditure of £60 million)

■ one WTE consultant per 180 medical students in training (of whom there are there are now 36,000)

■ three consultants per medical school (assuming that half of these hold academic contracts, implying that the expansion in consultant numbers will be predominantly in the NHS).

This figure requires an expansion in consultant numbers of at least 10% per annum over the next decade. Following the successful joint initiative of the NHS Executive and the Association of the British Pharmaceutical Industry, the number of trainees in clinical pharmacology has increased in the past few years. The scheme acknowledges the shortage of trained individuals and their importance to the future use of drugs in the NHS. Twenty-five SpRs expect to complete training by 2004.

CONSULTANT WORK PROGRAMME/SPECIMEN JOB PLAN

The following tables summarise the range of activities undertaken by consultant physicians in clinical pharmacology and therapeutics with responsibilities in GIM, alongside the recommended workload and the allocation of programmed activities (PAs) (considered to be a period of four hours). The job plan is based on a commitment of 10 PAs per week, although the typical working pattern of a clinical pharmacologist will involve a number of extra PAs. Suggested work programmes have been provided for a consultant working in a university teaching hospital and one in a DGH.

Academic clinical pharmacologists will normally hold a full-time university contract (the full-time salary being paid by the university) and an honorary (unpaid) NHS contract. The honorary contract will normally include not more than five NHS PAs, of which no more than 3.5 will be devoted to direct clinical care activities (as defined in the 2003 consultant contract). The award of these concurrent contracts recognises the contribution that academic consultants make, both directly and indirectly (eg medicines management, pharmacovigilance, safe and effective prescribing) to the NHS clinical service. This arrangement also recognises that the activities carried out on behalf of the NHS are valuable for the delivery of high quality teaching and research. The job plan of an academic clinical pharmacologist will be made by agreement between the consultant, the dean and the medical director of the NHS body (or their nominated representatives), and will take full account of the principles set out in the Follett Report concerning the relationship between academic and clinical workload.[7] The academic contract will include responsibilities for research, undergraduate teaching and administration relating to these and other NHS duties.

In some cases it will be the university department as a whole that makes a commitment to provide a fixed number of PAs to the NHS service, allowing for more flexible participation of individual academic consultants in clinical duties.

CONSULTANT WORK PROGRAMME/SPECIMEN JOB PLAN FOR AN ACADEMIC CLINICAL PHARMACOLOGIST WORKING IN A UNIVERSITY TEACHING HOSPITAL BASED ON 10 PROGRAMMED ACTIVITIES

Activity	Workload	Programmed activities (PAs)
Direct clinical care		
Emergency duties arising from acute receiving (24 hours)	10–15 patients	**0–1**
Inpatient (ward rounds, referrals, MDT meetings)	10–15 patients	**0–1**
Outpatient clinics	5–10 patients	**0–1**
Administration directly related to patient care (eg referrals, notes, complaints, correspondence with other practitioners)		**0.5–1**
Public health duties, eg medicines management: running drug and therapeutics committee, managing a formulary, developing prescribing policies, health technology assessment, drug information services		**0–2**
Supporting professional activities (SPA) Work to maintain and improve the quality of healthcare	eg CPD, postgraduate teaching and training, management of doctors in training, audit, job planning, appraisal, revalidation, contribution to service management and planning, clinical governance activities	**1.5 on average**
Other NHS responsibilities	eg Caldicott guardian, clinical audit lead, clinical governance lead, undergraduate and postgraduate dean, clinical tutor, regional education adviser, medical management responsibilities	**Local agreement with trust**
External duties	eg work for national NHS bodies, work for other external bodies (eg Medicines and Healthcare Products Regulatory Agency, CSM, NICE, Royal Colleges, General Medical Council, Postgraduate Medical Education and Training Board, British Medical Association), NHS disciplinary procedures, NHS appeals procedures, advisory appointments committees.	**Local agreement with trust**
Academic duties Teaching undergraduates		**1–2**
Research		**2–4**
University administration		**1**

CONSULTANT WORK PROGRAMME/SPECIMEN JOB PLAN FOR A NHS CONSULTANT CLINICAL PHARMACOLOGIST WORKING IN A DISTRICT GENERAL HOSPITAL BASED ON 10 PROGRAMMED ACTIVITIES

Activity	Workload	Programmed activities (PAs)
Direct clinical care		
Emergency duties arising from acute receiving (24 hours) including dealing with poisoned patients	20–30 patients	**1–2**
Inpatient (ward rounds, referrals, MDT meetings)	20–25 patients	**1–2**
Outpatient clinics	15–20 patients	**1–2**
Administration directly related to patient care (eg referrals, notes, complaints, correspondence with other practitioners)		**1–2**
Public health duties, eg medicines management: running drug and therapeutics committee, managing a formulary, developing prescribing policies, health technology assessment, drug information services		**1–2**
Supporting professional activities (SPA) Work to maintain and improve the quality of healthcare	eg CPD, teaching and training, management of doctors in training, audit, job planning, appraisal, revalidation, research, contribution to service management and planning, clinical governance activities	**2.5**
Other NHS responsibilities	eg Caldicott guardians, clinical audit leads, clinical governance leads, undergraduate and postgraduate deans, clinical tutors, regional education advisers, medical management responsibilities	**Local agreement with trust**
External duties	eg work for national NHS bodies, work for other external bodies (eg Medicines and Healthcare Products Regulatory Agency, CSM, NICE, Royal Colleges, General Medical Council, Postgraduate Medical Education and Training Board, British Medical Association), NHS disciplinary procedures, NHS appeals procedures, advisory appointments committees	**Local agreement with trust**

Note: The allocation of PAs worked by a consultant clinical pharmacologist will be variable. Most job plans are likely to involve extra PAs beyond the standard 10, allowing consultants to undertake other responsibilities and external duties (outlined above) in addition to the standard job plan. This is particularly important in clinical pharmacology where a relatively small number of consultants are strongly represented in national bodies such as the Medicines and Healthcare Products Regulatory Agency (MHRA), NICE, CSM and NPIS. There will be times in the career of a consultant when management and national duties increase to the extent that they will need to be reflected within the standard 10 PA job plan. Consultants who hold academic posts are likely to share NHS responsibilities with other academic colleagues, reducing the commitment to the clinical service when compared to full-time NHS colleagues.

References

1. Royal College of Physicians. *Clinical Pharmacology and therapeutics in a changing world.* Report of a working party. London: Royal College of Physicians, 1999.

2. The Federation of the Royal Colleges of Physicians of the United Kingdom. *Census of consultant physicians in the UK, 2003. Data and commentary.* London: RCP, 2003.

3. Federation of Royal Colleges of Physicians of the UK. *Acute medicine: the physician's role. Proposals for the future.* A working party report of the Federation of Medical Royal Colleges. London: Royal College of Physicians, 2000.

4. Royal College of Physicians. *Governance in acute general medicine. Recommendations from the Committee on General (Internal) Medicine of the Royal College of Physicians.* London: RCP, 2000.

5. Maxwell SRJ, Walley T. Teaching prescribing and therapeutics. *Br J Clin Pharmacol* 2003;**55**:496–503.

6. Federation of Medical Royal Colleges. *Census of consultant physicians in the UK, 2001. Data and commentary.* London: RCP, 2001.

7. Follett B, Michael Paulson-Ellis M. *A review of appraisal, disciplinary and reporting arrangements for senior NHS staff with academic and clinical duties.* A report to the Secretary of State for Education and Skills, September 2001.

Critical care

i   Description of the specialty and clinical needs of patients

In June 1999 the Specialist Training Authority granted specialty recognition to the discipline of intensive care medicine. This event represented the culmination of many years of development of the concept of intensive care, which emerged largely as a response to developments in medicine and surgery. Indeed, in some specialties (particularly neurosciences, cardiac and burns) intensive care units were developed specifically in order to provide high quality patient care in the post-operative period. High dependency units were introduced to provide step-down facilities between intensive and ward-based care, sometimes in dedicated areas associated with particular specialties. Overall, development was unplanned and haphazard, and relied largely upon the interest and enthusiasm of isolated groups of clinicians.

Consequently, in March 1999, an expert group was established by the Department of Health (DH) to propose a framework for the future organisation and delivery of adult critical care services. The group was asked to produce a national framework for adult critical care, which was to be evidence based, or at least based upon clear professional consensus, in setting out operational standards for intensive care and high dependency units.

The report was published in 2000 and made wide-ranging recommendations for the configuration and mix of general adult and neurological adult intensive care and high dependency care services.[1] The overarching principle of the report was that the modernised service must be based upon integration. Thus, a hospital-wide approach to critical care services, extending beyond the physical boundaries of intensive care and high dependency units, was envisaged to support, and interact and communicate with, the whole range of acute services. Critical care was to be provided in the context of an integrated network involving neighbouring trusts working to common standards and protocols, thereby providing a comprehensive range of services. Workforce development was planned (see below). Finally, the new service was to be underpinned by information and a data collection culture, promoting the development of an appropriate evidence base.

The implementation of this report in England is currently in progress under the supervision of the NHS Modernisation Agency.

ii   Organisation of the service and patterns of referral

Critical care services within trusts are now organised via delivery groups, rendered mandatory by a DH directive. Critical care delivery groups are to be composed of staff of all disciplines working within the spectrum of acute care and in services complementary to the field of critical care. Board level representation is required.

Twenty-nine critical care networks have been established in England, financed by the NHS Modernisation Agency. Each is led by administrative and clinical staff tasked with facilitating the development of a service integrated between neighbouring trusts to provide patients with the full range of specialties within a specified geographical area. This approach is designed to obviate the need for long-distance transfer of patients to access specialist services.

iii Working with patients: patient-centred care

Patient choice and involving patients in decisions about their treatment

Critical care has a long tradition of involving relatives in decisions about the treatment afforded to patients, and in being sensitive to patient choice where possible. Thus, the majority of patients with level 3 dependency (that is, traditionally necessitating admission to intensive care) are sedated and mechanically ventilated. The use of patient surrogates, developed more fully elsewhere in Europe and North America, is under active consideration in the UK.

The concept of the 'advanced directive', limiting the level of therapeutic intervention applied to patients according to their own wishes and desires, is particularly relevant to the critical care setting, especially given the need to provide appropriate care to patients for whom continued support is considered to be futile.

Access to information, patient support groups and the role of the expert patient

The NHS Modernisation Agency has started a work programme based on so-called 'discovery interviews' to learn lessons from patients' experiences within intensive care units that can be incorporated directly into clinical management protocols. The Intensive Care Society (ICS) (**www.ics.ac.uk**) is developing a patient liaison committee (CritPal) with a lay chairperson, specifically to address issues relating to patient involvement.

iv Interspecialty and interdisciplinary liaison

Multidisciplinary team (MDT) working is embedded within the philosophy of intensive care medicine for several reasons:

- Individuals may enter the clinical specialty from different base specialties, each bringing varying skills complementary to clinical practice.
- The very nature of the specialty concerns patients with the widest possible range of acute illness, which mandates the involvement of other specialists in the provision of care.
- The level of training and expertise among nursing staff is particularly high, giving weight to their role in the clinical decision-making process.
- Allied health professionals (especially physiotherapists and dietitians) have become increasingly necessary to effective clinical practice in recent years, often contributing to critical care outreach teams set up to assess patients at risk of clinical deterioration within the ward setting.
- The mandatory trust-wide critical care delivery group facilitates a multidisciplinary approach to service delivery.

v Delivering a high quality service

Critical care medicine has developed an impressive evidence base upon which the delivery of care is now based. This has been mandated by the government report, *Comprehensive critical care*[1] and facilitated by the establishment of the Intensive Care National Audit and Research Centre (ICNARC) in 1993. Thus, all trusts are now required to collect an ICNARC-compatible dataset for all patients of level 3 dependency, in addition to making national returns of the number of patients that require augmented care (those that have requirements in excess of routine ward dependency) on a daily basis.

Severity-of-illness scoring systems have facilitated effective audit between units by controlling for casemix, for example:

■ Acute Physiology And Chronic Health Evaluation score (APACHE) in the critical care unit

■ Patients At Risk Score (PARS) and Medical Early Warning score (MEW) in a ward setting.

The specialty has made significant contributions to a number of investigations initiated by the National Institute of Clinical Excellence (NICE) (**www.nice.org.uk**), principally via the ICS, and the Royal Colleges of Anaesthetists and Physicians.

The development of various specialised, competency-based training programmes designed to meet the needs of clinical staff from different base specialties is now complete, overseen by the Intercollegiate Board for Training in Intensive Care Medicine (IBTICM) (**www.rcoa.ac.uk/ibticm**).

Standards of staffing (clinical, technical and administrative) and physical facilities have now been established by the Intensive Care Society and are accepted by the DH.

vi   Quality standards and measures of the quality of specialist services

The Royal Colleges of Physicians and Anaesthetists have begun to establish minimum accepted criteria for the practice of intensive care medicine, relating particularly to immediate consultant review of patients admitted to intensive care units.

The ICS and the European Society of Intensive Care (ESICM) (**www.esicm.org**) have each developed guidelines covering aspects of administration of a critical care service and providing clinical protocols that are in widespread use.

The NHS Modernisation Agency has commissioned work in specific areas to evaluate the potential contribution of certain interventions (eg non-invasive ventilation) and to ensure they are made available via critical care networks.[2] Critical care networks are also used to disseminate best practice and act as a local educational resource for all staff.

CLINICAL WORK AND/OR LABORATORY WORK OF CONSULTANTS IN CRITICAL CARE

Appropriately qualified consultant clinical staff assume responsibility for directing the overall plan of patient care, for the direct supervision and teaching of trainee staff of many professions, and for the organisational (non-clinical) management and leadership of the service. The breakdown of time spent in each role varies depending upon the nature of the critical care unit, the level of other consultant and non-consultant medical staffing, and upon casemix, throughput and the range of services provided within the trust. Moreover, the breadth of responsibilities assumed by consultant staff is changing rapidly, and is likely to involve greater amounts of outpatient work (for example follow up of patients after intensive care discharge), supervision of clinical outreach within all areas of the hospital, and contributing to the assessment and management of a wide variety of acutely ill medical and surgical patients within and outside the confines of the critical care unit. There is a mandatory requirement to collect and analyse data.

The specialty requires a high degree of manual dexterity in performing a wide range of practical procedures. Expertise is needed in assessing and managing acutely ill patients, up to and including cardiopulmonary resuscitation. Out-of-hours commitments are onerous and involve a growing commitment to the provision of a consultant-delivered service at all times.

ACADEMIC MEDICINE

Academic intensive care medicine is established in continental Europe and North America, driven by the need to establish an evidence base for the delivery of care in what is a scarce and costly resource. The need for a strong academic base for the specialty in the UK has been recognised by the IBTICM, which has recently initiated a dialogue on this subject with the Academy of Medical Science and relevant Royal Colleges.

WORKFORCE REQUIREMENTS FOR CRITICAL CARE

The medical workforce requirements for critical care are currently unclear. A report from the Audit Commission noted that fewer than half of the intensive care units in the UK had a consultant presence on every weekday session.[3] This, and the progressive increase in the size and complexity of intensive care units, will lead to a need for additional manpower. Work is likely to be commissioned to assess the medical workforce needs in the context of the document *Comprehensive critical care*, and not just intensive care medicine.[1] The consultant Census 2003 identified 44 WTE consultant physicians in critical care in the UK. If the long-term aim per 250,000 population was to have one consultant physician with another specialist interest spending five programmed activities (PAs) per week in critical care, this would require 97 WTE in England, 117 across the UK.[4]

CONSULTANT WORK PROGRAMME/SPECIMEN JOB PLAN

The multidisciplinary nature of intensive care medicine, coupled with the requirement for the practice of the specialty to the exclusion of other clinical activity over relatively prolonged periods (eg seven days) to ensure continuity of care makes the production of a typical job plan difficult. However, the ICS is attempting to undertake this task in the light of the new consultant contract in England.

References

1.   Department of Health. *Comprehensive critical care: A review of adult critical care services.* London: DH, 2000

2.   Department of Health, Critical Care Programme. *Weaning and long-term ventilatory support.* London: DH, 2002.

3.   Audit Commission. *Critical to success: The place of efficient and effective critical care services within the acute hospital.* London: Audit Commission, 1999.

4.   The Federation of the Royal Colleges of Physicians of the United Kingdom. *Census of consultant physicians in the UK, 2003. Data and commentary.* London: The Federation of the Royal Colleges of Physicians of the United Kingdom, 2003.

Dermatology

i Description of the specialty and clinical needs of patients

Dermatologists manage skin diseases in people of all ages. Most dermatologists are skin surgeons as well as physicians and take the lead in the organisation and delivery of services for skin cancer. Skin cancer is increasingly common and is a significant cause of mortality in young adults in particular. Inflammatory skin diseases are disabling, disfiguring, distressing and highly symptomatic. Chronic inflammatory skin diseases significantly reduce quality of life and they impose a considerable burden on sufferers both in their personal lives and in their careers.[1,2,3] About one in four of the population are affected by skin disease that would benefit from medical care. In the UK, skin diseases are among the most common certified causes of incapacity to work.

Between 1981 and 1991, consultations for skin disease in general practice rose by almost 50%. Referrals to secondary care rose by 10% between 1996 and 2002. These increases reflected a growing prevalence of common problems such as atopic eczema, venous leg ulcers and skin cancer, together with widespread availability of effective treatments, and greater patient demand for specialist opinion.[3] GPs refer 1–2% of the population to dermatologists as new patients each year.

A major part of the work of dermatologists is teaching and training medical students, postgraduates, GPs and nurses. Although about 15% of GP consultations relate to problems with the skin, only 20% of GP vocational training schemes contain a dermatological component, and undergraduate curricula contain, on average, only six days of dermatology. Newly appointed GPs, therefore, have little experience of dermatological problems.

ii Organisation of the service and patterns of referral

Primary, secondary and tertiary levels

Primary care and community dermatology   Delivery of dermatology services in England has been reviewed within the government programme *Action On Dermatology*. It is planned that more care will be provided in the community by liaison dermatology nurses, and within intermediate care clinics and clinics for chronic disease management.

Some GPs with expertise in dermatology provide an intermediary service for colleagues in primary care, and there is a specific government initiative to extend this programme. The British Association of Dermatologists (BAD) recommends that such services should be developed according to the recommendations outlined in the Department of Health document *General practitioners with a special interest in dermatology* (**www.gpwsi.org**).[4] Such services should be developed in collaboration with local dermatologists, integrated with local services in secondary care and provided in adequately equipped and staffed facilities.[5]

Secondary care   Dermatologists provide a hospital-based service in departments with facilities for outpatients, skin surgery, day care and inpatients. Consultants with appropriate support staff work chiefly in outpatient clinics or outpatient operating theatres. They supervise their own inpatients and provide significant support to other disciplines' inpatient workload. They provide on-call cover for urgent dermatological problems.

Most full-time consultant dermatologists spend seven and a half clinical sessions each week on activities related to direct patient care. This includes time spent in outpatient departments (including surgical sessions) or on the wards; administrative tasks such as screening and prioritising referral letters, reviewing and acting upon laboratory results; and communicating with colleagues about patients in writing, by telephone or email. Dermatologists supervise the care of patients attending day care treatment. Consultants with expertise in subspecialties such as photobiology, paediatric dermatology, dermatopathology or contact allergy testing may have one or more sessions for this work.

Surgery is an increasing part of the workload because of the rise in incidence of skin cancer and the two-week waiting list imperative for cancers. The rules governing the organisation of cancer services, data collection within these services, and the intervals between diagnosis and treatment continue to change. Such rules inevitably alter service delivery and the staffing required to meet imposed targets. A limited number of surgical procedures such as cryosurgery, curettage, simple excisions and biopsies may be done in the outpatient clinic, provided that time and facilities are appropriately allocated. More complex surgical procedures are performed in a dedicated theatre session. Most dermatologists perform significant amounts of surgery but many larger departments appoint a dermatological surgeon specifically for complex cancer surgery such as Mohs' surgery and laser surgery. Dermatological surgeons may devote most of their sessions to cutaneous surgery.

Most consultants undertake regular ward rounds, including review of ward referrals from hospital-based colleagues. Dermatologists supervise the care of inpatients involving:

- those with severe skin diseases that require intensive management, of whom many have concomitant disease and may be elderly or socially deprived
- children on paediatric wards under the care of dermatologists and/or paediatricians
- those with life-threatening problems (eg severe drug reactions) who may require admission to an intensive care unit or burns unit.

Some consultants spend considerable time travelling from one hospital to another and may be expected to provide an on-call service for ward referrals and emergencies in a number of different hospitals. Consultants based in one hospital with colleagues and good support staff have a less onerous on-call commitment. The need for domiciliary visits varies between communities.

Dermatologists should not practise single-handedly. Hospitals serving a population of 250,000 need at least three consultant dermatologists with appropriate support staff, including specialist nurses (see workforce requirements, below). It is essential that they have regular meetings with colleagues in surrounding units for audit, continuing medical education (CME) and continuing professional development (CPD). Many consultants work in more than one district general hospital (DGH), or provide outreach clinics in community hospitals in country areas with dispersed populations and poor transport. Specialist services and inpatient facilities are provided in the central unit and consultants have sessions in both central and peripheral hospitals. There must be means of ensuring that patients are properly prioritised, that urgent patients are seen quickly and that all patients can get the advice and treatment they need when they need it.

Tertiary care   In larger centres, one dermatologist may be appointed to develop a specialised regional service, for example specialised dermatological surgery, complex medical dermatology, paediatric dermatology, photodermatology, the investigation of contact dermatitis and industrial skin disease, immunopathology or dermatopathology. Such centres may receive clinical referrals or requests for specific investigations.

Special patterns of referral

Urgent referrals Patients with suspected skin cancer (squamous cell carcinoma, malignant melanoma) must be seen within two weeks of referral.[6] Life-threatening inflammatory skin diseases (eg severe drug reactions) must be seen immediately. Dermatological problems are common among patients admitted to hospital wards and dermatologists receive requests for urgent opinions from colleagues in many specialties.

Telemedicine This may prove useful in some areas with geographically remote communities but should be developed only as part of an integrated local service. The cost-effectiveness of telemedicine is still to be validated.

Clinical networks and community arrangements

Dermatology departments tend to be relatively small in terms of staffing numbers but have high activity levels, particularly in outpatient areas. Good data collection and managerial support are required if the service is to be effective. Dermatology is often incorporated into medical directorates with other acute and/or non-acute medical specialties. Dermatology departments must have dedicated senior managerial support within trusts and primary care trusts (PCTs). There should be a regular forum for dermatology staff to meet with trust and PCT management to address problems and plan strategy and developments. Dermatology is a specialty with an *Action On* programme from the Modernisation Agency (**www.modern.nhs.uk**), therefore modernisation within strategic health authorities (SHAs) should involve dermatology in each locality.

Managed clinical networks Some areas, particularly large, densely populated conurbations, have developed managed clinical networks to integrate care between central 'hubs' and peripheral 'spokes' to enhance provision of care. In this model, one large dermatology unit, usually in a teaching hospital, is linked to a number of local DGHs and community-based centres usually organised around a GP with a special interest (GPSI). Dermatologists who do not have a dermatology colleague in their base hospital should have links with a larger central unit. Communication pathways and rapid referral routes must be available to these integrated systems.

Community arrangements These are variable, but integration between primary and secondary care has been strengthened in some areas by the work of community liaison nurses and GPs who have been appointed to work in hospital dermatology clinics, and the development of specialist services in the community (see section on primary care above).

Relationship with other services/agencies

Patients of all ages, races and social groupings use dermatology services. The dermatology team has regular contact with social services, school medical services, and community liaison services on behalf of patients. Considerable assistance is gained from patient support groups. Their literature should be readily available and departments should display addresses and points of contact. The Red Cross and other volunteers provide a skin camouflage service.

Other hospital-based services

These include:

- dermatopathology and immunopathology
- medical photography, medical physics, vascular technology

- chiropodists, psychologists, tissue viability nurses
- community leg ulcer clinics, patient support groups.

iii Working with patients: patient-centred care

Patient choice and involving patients in decisions about their treatment

Involving patients in decisions about their care is improved by allowing adequate time for consultations with specialist doctors and nurses and by providing good quality written information or details of websites. Some interactive programmes have been developed which could be made available to patients in hospital departments or GP surgeries where appropriate equipment is available.

Patients with chronic conditions, opportunities for education and promoting self-care

Recommendations:

- Short videos about skin disease, treatments and phototherapy are readily available. A suitably equipped quiet area and access to a health professional to discuss the information received are required.
- Patients should be involved in service planning through involvement in local forums that bring together trusts and PCTs.
- Day treatment units and nurse-led clinics are valuable sources of practical advice and training on how to use therapies effectively.
- The facility for patients to self-refer back to day treatment or phototherapy during relapse of chronic skin diseases such as psoriasis and eczema should be in place.
- There should be dedicated telephone consultation times with specialist nurses.
- Well-supported self-management by patients is particularly appropriate for patients with chronic skin conditions and dermatology professionals should support its development.

Patient support groups

Information about patient support groups should be available in all dermatology departments. Printed information about dermatological conditions should include the contact details for relevant support groups.

iv Interspecialty and interdisciplinary liaison

Multidisciplinary clinical networks in secondary care

Many patients require the services of a number of different specialties and disciplines. Dermatologists work regularly with histopathologists with expertise in skin pathology and immunopathology, plastic surgeons, vascular surgeons, gynaecologists, genitourinary physicians, paediatricians, general physicians and rheumatologists. The role of multidisciplinary teams (MDTs) to integrate care between such units is crucial. Teams may not all be based on a single site so team meetings may be virtual using teleconferencing. Electronic communication between sites with tele-dermatology is becoming more common for individual patient management. Staff and associate specialist grade doctors or clinical assistants support dermatologists in many hospital units.

Multidisciplinary clinics may consist of:

- rheumatology, immunology, dermatology (for connective tissue diseases, psoriasis)
- gynaecology, genitourinary medicine, dermatology (for vulval diseases)
- paediatrics, dermatology (for atopic eczema, genodermatoses and others)
- plastic surgery, radiotherapy, dermatology (for skin cancers)
- oral medicine, dermatology (for muco-cutaneous disorders)
- vascular surgery, dermatology (for leg ulcers)
- psychology, psychiatry, dermatology
- infectious diseases, dermatology (for HIV)
- medical genetics, dermatology (for inherited diseases).

Dermatology nurses

Nurses with expertise in dermatology are key members of the team.

- Nurses counsel and treat patients in day care units and on the wards, provide and supervise phototherapy (PUVA and UVB), carry out contact allergy testing (patch testing), and care for wounds and chronic leg ulcers.
- Specialist nurses working in outpatient departments may provide information to patients, demonstrate and apply treatments (in children and adults), dress wounds, remove sutures or review follow ups.
- Nurses with training in skin surgery assist in operating theatres and provide advice to patients undergoing surgery. In some units appropriately trained nurses perform skin biopsies or other surgical procedures such as cryosurgery.
- Dermatology nurses may advise professional colleagues who are caring for patients with skin problems in the hospital and the community.
- Dermatology nurses trained in paediatrics provide outreach services for children with problems such as atopic eczema.
- Liaison nurses who work in the dermatology department and in the community can help to provide a seamless service and assist with the training of practice nurses.
- Liaison nurses may advise on the management of leg ulcers or attend community leg ulcer clinics.
- Specialist nurses are increasingly involved in the establishment and supervision of nurse-led clinics based in primary care.

v   Delivering a high quality dermatology service[5]

Characteristics of a high quality service: requirements for consultant dermatologists

Consultant dermatologists should have completed an accredited training programme, possess a Certificate of Completion of Specialist Training (CCST) in dermatology and be on the specialist register of the General Medical Council (GMC). Applicants from outside the UK and Eire will be expected to demonstrate comparable quality of training as assessed by the Joint Committee on Higher Medical Training (JCHMT) of the Royal College of Physicians. Dermatologists should not work in isolation. They must have appropriate support staff including specialist dermatology nurses.

Quality in the dermatology contract

The concept of a quality driven service, with standards of care clearly defined in contracts, provides a framework in which the dermatology care in a community can be improved.

Standards should be set in relation to the following:

■ *The referral system* There should be sufficient consultant staff to provide 24-hour (on-call) dermatological advice for inpatients and the admissions unit, and dedicated administrative support staff. Referral letters should be prioritised by the dermatologist. Explicit standards should be set for the time from referral to first appointment for urgent and non-urgent patients.

■ *Outpatient clinics appointment system* In any clinic, time should be allowed for the doctor to read referrals, review and act on results, dictate letters, and to spend sufficient time with patients and their families as part of the consultation. The flexibility to spend an extended time with the family of a child with atopic eczema should have a greater priority than the need to keep strictly to outpatient waiting time guidelines.

■ *Dermatological surgery* There should be an agreed definition of a day case and recognition of the time required to perform the various surgical procedures.

■ *Outpatient/day patient treatment*

■ *Inpatient care*

■ *Discharge from the dermatology service* GPs should be informed of a patient's status when they are discharged from either inpatient or outpatient care, and receive advice on further management, including follow up.

■ *Training of medical and nursing staff*

■ *Availability of appropriate facilities and equipment*

■ *Secretarial, administrative and managerial support* Secretarial staff should be adequately trained in dermatological terms and policies and be provided with appropriate word-processing and data collection facilities to allow proper clinical audit.

■ *Information for, and education of, patients*

■ *Storage and handling of medical records.*

Contracts should incorporate protocols for referral and shared care, treatment guidelines, standards for audit and quality control. Other outcome assessments that might be used are quality of life and patient satisfaction.

Resources required for a high quality service

Integrated facilities should be the goal for all departments. The physical proximity of inpatient, outpatient, and day care facilities helps efficient working.

Outpatient facilities

■ dedicated outpatient area with consultation and examination rooms large enough for patients and accompanying persons, consultant and medical students or other trainees and nurse-led clinics

■ natural and additional lighting

- examination couches
- private area for undressing
- wound-dressing area
- treatment rooms with facilities for adults and children
- facilities for contact allergy testing, including appropriate storage of allergens
- rooms for patient education and educational material
- medical photography services
- access to a pharmacy service able to meet needs identified in the clinic, including the preparation of topical medicaments and allergens for contact allergy testing
- accommodation within the paediatric department for dermatology clinics and outpatient treatment for children.

Surgical facilities

- well-lit and ventilated operating rooms with couches
- surgical packs of appropriate instruments
- equipment for electrocautery, diathermy and hyfrecation
- equipment for cryosurgery and storage for liquid nitrogen
- facilities for freezing biopsies and storing frozen samples
- laser-safe areas where required
- facilities for Mohs' surgery, eg cryostat and histopathology equipment in some specialist units.

Day care centres and phototherapy

- day care centres staffed by dermatology nurses to provide an out-of-hours service, including phototherapy, to complement inpatient care
- a personal treatment plan made with each patient
- accommodation with privacy for changing, bathing/showering, application of creams and discussions about therapy
- a phototherapy area with TLO1 and PUVA, run by specialist dermatology nurses who can provide skincare rather than physiotherapists
- supervision of all phototherapy units by a named consultant, thus ensuring accuracy of dosimetry, record keeping and the training and monitoring of the staff who administer treatment
- a medical physicist to monitor UV output of units (likely to be simplified and standardised in the near future with computerised national managed clinical networks as in Scotland).

Inpatient unit

- All dermatologists should have admitting rights to a dedicated inpatient dermatology unit staffed by trained specialist nurses. Consultants and/or senior house officers (SHOs) and specialist registrars (SpRs) provide medical cover for these units.
- Patients with widespread chronic inflammatory skin diseases benefit from admission and are aided by the mutual patient support provided on a dermatological unit.
- Dedicated inpatient beds, some with facilities for reverse barrier nursing, are required for patients with severe and life-threatening skin conditions.

- Teaching hospitals need dedicated inpatient dermatology units for managing tertiary referrals of patients with complex diseases, and for training of undergraduates and SpRs.

- Two dedicated dermatological beds per 100,000 population are the minimum requirement, but a minimum of eight beds is necessary to support appropriate staffing for a self-contained unit.

- The inpatient unit should be geographically close to the outpatient unit, and staff should be able to operate flexibly between the two. The 'hub-and-spoke' arrangement referred to previously is often the most appropriate way of ensuring that patients have access to a suitable dedicated dermatology inpatient facility.

- Dermatological beds in general medical wards are satisfactory only where there are appropriate facilities for bathing and treatment and where patients receive care from specialist dermatology nurses.

- Patients with multisystem disorders who require both specialist dermatological care and care of their medical and surgical problems should be in the area defined by their most serious problem. Outreach by dermatology trained nursing staff is essential for patients with significant skin disease being cared for on general wards.

Support services

- Dermatology requires the same support services as many other general medical specialties, for example chemical pathology, haematology, X-ray, microbiology including mycology. The specialty particularly requires services in immunology, immunopathology and histopathology.

- Dermatology patients require access to other hospital specialties, including histopathology with specific expertise in dermatopathology, plastic surgery, radiotherapy, immunology, and psychiatry.

VI **Quality standards and measures of the quality of specialist services**

Specialist society guidelines

Clinical and service guidelines are produced and updated regularly by the BAD. Completed and draft guidelines are available on their website (**www.BAD.org.uk**).

National Institute for Clinical Excellence (NICE) guidelines

A limited number of guidelines relevant to dermatology are available at **www.NICE.org.uk**. NICE appraisals relevant to dermatology are increasingly available at the same web address.

Clinical governance

A working party of the BAD produced guidance on clinical governance for dermatology (also available on their website). This is being expanded and updated.

CLINICAL WORK OF CONSULTANTS IN DERMATOLOGY

Contributions made to acute medicine

Dermatologists provide a consultation service for urgent problems at all times. Some patients, such as those with cellulitis or drug eruptions, may be admitted directly to the dermatology unit from the acute medical take. Dermatologists do not participate in the on-call rota for general medicine. A significant number of patients benefit from joint care with other specialties.

Direct clinical care

Inpatient work

Two ward rounds with specialist nurses and other members of the healthcare team are required per week. Teaching and training are an important component of ward rounds.

Requests for a dermatological opinion are common. Ward referrals are seen on the wards or in outpatient clinics as required.

Outpatient work

The greater part of the work of consultant dermatologists takes place in outpatient clinics. The activities of these clinics are summarised below.

General dermatology clinics

▪ Ratio of new to follow-up patients per clinic:

Between 8–12 new patients or 12–16 follow-up patients, or a combination of the two (varies depending on the complexity of the cases seen, the time allocated to each patient, and the balance of new, follow-up, complex and simple cases).

Some patients, new or follow up, with complex disease may require longer appointments. Some skin cancer screening clinics may allocate shorter appointments to each new patient, but see-and-treat clinics will require considerably longer. Flexibility is essential.

▪ Average number of patients seen per clinic:

Without trainees or teaching commitments

8–16 patients per consultant per general clinic, depending on casemix and ratio of new to follow-up patients.

If the consultant carries out one-stop skin surgery within the clinic appointment, times must be adjusted accordingly.

Thirty minutes may be required for a surgical procedure.

With trainees, non-training grades or teaching commitments

There should be a one-third reduction in patient numbers for teaching to be effective; 6–12 might be appropriate for each consultant.

Patient numbers for the trainee should be approximately two-thirds of those allocated for the consultant.

Consultants in both DGHs and teaching hospitals train doctors (GPs, GPSIs, SHOs, SpRs), nurses and medical students within outpatient clinics.

One consultant can supervise a maximum of two trainees or non-training grades per clinic but must allocate extra time to review the patients and to teach.

Special clinics within dermatology

▪ tumour clinics, ideally with facilities for immediate skin surgery (one-stop clinic)

▪ vulval clinics with facilities for colposcopy

▪ paediatric dermatology clinics in suitable paediatric facilities with paediatric-trained nurses

▪ other multidisciplinary clinics, particularly for psoriasis and atopic dermatitis, depending on the expertise of the consultant dermatologist, other specialist colleagues and hospital resources.

Specialised investigative and therapeutic procedure clinics

▪ dermatological surgery clinic including Mohs' micrographic surgery with dedicated surgical facilities suitable for day surgery (access to cryostat and trained histopathology technician required for Mohs' micrographic surgery)

continued over

■ laser-surgery clinic, requiring a laser-safe area, general anaesthetic facilities for treatment of children with vascular naevi

■ contact allergic dermatitis and occupational skin disease clinics involving work place visits and allergy testing in the hospital department.

■ photobiology clinics with facilities for phototesting and 'hotel' facilities for patients

■ wound care (leg ulcer) clinics, with vascular surgeons and specialist nurses.

All clinics will require adequate support staff including specialist nurses. The number of patients seen depends on the complexity of the procedure or investigation.

Specialist on-call

Consultants with highly specialised practice would expect to provide a reasonable on-call service for these patients.

Other specialist activities including activities beyond the local services

Consultant dermatologists are involved in MDTs, cancer networks and community services.

Clinically related administration

This includes tasks such as screening and prioritising referral letters, reviewing and acting upon laboratory results, communicating with and about patients with colleagues in writing, by telephone or email. A reasonable balance between direct patient contact and clinical administration for dermatologists appears to be 1:0.5. This is based on clinicians' diaries and reflects the large number of outpatients seen in the specialty.

Work to maintain and improve the quality of care

Leadership role and development of the service

Dermatology falls within the Long Term Conditions Care Group (LTCCG) and has a specific subcommittee considering service delivery and workforce planning. Representatives of the specialty are essential in this process. Specialty representatives have been involved in the *Action On* programme with the NHS Modernisation Agency to lead and disseminate good practice in service delivery.

Medical education, training and appraisal of trainees

Almost all consultant dermatologists are involved in education and training of individuals ranging from medical undergraduates to pharmacists, hospital doctors, GPs and nurses. In teaching hospitals and, to a lesser extent, in hospitals to which medical students are seconded, the design and delivery of teaching to students requires a significant amount of time within the consultant's week. Students may be present within dermatology continuously throughout the year, or attachments or teaching periods may be intermittent. If medical students are taught within 'working' clinics (as opposed to special clinical sessions purely for teaching) the number of patients that can be seen by the consultant during one programmed activity (PA) will be reduced by 10–25%.

Units that have SpRs create an additional workload for the consultant. A consultant dermatologist might spend between one half and two PAs each week on teaching and training, according to local circumstances. The education committee of the BAD, together with the specialist advisory committee

(SAC) for dermatology, is developing competency frameworks to underpin the new postgraduate curriculum. The LTCCG is coordinating consistency between these developments and the task-related competencies being developed by other professional groups such as nurses.

Mentoring and appraisal of medical staff and other professional staff

These procedures are carried out at a local level, sometimes with the involvement of the regional representatives of the BAD.

Continuing medical education

Dermatologists and trainees are involved in the Royal College of Physicians programmes for CME. A consultant is expected to spend an average of 50 hours each year on CME (at least one half PA each week).

Clinical governance

Some senior consultants undertake a lead role in governance, but all consultants should be aware of the issues relating to their specialty and have time to document these in preparation for annual appraisal. Formal meetings to discuss outcomes and review departmental data should be included in the work programme as part of the audit process. They may be taken in conjunction with teaching and training. Protected time should be allowed for audit. A working party of the BAD produced guidance on clinical governance for dermatology (available on their website).

Clinical and scientific research

There is a strong research base to dermatology. Basic science research is carried out in both teaching and district general hospitals; much of this work is funded by the British Skin Foundation. The BAD Clinical Trials Network develops ideas for trials and identifies sources of funding. Around one-third of British dermatologists are involved in this enterprise. A teaching hospital consultant might be expected to spend one PA each week in research.

Local management duties

Individual dermatologists may lead the clinical service or, at more senior levels, be involved in hospital management structures. Management duties might include clinical directorship and service planning.

Regional and national work

It is essential that there is medical representation on local, regional and national committees, and appropriate time should be allocated in the work programme. For some consultants, between half and one PA might be spent on such work. Individuals holding significant posts with national professional or governmental organisations may need to negotiate additional protected time. The BAD has elected officers and committees that require considerable input from individual dermatologists, and contribute significantly to national policies. Other roles include committee membership at the College and the British Medical Association (BMA), and involvement in preparing NICE appraisals and guidelines.

ACADEMIC MEDICINE

The NHS work of academic dermatologists depends on their academic responsibilities and individual job descriptions, but most academic dermatologists make a strong contribution to the routine work of the NHS department, in addition to setting up tertiary services. Major advances in clinical research come from the close collaboration of dermatologists, laboratory scientists and patients. The teaching role of all dermatologists continues to expand, particularly with the development of the new medical schools. Some academic dermatologists in large centres make a significant contribution to the broad academic community within their institution.

WORKFORCE REQUIREMENTS FOR DERMATOLOGY

Dermatology is predominantly an outpatient specialty and the following calculations are based on the workload in the outpatient department.

For a population of 100,000

If 1.5% of a population of 100,000 is referred per annum this generates 1,500 new patients. With a ratio of one new to two follow-up patients per general clinic, 1,500 new patients plus 3,000 selected follow-up patients gives 4,500 patients per year.

A PA lasts four hours under the new contract in England, and 3.5 hours in Wales. Assuming a consultant has no travel to other centres, no inpatients, no ward rounds, no on call, no specialist clinics and no MDTs, he/she would be able to undertake two new patient, two follow-up and one skin surgery clinics per week.

Consultant working without an assistant and no trainees or students to teach

He/she can see 10 new patients (mix of neoplastic lesions and inflammatory rashes) per new clinic, 20 follow-up cases per follow-up clinic, and seven cases in a skin surgery clinic. Thus, in such a week, a consultant without assistance could see 20 new and 40 follow-up patients, and undertake seven surgical procedures. This allows an appropriate amount of time for in-clinic administration. Clinics mixing old and new cases would adjust numbers in a pro rata manner.

Activities related to direct clinical care such as reviewing and prioritising referral letters, checking and acting upon laboratory results and communicating with colleagues generate approximately 0.5 PA for each clinic. Thus, a consultant would work five PAs in the outpatient clinic with 2.5 PAs of supportive administration and management. Additional PAs are required for ward work, travel, teaching, MDTs, on call, or special interest clinics, otherwise the number of outpatient clinics should be reduced appropriately. Full details are shown in the specimen job plan.

Assume a consultant works 40 weeks per year (6 weeks annual leave, 6 weeks study leave/professional leave and bank holidays). In one year a consultant (with no supervisory duties nor special interest clinics), could see 800 new and 1,600 follow-up patients and perform 280 procedures. This does not allow for a special interest clinic, for teaching medical students, for supervision of any grade of staff, for ward work, on call, travel, or MDTs. These factors will reduce the number of patients it is possible to see. On this basis, for a consultant-only service for a population of 100,000, it would be necessary to have 1.9 consultants, that is, one consultant per 53,000 population.

Consultant working with an assistant or trainee

Non-consultant medical staff who support the dermatology service require variable supervision. A consultant working with a trained non-consultant doctor could together see an average of 16 new patients or 32 follow-up patients per clinic (or eight new and 16 follow-up for a mixed clinic). The calculation above indicates a requirement for 1.2 consultants plus 1.2 WTE assistants per 100,000 population. Trainees are regarded as supernumerary to the service, but will require time from the consultant for training within the clinic.

Notes on clinic size calculations

1. A ratio of one new patient to two follow-up patients can usually be seen in a mixed clinic, for example five new patients plus 10 follow-up patients. However, as follow-up numbers decline with changes in community service delivery, many follow ups are sufficiently complex to require longer appointments. Therefore, casemix is important in deciding clinic numbers and flexibility is essential.

    It is difficult to discharge more patients if GP referrals are appropriate and the needs of trainees are considered. Knowledgeable GPs only refer complex problems that need specialist management. It is not possible to discharge these patients after one or two visits.

    Trainees must follow their patients to learn how to manage disease. When trainees are present, the overall number of patients per clinic increases but this has little impact on the number of new patients seen because the consultant will see fewer patients and trainees bring back more follow ups.

    The ratio may approach 1:2.5 if phototherapy and patch testing are included.

2. 10 new patients can be seen per clinic (based on 20 minutes for each new patient). New patients who have difficult forms of common problems such as psoriasis or atopic eczema deserve appropriate consultation time. Flexibility in clinic booking is essential. It is possible to see more patients in a tumour clinic but only if surgery is not performed during the clinic.

3. Each consultant works with a maximum of two staff requiring supervision. These are trainee and/or non-training grades. No consultant should work in isolation from colleagues. All consultants responsible for a population of 100,000 should have assistance in clinics.

4. The pattern of work will depend on the specialist services provided by individual consultants and departments, eg skin surgery, contact allergy (patch) testing, wound healing, paediatric dermatology, phototherapy and dermatopathology.

CONSULTANT WORK PROGRAMME/SPECIMEN JOB PLAN

The standard contract for a consultant working full-time within the NHS will consist of 10 PAs. These will be divided into 7.5 PAs related to direct patient care and 2.5 related to supporting activities. The 7.5 PAs devoted to patient care should include time spent in outpatient clinics (including surgical sessions), time allocated to the supervision of the care of patients attending for day care, treatments or investigations such as phototherapy or patch testing, and regular ward rounds and review of ward referrals from hospital-based colleagues. Direct clinical care also includes time spent on administrative tasks that relate directly to patient care.

Activity	Workload	Programmed activities (PAs)
Direct clinical care		
Ward rounds, day care	Number of beds varies	**0.5–1**
Outpatient clinics	10 new for new clinic, 20 follow-ups (for a follow-up clinic)	**3–4**
Skin surgery	7 cases of average complexity	**0–1**
Skin cancer MDT	Variable	**0–1**
Dermatopathology	Variable	**0–0.5**
On call	Depends on number of colleagues	**0.5**
Administration and management	Direct patient care, review of results, communication with other healthcare professionals	**0.5–2**
Special interest clinic	eg patch testing, skin cancer, phototherapy, psoriasis	**0–2**
Travel	Variable	**0–1**
Total number of direct clinical care PAs		**7.5 on average**
Supporting professional activities (SPA)		
Work to maintain and improve the quality of healthcare	Education and training, appraisal, departmental management and service development, audit and clinical governance, CPD and revalidation, research	**2.5 on average**
Other NHS responsibilities	eg medical director/clinical director/lead consultant in specialty/clinical tutor	**Local agreement with trust**
External duties	eg work for deaneries/Royal Colleges/specialist societies/Department of Health or other government bodies etc	**Local agreement with trust**

Clinical elements of job plan

▪ clinics, surgery and supervision, for example day unit treatments, patch tests, phototherapy, lasers, histopathology review and ward work

▪ administration related to direct clinical care and travelling time, consisting of time allowed within clinics and additional PAs as identified by the analysis of work diaries (administrative time available is significantly reduced by teaching).

The balance between formal clinics, ward work and supervisory activity will vary. Direct patient contact time must be balanced by appropriate clinical administration time. Numbers in clinics should be adjusted to ensure completion within four hours including teaching and immediate clinical administration. Additional administrative responsibilities will require further time drawn from the 7.5 PAs allocated to patient care.

Work for national bodies should be acknowledged and programmed. This may require a negotiated reduction in the clinical elements of the annual job plan. The on-call commitment will vary with local policies and staffing levels. Those working part-time or in academic posts will still be required to complete the full complement of supporting activities, and should have no significant reduction in the 2.5 PAs allocated for this.

Job planning in teaching hospitals

Teaching hospital consultants will need additional time for teaching and supervision of research. This will reduce the clinical elements of the job plan.

Academic appointments

The job plan is likely to include, on average, five PAs for university-based activity (eg research) and five PAs for direct clinical care and supporting professional activities.

References

1. Williams HC. *Dermatology: health care needs assessment.* Oxford: Radcliffe Medical Press, 1997.

2. Harlow D, Poyner T, Finlay AY, Dykes PJ. Impaired quality of life of adults with skin disease in primary care. *Br J Dermatol* 2000;**143**(5):979–82.

3. Williams HC. Increasing demand for dermatological services: how much is needed? *J R Coll Physicians Lond* 1997;**31**:261–2.

4. Department of Health and Royal College of General Practitioners. *Guidelines for the appointment of general practitioners with special interests in the delivery of clinical services: dermatology,* April 2003. www.dh.gov.uk/ assetRoot/04/08/02/70/04080270.pdf

5. Provision of secondary care for dermatology within general practice. Guidelines for the Royal College of Physicians Dermatology Advisory Committee. *J R Coll Physicians Lond* 1999;**33**:246–8.

6. Department of Health. *The NHS cancer plan: a plan for investment, a plan for reform.* London: DH, 2000.

7. Quality in the dermatological contract. A report from the workshop on quality issues in dermatological contracting of the British Association of Dermatologists. *J R Coll Physicians Lond* 1995;**29**(1):25–30.

Diabetes and endocrinology

i Description of the specialty and clinical needs of patients

The specialty of diabetes and endocrinology deals with the diagnosis and management of a diverse range of hormonal and metabolic disorders. It encompasses a wide variety of conditions ranging from the most common (eg Type 2 diabetes), which are responsible for a large component of the chronic disease burden of healthcare, to those that are rare but eminently treatable (eg pituitary tumours). Most conditions are chronic, requiring long-term and often lifelong management. There is a strong evidence base for the management of disorders encountered within the specialty. Delayed, inadequate or inappropriate treatment leads to poor health, reduced lifespan and increased burden on the health service.

Type 2 diabetes is a common multifaceted disorder that is rapidly increasing in incidence. The demands of glucose control management are progressive and, almost invariably, concurrent management of hypertension and dyslipidaemia is also required. Type 1 diabetes often starts in childhood and the intrinsically unstable nature of the condition is often compounded by emotional and behavioural problems common to adolescent and young adult medicine. In either kind of diabetes, potential complications are protean. Untreated they lead to disability and early death.

Endocrine disorders range from the relatively common (eg polycystic ovarian syndrome (PCOS), hyperthyroidism and hypothyroidism) to rare and very rare conditions, which are nonetheless extremely important to identify because they are usually both eminently treatable (eg pituitary tumours, multiple endocrine neoplasia (MEN), Addison's disease) and devastating if neglected.

ii Organisation of the service and patterns of referral

Primary, secondary and tertiary care

Diabetes services These are largely outpatient based. A complex local network of services is required to encompass the needs of all people with diabetes throughout their lifelong pathway of care. Much of the routine work can be provided in primary care by nurses, dietitians, podiatrists and GPs. A core requirement for all patients is support for self-efficacy, which necessitates effective, ongoing patient education programmes. At various stages, however, specialist physician management is required: at the time of transitions (eg new diagnosis of Type 1 diabetes or the progression to more complex therapy for someone with Type 2 diabetes); for particular clinical scenarios (eg young people with diabetes, diabetic pregnancy, metabolic emergencies, serious intercurrent non-diabetic illness, psychosocial interactions); and for the identification and collaborative management of complications (eg severe diabetic foot disease, diabetic nephropathy, erectile dysfunction, painful and autonomic neuropathy, macrovascular disease). Because diabetes is so common, and because there are both ongoing and intermittent unpredictable components of management, the local organisation of an integrated diabetes care service is a complex exercise.

Rapid changes in the structure and delivery of services are occurring as a result of:

- treatment developments such as continuous subcutaneous insulin infusion
- technological developments such as remotely accessed blood glucose results, call-centre support, and electronic care records

■ workforce changes such as consultant nurses and podiatrists

■ the 2003 GP contract

■ general practitioners with a special interest (GPSI) in diabetes

■ changing primary/secondary care organisational relationships.

Endocrine services   For common conditions such as PCOS and thyroid disorders services are often organised on a multidisciplinary/multisector basis, which is much less complex but in other respects similar in structure to that for diabetes. Unusual endocrine disorders require sophisticated laboratory and clinical imaging support for diagnosis, and close liaison with highly specialised surgical services for treatment. Nonetheless, following diagnosis, management and initial stabilisation, the ongoing care of endocrine disorders is also beginning to change under the enabling influence of technologies that permit remote monitoring and electronic communication.

iii   Working with patients: patient-centred care

Patient choice and involving patients in decisions about their management

Treatment choices in diabetes and endocrinology are often complex and entail difficult risk assessments. Lengthy, well-informed negotiation between specialists and patients is necessary in order to achieve optimum outcome. Young people with diabetes and endocrine disorders require support and negotiated management appropriate to their stages of physical and emotional development. Long-term clinical records are indispensable; ideally, they should integrate information and results from all the healthcare providers and be accessible to both professionals and patients.

Access to information, opportunities for education and promoting self-care

Because diabetes is always chronic, and many endocrine disorders are also lifelong conditions, supported self-efficacy is a core part of delivering appropriate services. Patient education programmes are an essential component of management for Type 1 and Type 2 diabetes and feature increasingly in the management of endocrine conditions such as PCOS, pituitary disease and hypogonadism. National and local patient organisations are prominent and supportive in these areas as well.

iv   Interspecialty and interdisciplinary liaison

Multidisciplinary team (MDT) working and collaboration with other specialists is a characteristic of almost all aspects of diabetes and endocrine specialist care.

The diagnosis and ongoing care of children, young people and adults with Type 1 diabetes demands close collaboration between paediatricians, paediatric diabetes specialist nurses, physicians with a special interest in diabetes, adult diabetes specialist nurses, dietitians and, often, contributions from podiatrists, optometrists and psychologists. For Type 2 diabetes, primary care teams make the majority of the diagnoses and provide the ongoing care. Specialist services provide consultative advice at intervals and, at times, temporary ongoing care for particularly difficult metabolic or complicated management problems. Diabetic foot care requires an extensive MDT including community podiatrists and district nurses, hospital podiatrists, orthotists, microbiologists, vascular surgeons and orthopaedic surgeons, in addition to diabetes specialist nurses and physician specialists. Diabetes pregnancy care requires integrated team working with obstetric and midwifery colleagues. Other aspects of diabetes care involve collaborative management with ophthalmologists, nephrologists, stroke physicians, cardiologists, rheumatologists, emergency care teams, elderly care teams and every kind of inpatient hospital care for which people with diabetes are admitted. The need to involve such specialties is often concurrent with the need to reconfigure the metabolic care plan.

Both diabetes and endocrinology are heavily dependent on close collaboration with laboratories but this is particularly the case for endocrinology where access to specialist laboratory techniques may determine the ability to deliver service. Endocrinology is also dependent on a variety of sophisticated imaging techniques requiring close collaboration with specialist radiologists. For the management of pituitary disease endocrinologists work in teams with neurosurgeons and radiotherapists; for thyroid and adrenal disorders partnership with an endocrine surgical team is essential; while for reproductive endocrinology it is necessary to work closely with specialist gynaecologists. Several complex endocrine disorders have their origins in childhood (eg growth disorders, Turner's syndrome, congenital adrenal hyperplasia (CAH)) so liaison between adult and paediatric services during the vulnerable transition period is essential to effective continuing care. The management of genetically based endocrine disorders such as CAH and MEN will usually involve geneticists. The majority of specialist endocrine practice requires specialist nurse support.

v Delivering a high quality service

Characteristics of a high quality service

High quality diabetes services are managed on a cross organisational basis in 'natural health economies'. They deploy primary, intermediate, secondary and tertiary care facilities in an integrated programme that aspires to achieve all of the standards set out in the National Service Framework (NSF) for Diabetes. Services continually self-assess their structures and processes using systems such as DiabetesE, and monitor outcomes of care through national clinical audit.

In endocrinology, as for diabetes, common conditions need to be managed collaboratively between primary and secondary care according to local guidelines and with ongoing audit of satisfaction and outcome. Regional centres deal with the rarer endocrine conditions and should be co-located with the laboratory and imaging and surgical teams in order to provide a seamless, comprehensive, safe, high quality service.

vi Quality standards and measures of the quality of specialist services

Diabetes

- The National Service Framework for Diabetes: www.nelh.nhs.uk/nsf/diabetes/default.htm
- NICE health technology appraisals: www.nice.org.uk/catrows.asp?c=153
- Numerous NICE guidelines: www.nice.org.uk/catcg2.asp?c=20034
- A service assessment mechanism: www.diabetesE.net
- National audit and regional audits for specific aspects of care such as pregnancy.
- International guidelines: International Society for Paediatric and Adolescent Diabetes (www.ispad.org); American Diabetes Association (www.diabetes.org/for-health-professionals-and-scientists/cpr.jsp)

Endocrinology

- NICE health technology appraisals for the use of growth hormone: **www.nice.org.uk/ catrows.asp?c=153**
- Society for Endocrinology national guidelines that contain standards against which practice can be audited: **www.endocrinology.org/SFE/handbk.htm**
- International guidelines: American Association of Clinical Endocrinologists **www.aace.com/clin/guidelines**

CLINICAL WORK AND/OR LABORATORY WORK OF CONSULTANTS IN DIABETES AND ENDOCRINOLOGY

Contributions made to acute medicine

Most consultants with a specialist interest in diabetes and endocrinology work in acute hospitals. They contribute substantially to the provision of the acute general medical service. Usually they participate in a one in 10 to one in 14 acute take rota that includes post-take ward rounds on the emergency medical admissions unit. Additionally, they will lead a ward-based team responsible for about 16–20 unselected general medicine inpatients.

Direct clinical care

Work in the specialties

Specialty service provision varies between a strong or exclusive bias to diabetes or endocrinology or, most commonly in a district general hospital (DGH), a mix of diabetes and endocrinology. Some physicians in diabetes now work solely in the provision and management of diabetes services in the community (community diabetes physicians) and may be employed by primary care trusts. A few endocrinologists work exclusively to provide an endocrine specialist service from within a tertiary referral centre concentrating on pituitary disease, rare endocrine tumours and inherited endocrine disorders. A substantial number of hospital-based physicians with a special interest predominantly in diabetes provide a lead role for diabetes services throughout their local community.

Inpatient work

Very few patients will be in hospital because of their diabetes or endocrine disorder. Most endocrine investigations are conducted on an outpatient or day case basis. Diabetic foot disease is the most commonly admitted diabetes-related disorder and is increasingly managed on an outpatient basis with the support of community-based high-risk foot care teams and home intravenous therapy services. Inpatient consultation work varies considerably depending on the co-specialty profile of the hospital. Because of the high prevalence of diabetes as a co-morbidity among hospital inpatients (10–15%) there is a substantial workload in supporting colleagues in other specialties when their patients develop metabolic problems; this is increased substantially if there are tertiary referral maternity, renal, vascular or cardiac services. For endocrinology, the workload is greater where a hospital has neurosurgery, a cancer centre or a specialist endocrine surgical service.

Outpatient work

General internal medicine (GIM)   The GIM load varies considerably: Thirty minutes should be allowed for new patients and fifteen minutes for follow-up patients.

Diabetes services   New patient consultations for people with diabetes are generally complex and require about thirty minutes of consultation time. Review diabetes patients require about twenty minutes but may require more time (30 minutes for diabetes renal service) or slightly less time (15 minutes for diabetic foot disease or antenatal care). Many of these consultations will need to be organised jointly or coordinated with other specialists, for example renal services with nephrologists, foot services with podiatrists, vascular surgeons with microbiologists, antenatal services with obstetricians.

Endocrine services   New endocrine patients require about 30 minutes of consultation time and review patients about 15 minutes. Complex reviews for pituitary patients or endocrine tumours, paediatric transition or genetic consultations may take longer and require joint or co-consultation arrangements with colleagues from other specialties.

Work to maintain and improve the quality of care

This work encompasses continuing professional development (CPD), clinical governance, professional self-regulation, education and training. For many consultants at various times in their careers it may also include research, management and providing professional advice. Management is a common component of diabetes service provision. The role typically involves providing 'whole systems' clinical and organisational leadership across a care community usually comprising about 250,000 people and includes responsibility for the education, development and quality assurance of primary care and community staff and those working from a hospital base.

ACADEMIC MEDICINE

Physicians in the specialty who have university contracts generally divide their time equally between research and a work programme similar in configuration but reduced by 50% of the volume to their NHS colleagues. Quite frequently, the clinical contribution will be restricted to the specialty (for example, no GIM or only endocrinology). The academic component of such posts is normally orientated primarily towards research productivity but there is likely to be a substantial teaching load and other academic, administrative and managerial responsibilities attached.

WORKFORCE REQUIREMENTS FOR DIABETES AND ENDOCRINOLOGY

Current workforce numbers

The 2003 annual Royal College of Physicians/Diabetes UK Survey identified 501 whole time equivalent (WTE) consultants in diabetes and endocrinology in England and Wales (522 individuals) on 30 September 2003. This is a provision of one consultant per 81,000 population in England and one per 96,000 in Wales. Long-term (over six months) vacancies had increased substantially from the previous year's survey, from three to 17.

Sixty-five hospitals in England and seven in Wales had single-handed consultants in diabetes and endocrinology. Of the appointments to consultant posts in the preceding year, 42% came from previous holders of consultant posts, as opposed to 27% in 2002 and 10% in 2001. Of advertised posts, 40% had failed to result in an appointment.

Estimate of number of consultant physicians necessary to provide a specialist service to a population of 250,000

This is a difficult exercise. There has been a considerable increase in the numbers of patients with Type 2 diabetes and the prospect of formal screening for diabetes is likely to result in a very steep increase in demand for diabetes care; epidemiological studies suggest that screening may double the number of those identified as having diabetes. However, the National Service Framework for Diabetes and other initiatives such as the College advocacy of the Chronic Disease Model are encouraging the development of ongoing primary and intermediate care diabetes services. The combination of these factors makes accurate prediction of the need for specialist and secondary care diabetes care a complex calculation. The best current estimate is that the increased prevalence and longevity of people with diabetes, the increased complexity of care, and the provision of new care models will mean no net change in the diabetes specialist workload. However, the nature of that work is likely to change quite radically with more time devoted to problem solving and support of primary and specialist colleagues. Similarly, for endocrinology it is expected that the devolution of more routine care will be balanced by the increased complexity of treatment options for rare conditions.

Table 1 is a calculation based on currently available information from central sources and clinical centres. This is a detailed analysis of the present position based on current work patterns but it is recognised that these are likely to change substantially during the period up to the projection for 2009. Nonetheless, as explained above, it is anticipated that overall workload can be reasonably calculated using the current position.

Table 1. Calculation of the need for consultant physicians with specialist training in diabetes and endocrinology in a district of 250,000

	2004	2009
District population[a]	250,000	253,773
Diabetes Prevalence at 0.3% increase/year[b]	3.5%	5%
Number of people with diabetes:	8,750	12,689
Number with Type 1 diabetes	875	1,000
Number with Type 2 diabetes[c]	7,875	11,989
Diabetes outpatient work for district		
Assume all Type 1 diabetes seen in hospital	875	1,000
Assumed % of Type 2 diabetes seen in hospital[d]	30	25
Estimated patients with Type 2 diabetes seen in hospital	2,363	2,997
Estimated total diabetic clinic population	3,268	4,022
Number of patients seen as new in diabetes clinic[e]	300	300
Hours/year at 30 minutes/patient	150	150
Mean hours/week	2.9	2.9

	2004	2009
Number of annual reviews in diabetes clinic	3,268	4,022
Hours/year if allow 20 minutes/review	1,089	1,341
Mean hours/week	20.9	25.8
Assume 33% of patients are seen >1/year[f]	1,078	1,327
Hours/year if allow 20 minutes/appointment	359	442
Mean hours/week	6.9	8.5
1 x 2.5 hour diabetes antenatal clinic/week	4	4
1 x 4 hour foot clinic/week	4	4
1 x 2 hour adolescent clinic/week	2	2
1 x 4 hour renal clinic/week	4	4
Total diabetes outpatient activity with supporting admin time at + 50% (hours/week)	67.1	76.8
Endocrine outpatient activity		
Endocrine new referrals (assume 0.12% of population/year)[f]	300	305
Hours/year if allow 30 minutes/new patient	150	152
Mean hours/week	2.9	2.9
Endocrine follow up appointments(n)[g]	1,250	1,268.9
Hours/year if allow 15 minutes/follow up	312.5	317.2
Mean hours/week	6.0	6.1
Total endocrine outpatient activity with supporting admin time at + 50% (hours/week)	13.3	13.5
General medical outpatient activity		
General medical new patient referrals hours (2 patients/week at 30 mins)[h]	1	1
General medical/ward follow-ups hours assume 10 patients/week at 15mins	2.5	2.5
Total general medical outpatient activity with supporting admin time at + 50% (hours/week)	5.3	5.3
Diabetes + endocrine + general medical outpatient activity (hours/week)	85.7	95.7
Diabetes community work hours/week to include NSF implementation/ retinal work/LDSAG/training GPSI etc	4	8
Inpatient work (assumes sharing one firm on 1 in 10 rota)		
Allow 8 hours/week for care of existing inpatients	8	8.1
Allow 4 hours/week for emergency work	4	4
Allow 6 hours/week for referrals/surgical support	6	6
Inpatient hours/week	18	18.1
Allow admin time to support inpatient work at 20% of total	3.6	3.6
Inpatient total hours/week	21.6	21.7
Total clinical hours	111	125
Total clinical programmed activities (PAs)	27.8	31.4
Total PAs corrected to 7.5/2.5 CPA/SPA ratio (at 10 PA contract)	37.1	41.8
Total PA needs for 250,000 population corrected for 8 weeks absence/consultant/year[j] to give	**43.8**	**49.4**
Worked out as 1 consultant per x population	**57,018**	**51,368**

Notes

a   Increases by 0.3% pa: Government figures.

b   International Diabetes Federation (IDF) estimates and data from centres. IDF suggest prevalence of 6% by 2010. This does not take account of any NSF screening programs.

c   Rate of rise much faster in Type 2 than in Type 1 diabetes.

d   Assumed to decrease over time with increased primary care involvement.

e   May well increase with time as prevalence increases; will depend on local care pathways.

f   Mean estimate from current practice; may well increase as complexity of hospital patients is likely to increase.

g   Data from centres: new patient referrals at 0.12% of population per year.

h   Data from centres.

j   Annual leave and study/professional leave.

LDSAG = local diabetes service advisory group

SPA = supporting professional activities

This analysis would suggest a current need for approximately 4.5 WTE consultants for a district of 250,000, rising to 5 WTE consultants by 2009.

This analysis is for a consultant-provided service and does not take outpatient activity by other grades into account. The demands of acute medicine on specialist registrars and the need to supervise junior doctors when in the clinic mean that most consultants feel it is not possible to quantify their input. Some centres run parallel nurse-led clinics, which are not included in the calculations; these need medical supervision and could be seen as balancing the input from non-consultant medical staff.

National consultant workforce requirements

Based on the above estimate of one consultant physician per 57,000 population, and one per 51,500 in 2009, this would give a current WTE requirement for England and Wales of 931, rising to 1,030 in 2009. This should be contrasted to the estimate of 426 from last year's specialty survey.

CONSULTANT WORK PROGRAMME/SPECIMEN JOB PLAN

The programme below assumes the above estimated number of physicians sharing a general medical commitment and working a 10 PA contract. This would fit a typical DGH in diabetes and endocrinology and would be different for more specialised or academic posts.

Activity	Workload	Programmed activities (PAs)
Direct clinical care		
Inpatients		
Ward rounds, referrals and other associated activities	20–25 patients	**1.5–2**
Outpatient clinics		
Diabetes	4 new and 6 follow up or 12 follow up*	**2–4.5**
Endocrinology	4 new and 8 follow up or 16 follow up*	**0.5–2**
General medical	4 new and 8 follow up or 16 follow up*	**0.5**
Patient related and supporting clinical administration		**1.5–2.5**
Total number of direct clinical care PAs		**7.5 on average**
Supporting professional activities (SPA)		
Work to maintain and improve the quality of healthcare	Education and training, appraisal, departmental management and service development, audit and clinical governance, CPD and revalidation, research	**2.5 on average**
Other NHS responsibilities	eg medical director/clinical director/lead consultant in specialty/clinical tutor	**Local agreement with trust**
External duties	eg work for deaneries/Royal Colleges/specialty societies/Department of Health or other government bodies etc	**Local agreement with trust**

*for a four-hour clinic session

Gastroenterology

i Description of the specialty and clinical needs of patients

The specialty of gastroenterology and hepatology cares for patients with both benign and malignant disorders of the gastrointestinal tract and liver. The specialty encompasses a wide range of conditions from common disorders to highly complex problems and specialised procedures such as transplantation.

Common problems include indigestion, irritable bowel syndrome, constipation and inflammatory bowel disease, chronic viral hepatitis and problems with liver function. Much of the work is outpatient based, to exclude organic disease in the symptomatic patient. Investigations often include endoscopy and imaging. An acute inpatient service is needed for common problems such as gastrointestinal haemorrhage, acute inflammatory bowel disease, jaundice and abdominal pain.

Although initial investigation of gastrointestinal cancer is part of the work of all gastrointestinal units, the Department of Health clinical outcomes group (COG) guidelines recommend referral of oesophageal and upper gastric cancers to specialist units serving a population of more than one million.[1] Similarly, pancreatic and biliary cancer are referred to specialist units serving a population of two million or more. Other conditions that may be referred to tertiary referral units include complex hepatobiliary disease, complex nutritional problems requiring total parenteral nutrition, and complex non-malignant gastrointestinal (GI) surgery. Transplantation of the liver and small intestine are referred to the small number of units undertaking organ transplantation.

ii Organisation of the service and patterns of referral

Most symptomatic patients are looked after by their family practitioner, and the majority of problems are resolved by discussion, advice and medical treatment. Most other problems can be resolved by appropriate outpatient medical or surgical referral. Some patients require emergency inpatient care, particularly those with abdominal pain, gastrointestinal haemorrhage or acute colitis, and a smaller number require admission for evaluation of persistent symptoms.

While much of the inpatient work is broad based there is increasing specialisation within gastroenterology. There is co-location of medical and surgical teams working in treatment of disorders of the oesophagus and stomach, hepatobiliary and pancreatic disease, disorders of the liver, small bowel disease and of medical and surgical groups concerned with the treatment of colorectal disease. Each of these groups plays a major role in the investigation, diagnosis and treatment of cancer at each of these specific sites. The National Service Framework (NSF) for Cancer and the COG guidelines on upper GI cancer have led to a major restructuring of cancer services, the integration of all disciplines involving cancer care and the initiation of multidisciplinary team (MDT) working. Most departments will participate on a weekly basis in team meetings involving surgeons, physicians, radiologists, pathologists and oncologists with their supporting teams.

Outpatient referral is now more targeted. There are clinics for patients with specific symptoms such as dysphagia, jaundice, rectal bleeding or abdominal pain. Primary care referral to hospital-based open-access endoscopy is also a common pattern of referral.

iii   Working with patients: patient-centred care

Patient choice and involving patients in decisions about their treatment

Much of the outpatient work in gastroenterology relates to the management of chronic conditions such as chronic liver disease and inflammatory bowel disease. Success depends on a working relationship with the patient whereby the patient has full understanding and participates in the management of his/her condition. It must be clear where responsibility lies in patient care between the specialist, patient and GP. Inflammatory bowel disease is one example where patients will often initiate a change in their treatment in the face of a relapse of their disease, usually in close liaison with the specialist team and/or their GP. The increasing number of specialist GI and hepatology nurses provides easy access to advice through telephone helplines and often obviates the need for outpatient visits.

Opportunities for education and promoting self-care

Specialist GI nurses can expand the opportunities for patient education through discussion, leaflets and videos.

There are many opportunities for improved patient care, including clear guidelines for the management and primary care of patients with peptic ulcer and non-ulcer dyspepsia. Targeted outpatient clinics, groups for patients with suspected malignancy, and joint medical and surgical assessment and management are increasingly being developed in all areas of the specialty. Other major advances have been made in diagnostic and therapeutic endoscopy and imaging, particularly the use of magnetic resonance imaging (MRI) and endoscopic ultrasound. Some invasive diagnostic procedures such as endoscopic retrograde cannulation of the pancreas are being replaced by MRI techniques. All these developments need to be underpinned by first class teaching and training. The identification of *helicobacter pylori* as the cause of peptic ulcer, and treatment for one week by triple antimicrobial therapy as the cure, have been remarkable examples of such progress.

Access to information and patient support groups

There are various patient support groups in gastroenterology: the National Association for Crohn's and Colitis (NACC), the Ileostomy Association of Great Britain and Coeliac UK. There is usually close integration between the specialist services team and these patient self-help groups.

iv   Interspecialty and interdisciplinary liaison

Multidisciplinary team working and working with other specialists

The practice of gastroenterology involves many specialties and there is perhaps a greater overlap between medical and surgical practice than in any other specialty. For this reason, well-organised MDT working is essential. This is coordinated through MDT meetings which, following the NSF for cancer, are usually held twice a week. The MDT meeting for GI cancer involves pathologists, oncologists, surgeons and physicians. The MDT meeting for gastroenterological services in general involves radiologists, pathologists, GI surgeons, physicians and supporting teams.

Close liaison with tertiary referral centres is an integral part of the management of complex GI problems, for example complex liver disease, pancreatic cancer, liver/small bowel transplantation and complex nutritional problems requiring home parenteral nutrition. Specialist nurses in nutrition, stoma care, GI oncology, general gastroenterology, management of viral hepatitis therapy and others play an increasingly valuable role in improving quality of service, communication and liaison between disciplines within the team.

Working with GP specialists

Close links with primary care are of the greatest importance, particularly as much gastroenterological practice relates to the management of chronic disease. Shared responsibility between the GP, patient and specialist is essential to good management of the patient's problems.

v Delivering a high quality service

Characteristics of a high quality service

While most patient care takes place in the outpatient department, this must be supported by a combined medical and surgical inpatient unit for acute and elective problems within gastroenterology, particularly acute abdominal pain, GI haemorrhage and acute colitis. Specialist units have been developed at both district and teaching hospital level, with some regional and national centres for specific problems.

The main service groupings are units for upper gastrointestinal disorders (including the oesophagus and stomach), hepatobiliary and pancreatic units, and colorectal units. Regional and national units include those for acute and chronic liver failure and transplantation, particularly of the liver and small intestine.

A high quality service in the specialised units requires co-location of the medical and surgical practice, with a team approach from specialists, dietitians and nutrition specialists, and close collaboration with colleagues in imaging, histopathology and laboratory services.

Resources required for a high quality service

Specialised facilities

These have been clearly described in the British Society of Gastroenterology (BSG) working party report of 2001, *Provision of endoscopy-related services in district general hospitals.*[2] Specialised facilities include a diagnostic and therapeutic endoscopy unit, facilities for parenteral nutrition, operative, anaesthetic and intensive therapy unit support and interventional radiology. There must be arrangements to support close collaboration with colleagues in oncology.

Workforce requirements: clinical and support staff

Workforce requirements are considered in detail later in this chapter. Those relating to endoscopy services are detailed in the BSG working party report referred to above.[2] Adequate secretarial support for every consultant is essential to the smooth running of a gastroenterology department. The complex working pattern of specialists/consultants necessitates each having their own office. Communication is central to safe management of patients and good IT support is necessary for auditing standards of practice within the department. At the very least there should be computer terminals at all workstations, and in endoscopy rooms and offices.

vi **Quality standards and measures of the quality of specialist services**

Specialist society guidelines

The BSG has produced guidelines of the highest standard in all areas of clinical practice in gastroenterology. These have been published by Gut and are available on the BSG website (**www.bsg.org.uk**).

The liver section of the BSG and the British Association for the Study of the Liver (BASL) are developing a standards document for the provision of liver services at district general hospital (DGH) and tertiary level.

National Institute for Clinical Excellence (NICE) guidelines

Guidelines relating to certain key areas of gastroenterological practice have been produced by NICE. These include guidance on the use of ribavirin and interferon for hepatitis C, the use of pegylated interferon for hepatitis C, the use of proton pump inhibitors, treatment of dyspepsia, and the use of infliximab for Crohn's disease. These are available on the NICE website (**www.nice.org.uk**).

Clinical governance

It is an essential requirement that clinical governance is an integral part of the workings of a gastroenterological department. A monthly or bimonthly meeting of all members of the department is held to discuss all important areas of clinical governance.

CLINICAL WORK AND/OR LABORATORY WORK OF CONSULTANTS IN GASTROENTEROLOGY

Contributions made to acute medicine

Most gastroenterologists are general physicians with a specialist interest in gastroenterology and, therefore, commit a major part of their time to the management of patients with general medical problems as part of the unselected acute medical take, ward work and outpatient work.

The range of clinical commitments includes providing inpatient and outpatient services in general medicine, gastroenterology and hepatology, a specialist diagnostic and therapeutic endoscopy service, and facilities for nutritional support. Gastroenterology is characterised by high volume, frequent outpatient consultations, several sessions per week in diagnostic and therapeutic endoscopy, and the inpatient care of patients within acute medicine and the specialty. There are regular collaborative meetings to discuss clinical problems. Other tasks include contributions to the teaching and appraisal of medical staff, teaching medical students, continuing medical education (CME), clinical audit, clinical research, administration and management.

Multidisciplinary working

The workload is shared with a wide variety of colleagues in nursing, dietetics, nutrition, imaging and histopathology. This team effort is a hallmark of the specialty.

Since the last edition of this document there have been added demands on the work expected to be delivered by consultant gastroenterologists. Acute medicine has become more onerous and supervision and training of junior doctors occupies more time. In most units cancer services are up and running, often demanding much time spent managing these services and in multidisciplinary meetings. In spite of all this, gastroenterologists continue to work as previously defined in the second edition of *Consultant physicians working for patients*.[3] There is, perhaps, increased pressure from managers wanting ever faster turnaround times for inpatients, meaning that endoscopic services have to be delivered more promptly. In addition, colorectal cancer screening is to be developed and this will lead to an increased workload. The surveillance work will throw up a large number of polyps, which in turn require further colonoscopy.

Direct clinical care

This section describes the work of a consultant physician providing a service in acute general medicine and gastroenterology and recommends a workload consistent with high standards of patient care. It sets out the work generated in gastroenterology by a population of 250,000 and gives the consultant workload as programmed activity (PA) for each element of such a service.

The Royal College of Physicians gastroenterology committee and the BSG have published several studies concerned with the provision of a combined general medical and gastroenterology service.

The following account will apply to most consultant physicians in gastroenterology, although the pattern may be different in specialist centres. The guidelines and recommendations on the appropriate workload for each element of the consultant's work have been drawn up following extensive consultation within the specialty.

Inpatient work

A consultant-led team should look after no more than 20–25 inpatients at any time. Most are admitted on emergency 'take' days, with various general medical problems. A minority are admitted, either urgently or electively, for evaluation of gastrointestinal problems. Programmed activities need to be allocated for two routine ward rounds and one post-take ward round per week per consultant.

Outpatient work

New patient clinic   A consultant physician in gastroenterology working alone in a new patient clinic sees six to eight new patients in a session of one PA (the exact number is dependent on experience and the complexity of the problem). Each new patient should be given 20–30 minutes. Endoscopy procedures should normally be carried out at a different time, except where facilities are available for flexible sigmoidoscopy, which may, in appropriate cases, be performed at the same visit.

Follow-up clinics   A consultant physician working alone in a clinic for selected patients following acute medical admission sees 12–15 patients in a session of one PA. A physician working alone in a specialist follow-up clinic for chronic gastrointestinal and liver disease sees 12–16 patients in one PA. In practice, most gastroenterologists will run clinics which are a mixture of new and old patients.

Junior medical staff support   Outpatient clinics are often run with doctors in training, either senior house officers (SHOs) or specialist registrars (SpRs), and the consultant must allocate time to review the patients seen by them. The number of patients that junior staff see depends on their experience. For each junior doctor, the outpatient workload is increased by about 50% of that undertaken by the consultant. It should be noted that this only creates a potential saving in outpatient and endoscopy consultant sessions and not in the other components of the consultant's work. Moreover, this saving (amounting to perhaps one session) is counterbalanced by the need for the consultant to devote time to training (including training in endoscopy). A SpR should be able to see six new patients or 10 follow-up patients or some combination of the two. Time must be allowed for training and amounts to approximately half an hour during a three-and-a-half-hour clinic.

Diagnostic and therapeutic endoscopy service   The workload of a consultant physician undertaking endoscopy depends on the procedure.

▮ Diagnostic upper GI endoscopy/diagnostic flexible sigmoidoscopy: A maximum of 10–12 procedures should be carried out in a session of one PA allowing 15–20 minutes per procedure. For a teaching session six patients should be allocated.

▮ Therapeutic upper GI endoscopy: This includes injection sclerotherapy and banding of oesophageal varices, injection of bleeding ulcers, palliative treatment of oesophageal cancer, and placing feeding tubes (percutaneous endoscopic gastrostomy (PEG)). Such procedures take twice as long as routine upper GI endoscopy and five to six might be undertaken in a session allowing 30–40 minutes per procedure (four to five if a teaching session).

▮ Therapeutic flexible sigmoidoscopy: This usually involves polypectomy and takes twice as long as routine flexible sigmoidoscopy; five to eight might be undertaken in a session.

▮ Diagnostic and therapeutic colonoscopy: There should be a maximum of six colonoscopies per session of one PA (three if a teaching session) allowing 30–40 minutes per procedure.

Training endoscopy lists   It is essential that adequate time for proper training is allowed and that special endoscopy training lists are scheduled into the programme. Training sessions inevitably reduce the service throughput and this must be taken into account. Hands-on training cannot be adequately carried out during the course of a busy standard service endoscopy list.

Diagnostic and therapeutic endoscopic retrograde cholangiopancreatography (ERCP)   A maximum of five procedures should be carried out in one PA.

On call for gastroenterological emergencies

Sessional time must be allocated for emergency out-of-hours endoscopy work, predominantly the management of gastrointestinal haemorrhage. In larger units with more trained endoscopists, 24-hour, seven-day-a-week emergency cover should be the aim. This is much harder to achieve in smaller units with fewer staff. As far as possible, the aim should be to have scheduled sessions during the week and at weekends to manage those patients admitted with acute GI haemorrhage. Such rotas should include all those with appropriate skills, particularly members of the medical and surgical GI teams.

Nutrition service

Consultant physicians with an interest in gastroenterology are usually responsible for leading the enteral and parenteral feeding service. Supervision of home-based parenteral nutrition is usually provided from specialist centres. Nutritional rounds need to be regular and would be expected to account for two hours per week for the gastroenterologists taking responsibility for the nutritional service.

ACADEMIC MEDICINE

The clinical contribution of academic gastroenterologists varies widely, depending upon other responsibilities. However, many clinical academics provide a substantial contribution to the clinical service and often provide a specialist tertiary advice.

The majority of academic gastroenterologists have an honorary consultant contract with their local NHS trust and the usual proportion of academic to service work is approximately 50:50. There are wide variations and great flexibility in practice, but with the advent of job planning under the auspices of the 2003 consultant contract greater clarity will be necessary. This will potentially make the planning of service provision easier and it will be clearer to all parties what is expected.

With such an honorary consultant contract, the academic gastroenterologist would expect to provide proportional input into the gastroenterology service. It should be stressed that this will be proportionate for all activities in a gastroenterologist's job description, including support, training, governance, teaching and administrative roles, as well as direct patient-related activities.

Since local circumstances permit the negotiation of a different proportional contract, these may vary from centre to centre. An academic, for example, may be leading a very active research group and would require 70–80% time for this activity. The university (or other academic employer) would agree the proportions (including funding) with the local trust.

The academic employer is responsible for the academic time of the clinical academic. Inevitably, clinical academics develop national and international roles and, consequently, these activities should be allocated between academic and clinical time by local negotiation. Since academic gastroenterologists are often research leaders or leaders in the organisation and development of clinical education, they are an important resource for their clinical colleagues. Within a gastroenterology unit, therefore, good relationships are vital so that academic input can support the development of the clinical service and the clinicians can be involved in up-to-date academic developments.

WORKFORCE REQUIREMENTS FOR GASTROENTEROLOGY

Current workforce numbers

As of 30 September 2003 there were 643 consultant gastroenterologists in England, an increase of 43 over the previous year. This represents an annual expansion rate of 7.2%.

Consultant PAs required to provide a service in gastroenterology for a population of 250,000

The consultant requirement, measured as the number of consultant PAs needed to provide a service, depends on the volume of inpatient, outpatient and endoscopic work, and can be calculated for any given workload. This paper gives a calculation of the consultant PAs required to service the average workload of a DGH serving a population of 250,000. Although it is not yet universal practice, it is assumed that consultant physicians with an interest in gastroenterology work together to run a single inpatient service. Increasingly, one or more consultants will specialise in providing hepatology services. An important component of the outpatient workload will involve the investigational management of viral hepatitis. Maintaining liaison with a regional liver centre for the appropriate management of acute liver failure and some of the complications of cirrhosis will be another major role.

Inpatient service   Three consultant PAs per week should be allocated for inpatient rounds, discharge letters and other related administration, with an additional consultant PA per week for a post-take ward round.

Outpatient service   Outpatient services are often provided by the consultant staff and team in training. The reduction of junior doctors' hours and the commitment to run the emergency medical service often means that the junior medical staff cannot attend outpatient clinics regularly. In this example it is assumed that the consultant physician is working alone in outpatients.

New outpatient referrals   A DGH serving a population of 250,000 should see at least 4,100 new GI patients each year, made up of approximately 3,600 urgent cancer referrals, as estimated in the two-week cancer referral guidelines, and about 500 additional GI and hepatology cases. A variable proportion of this workload – around 1,500 cases – will be seen by gastrointestinal surgeons. The remaining 2,600 requires eight to 10 consultant PAs per week for consultants working alone in the outpatient clinic. Depending on the area, up to 0.7% or more of the population may be carriers of hepatitis C or B, and the workload associated with this is likely to rise.

General medical outpatient follow up post-discharge   Up to three consultant PAs are required per week to provide this service.

Outpatient specialist follow-up clinic per week   Three consultant PAs per week are required for this service.

Diagnostic and therapeutic endoscopy service

■ Diagnostic upper GI endoscopy and flexible sigmoidoscopy: The requirement for upper GI endoscopy in the general population is 1.5:100 population per annum. This gives an annual workload of 3,750 examinations in a DGH serving a population of 250,000. On the conservative assumption that at least two-thirds of urgent lower GI cancer referrals will require flexible sigmoidoscopy or colonoscopy, the requirement for flexible sigmoidoscopy gives a workload of $\frac{2}{3} \times 2,375 = 1,500$ examinations per year, of which 900 are likely to be provided by GI physicians. Therefore, seven to nine PAs per week are required for these procedures.

■ Diagnostic and therapeutic colonoscopy and ERCP: Workload figures for the average DGH indicate that at least two PAs per week are needed for diagnostic and therapeutic colonoscopy. One PA is needed for diagnostic and therapeutic ERCP.

■ Cancer screening and surveillance programmes: The need for screening high-risk groups within the population and the move towards more general population screening to identify those with cancer is now being more clearly defined. There is no doubt this will lead to a substantial increase in endoscopic workload, particularly flexible sigmoidoscopy and colonoscopy. Some of this work will be undertaken by specialist nurse endoscopists but a substantial proportion of the work will be undertaken by consultant gastroenterologists and will probably amount to two additional colonoscopy sessions per department per week.

Out-of-hours endoscopy service   This service requires up to one consultant PA per week.

Nutrition service   This service requires up to two consultant PAs per week

Monitoring service   This service requires up to one consultant PA per week.

Consultant PAs required per week to provide a service in gastroenterology and general internal medicine in a district general hospital with an average workload

Direct patient care   Where junior medical staff provide support for the inpatient service and consultants provide the outpatient and endoscopic service, about 38 PAs are required. The number of PAs required to run the service is reduced if part of the work is undertaken by consultant colleagues, for example those in radiology or surgery might share the endoscopic workload. Regular help in outpatients by junior medical staff, each of whom might contribute to the work done by around 50% of that recommended for a consultant PA, will also reduce that consultant sessional requirement. It should be noted that commitments may change with the development of outreach clinics in primary care and endoscopic services outside the specialist centres.

Work to maintain and improve the quality of care   Additional PAs for each consultant are required for this work. Time must be allocated for each consultant for: CME (one PA per week); teaching junior medical staff, nursing staff and medical students (one PA per week); administration and management (one PA per week); clinical research (one PA per week); and clinical governance (one PA per week).

On the basis of these conditions and recommendations, the number of PAs required by a DGH serving a population of 250,000 to provide a clinical service in gastroenterology and general medicine can be calculated. Allowing five PAs for each consultant for the supporting activities given above, the total is 61 PAs (this assumes six consultants).

Table 1 summarises the work programme of consultant gastroenterologists providing a service for a population of 250,000, giving the recommended workload and allocation of PAs.

Table 1. The work of consultant gastroenterologists generated by a population of 250,000 (PAs per week)

Activity	Workload	PAs per week for 250,000 population
Direct patient care		
Ward rounds (except on-take and post-take)		4
Outpatient clinics		
New patients	6–8 patients per clinic	8–10
Follow-up patients		} 12–14
General medical	12–15 patients per clinic	3
Specialist	12–15 patients per clinic	3
Diagnostic and therapeutic endoscopy		
Diagnostic upper GI endoscopy	10–12 patients per clinic } 3,750 pa	5–7
Therapeutic upper GI endoscopy	5–6 patients per clinic	
Diagnostic flexible sigmoidoscopy	10–12 patients per clinic } 1,000 pa	2 } 10–13 (+2 training)
Therapeutic flexible sigmoidoscopy	5–8 patients per clinic	
Diagnostic and therapeutic colonoscopy	6 patients per clinic	2–3
Diagnostic and therapeutic ERCP	5 patients per clinic	1

Continued

Activity	Workload	PAs per week for 250,000 population
Nutrition service (usually in a specialist unit)		2–3
Monitoring service		
On-take, and mandatory post-take rounds	Rota 1:10 for this example	1–2
On-call for emergency endoscopy *(assuming some registrar input to the rota)*		4
Total direct patient care		34–44
Work to maintain and improve the quality of care (6 consultants) Including new MDT cancer meetings		30
Total		65–74

This number of PAs indicates that six consultants with 10–12 PAs per week would be required.

National consultant workforce requirement

The calculation above allows an estimate of the consultant requirement to be made. Assuming that teaching hospitals serve a population 13,478,000 and non-teaching hospitals a population of 38,251,000, the total need in England and Wales is for 1,476 whole-time consultants in gastroenterology (with general medicine). Currently there are 643. The NHS Cancer Plan states that 208 additional consultant posts would be provided over the next six years but even this increase leaves a major shortfall.[4] With 7% expansion it is unlikely that these numbers of gastroenterologists will be achieved before 2014.

These calculations do not take into account an increasing demand for colorectal screening for cancer, already introduced for high-risk individuals. It has been estimated that introduction of a screening programme for individuals who are not at increased risk would generate a requirement for an additional 50–160 consultants. The calculations also do not include the extra staffing required in hospitals with a major regional referral practice (eg regional liver units) or national centres (eg transplant units).

Finally, working patterns appear to be gradually changing so that there are more part-time workers and increasing numbers intending to work flexibly. Thus, although calculations should be done on a whole-time consultant basis it is likely that the number of heads in the jobs will be substantially greater.

CONSULTANT WORK PROGRAMME/SPECIMEN JOB PLAN

The following is an example of the work programme of consultant physicians undertaking gastro-enterology and acute general medicine, giving the recommended workload, and allocation of PAs.

Activity	Workload	Programmed activities (PAs)
Direct clinical care		
On-take, and mandatory post-take rounds	According to numbers of admissions, rota and non-consultant support*	**1–4**
On-call for emergency endoscopy		**0–2**
Ward rounds and other inpatient work (except post-take rounds – see above)		**2**
Referrals and specialist services, eg nutrition rounds, monitoring service		**1**
Diagnostic and therapeutic endoscopy	Diagnostic upper GI endoscopy: 10–12 Therapeutic upper GI endoscopy: 5–6 Diagnostic flexible sigmoidoscopy: 10–12 Diagnostic and therapeutic colonoscopy: 6 Diagnostic and therapeutic ERCP: 5**	**1–2**
Outpatients (general medical or specialist)	New: 6–8 patients per clinic Follow-up: 12–15 patients per clinic	**1–2**
Clinically related administration		**1.5–2.5**
Total number of direct clinical care PAs		**7.5 on average**
Supporting professional activities (SPA)		
Work to maintain and improve the quality of healthcare	Education and training, appraisal, departmental management and service development, audit and clinical governance, continuing professional development and revalidation, research	**2.5 on average**
Other NHS responsibilities	eg medical director/clinical director/lead consultant in specialty/clinical tutor	**Local agreement with trust**
External duties	eg work for deaneries/Royal Colleges/specialist societies/Department of Health or other government bodies etc	**Local agreement with trust**

*It is recommended that all other activities are cancelled for a large proportion of the time when a consultant is on take for acute medicine, which will clearly have an impact on the routine clinical workload that can be undertaken by a consultant.
**Numbers = patients per four hour list. List sizes will be reduced proportionately if training is included.

The figures given in this document are the best estimate of consultant requirement from available evidence at the present time. They will need to be reviewed to assess the impact of both the European Working Time Directive and the implementation and interpretation of the new consultant contract, about which much uncertainty remains.

References

1. Department of Health. *Guidance on commissioning cancer services: improving outcomes in upper gastrointestinal cancers.* London: DH, 2001. www.dh.gov.uk/assetRoot/04/08/02/78/04080278.pdf

2. British Society of Gastroenterology. *Provision of endoscopy-related services in district general hospitals.* Report of a working party. London: BSG, 2001.

3. Royal College of Physicians. *Consultant physicians working for patients.* 2nd edition. London: RCP, 2001.

4. Department of Health. *The NHS cancer plan: a plan for investment, a plan for reform.* London: DH, 2000.

Genitourinary medicine

i Description of the specialty and the clinical needs of patients

Genitourinary medicine (GUM) encompasses many aspects of sexual healthcare provision principally in the fields of sexually transmitted infections (STIs) and HIV disease which are of major public health concern. The Department of Health (DH) has published papers on the National Strategy for Sexual Health and HIV (NSSHH)[1] and its implementation.[2] The strategy envisages a greater involvement of primary care, with consultants providing secondary and tertiary services, training and governance for GPs. The success of the strategy is dependent on commitment from the Government and the provision of adequate numbers of consultants and facilities.

The House of Commons Select Committee (HCSC) report on sexual health concluded that there was a crisis in the sexual health of the nation.[3] MPs were appalled at the lack of support for provision of services and the poor fabric of many clinical facilities. They concluded that this was a consequence of several factors:

- a failure of local NHS organisations to recognise and deal with this major public health problem
- a lack of political pressure and leadership over many years
- the absence of a patient voice
- a lack of resources
- a lack of central direction to suggest that this is a key priority
- an absence of performance management.

These and many other issues need to be resolved if the aims of the national strategy are to be achieved.

Genitourinary medicine is primarily outpatient based. The largest group of patients are those with STIs and a wide range of other sexual health conditions. The number of attendances has been rising in recent years. In 2002 there were 1.5 million attendances at GUM clinics in England, Wales and Northern Ireland; an increase of 15% since 2001.[4] These increases are in all STIs, with a number of outbreaks of syphilis reported. Diagnosis of early syphilis rose from 137 cases in 1996 to 1,167 in 2002.[5] Failure to treat STIs in the early stages can lead to serious costly sequelae. Management of STIs is important in the control of human immunodeficiency virus (HIV) infection. Epidemiological evidence indicates that STIs predispose to the transmission of the virus and this is supported by reports of increased viral load in infected genital secretions.[6,7]

Patients with HIV infection form a rapidly increasing and more time-consuming group who develop a wide variety of medical, social and other problems and provide the inpatient work of GUM. Newly diagnosed HIV infections continue to increase.[4] Highly active antiretroviral therapy (HAART) has improved survival, further adding to caseloads.[8]

ii   Organisation of the service and patterns of referral

Patients are free to attend GUM clinics without referral from another provider. Historically, clinics provided an open access walk-in facility. Recently, higher numbers of patients and limited resources have led to increased use of appointment systems. This has led to many clinics having unacceptable waiting lists. Patients still attend the clinic of their choice – this may be near where they live or work for ease of travel or may not because of concerns about confidentiality. A proportion are referred from general practice, family planning, A&E departments and other providers.

Patients with HIV infection may prefer to seek treatment at major centres in conurbations. This pattern of care was facilitated by the principle that funding should follow patients. Currently, the NHS is moving to district-of-residence-based funding for STIs and HIV infection, which will encourage care within the district of residence but may restrict patient choice and comfort. Referral patterns may be affected by the development of clinical networks for HIV-infected patients.

Primary, secondary and tertiary levels

Primary care   An unknown number of patients are managed in primary care, but there is evidence of increased screening for chlamydia trachomatis and referral to GUM clinics.[9] This follows the report of the Chief Medical Officer's (CMO) expert advisory group on chlamydia trachomatis, which recommended community-based screening.[10] The NSSHH has outlined the increasing role primary care is expected to take in screening for STI. This will inevitably result in increased referral to GUM clinics. The strategy has set standards for those providing care at this level, and GUM will collaborate in developing protocols, training and clinical governance.

Secondary care   GUM specialists provide a service for the community in designated departments. These may be based in acute hospitals but increasingly clinics are situated in non-acute sites. There should be facilities for outpatients, and any service with HIV-infected patients should have access to day care and beds. Although consultants work primarily in outpatient clinics, they are on call for urgent problems and provide support for other specialists. At least two consultants with appropriate support staff are required for a hospital serving a population of 250,000 although all too frequently this is not the case. It is essential that single-handed consultants have regular meetings with GUM colleagues from surrounding units for audit and continuing professional development (CPD).

Tertiary care   This is provided in GUM clinics by specialists with special skills and training. Examples include complex HIV disease, sexual problems and vulval disorders.

Clinical networks and community arrangements

Most patients with STIs and allied conditions are managed within the clinics. Those with conditions such as infertility require referral to other specialists. Genitourinary medicine clinics collaborate when managing patients who travel to other clinics for care, when undertaking partner notification, or recalling patients who fail to attend for follow-up. Informal networks are maintained for this purpose.

HIV-infected patients require integrated care between hospital and general practice. This requires collaboration between primary and secondary care and community health services such as nursing, social services and voluntary agencies. The NSSHH and the Medical Foundation for AIDS and Sexual Health (MedFASH) has recommended the development of clinical networks, as in cancer care, to manage HIV infection.[1,11]

Relationship with other services/agencies

Relationships with other services in the area of sexual health include obstetrics and gynaecology, urology, pathology, family planning, psychology, termination and forensic medicine services. For HIV medicine, relationships with many services, for example infectious diseases, palliative care and multiple statutory agencies, are essential. Voluntary agencies provide invaluable links for HIV care and education. Close links with the Health Protection Agency (HPA) have been forged over recent years and have yielded enormous benefits in the epidemiological surveillance and targeting of health promotion.

Complementary services

Complementary medicine has, to date, had little role in the field of STIs. On the other hand these services are valued by patients with HIV disease, particularly aromatherapy and reflexology. These are sometimes supplied by the statutory sector but more usually by the voluntary.

iii   Working with patients: patient-centred care

Patient choice and involving patients in decisions about their treatment

It is essential that patients are involved in decisions about their treatment. This is especially true for successful HAART where it has been shown clearly that the doctor-patient relationship and understanding of treatment are key components for long-term adherence to, and success of, therapy.[12] For prevention of onward transmission of STIs, patients need a clear understanding of the aims of therapy and the importance of partner notification. The specialty sets great store by these principles.

Cultural sensitivity is extremely important in the field of sexual health. There is a considerable amount of information for patients published in many languages. Intimate examinations need to be carefully explained and understood by all patients, especially those who may have cultural taboos in respect of female examination. Patients with HIV from developing world countries will often have beliefs in traditional medicine or disease causation which need to be addressed. Sensitivity to the patient's sexual orientation is an integral part of care.

Opportunities for education and promoting self-care

Education is a cornerstone of the practice of GUM for the the prevention of transmission of infection. Verbal explanations and written materials are provided for all patients with STIs/HIV during consultations. Health advisers provide an extra level of education for those with serious or recurrent disease for example, syphilis, chlamydia trachomatis, gonorrhoea, genital herpes, hepatitis B/C and HIV infection.

Both in the specialty and in health promotion campaigns emphasis is placed on prevention (use of condoms, limiting the number of sexual partners, safer sex, healthcare seeking behaviour etc). The relatively low incidence of HIV in the UK has been partly attributed to these interventions. Gay men are routinely advised to have vaccination against hepatitis B.

Patients with chronic conditions

Of principal concern are those patients with HIV, hepatitis B and C, relapsing herpes genitalis, genital warts and the sequelae of pelvic inflammatory disease. By the nature of these conditions many patients opt for continuing care by the GUM team. Facilities for support and psychological services are often required but are underprovided in the majority of clinics.

The role of the carer

Patients attending for care of STIs and HIV may be extremely nervous. A partner or other carer sitting in on the consultation can help to ensure information and advice is understood, providing issues of confidentiality are considered. Carers frequently accompany patients with HIV disease and can be vital to adherence to HAART and care in the community.

Access to information, patient support groups and the role of the expert patient

Patients have ready access to information on infection and other areas of sexual health from freely available written material, and from health advisers, nurses and doctors. Information leaflets outlining the service and what the patient should expect is provided on registration, and should include mechanisms for complaints. Many clinics have websites providing clinic information and general information on STIs. Details of clinics and general information are also available on the British Association for Sexual Health and HIV (BASHH) website.[13]

Although patient support groups such as the Terrence Higgins Trust have been key to good services in HIV medicine, similar groups are much less in evidence for other STIs due to perceived stigma. The Herpes Association and Vulval Pain Society provide sources of support and information.

The expert patient has been a long established and valuable feature of HIV care. They are useful for individual or group support and bring their experience to educational events. In the field of STIs the expert patient is notable by their rarity and should be encouraged.

Availability of clincial records/results

Genitourinary medicine/HIV outpatient records and computer registration are kept on site, separate from the general hospital records for reasons of confidentiality and ease of access. Access to test results is linked increasingly to service laboratories by computer. Tests should be anonymised by coded identifiers. These systems should be 'firewalled' from users outside the clinic and laboratories. Access to the notes by patients or for medico-legal reasons is as for other specialities.

iv Interspecialty and interdisciplinary liaison

Multidisciplinary team working

The modernisation of practice has been embraced by GUM.[14] The standards for NHS HIV services recommend the establishment of clinic networks as many smaller clinics cannot meet these standards on a stand alone basis.

Multidisciplinary work is key to quality service delivery. Nurse-led clinics and nurse practitioners are increasingly common, and health advisers are important within teams. Close links with microbiologists and virologists are essential and many departments have the services of a medical laboratory scientific officer (MLSO) in microbiology within the clinic.

Services with many HIV-infected inpatients hold a weekly clinical meeting or round attended by clinicians from all the disciplines involved, and all inpatients and problem outpatients are discussed.

Clinicians from the investigation departments make useful contributions. Other providers such as pharmacists, dietitians, physiotherapists and clinical psychologists attend. If regular meetings cannot be held there should be alternative arrangements to serve a similar purpose. These meetings have an important training role.

Later stages of HIV infection require close collaboration between many hospital specialists and between secondary care, primary care and community nursing, social services, dietetics, obstetrics and gynaecology, home helps, residential and hospice care, and voluntary organisations.

Working with other specialists

Joint clinics are held with other specialists such as dermatologists for patients with genital skin disease and gynaecologists for patients with vulval pain syndromes. There are many overlapping areas of interest with family planning specialists. It is of particular importance for future developments that specialties work together. For HIV, working with other specialists across the spectrum of medicine and surgery is routine. The joint care of pregnant women and children with HIV infection is recommended.

Working with other GP specialists

Many GPs do sessional work in GUM clinics. These GPs have a high level of expertise and are ideally placed to take the NHHSS implementation forward. Sexual health has been identified as one of the priorities for the development of general practitioners with special interests (GPSI).[15,16] The specialty is committed to working closely with the Royal College of General Practitioners (RCGP) and primary care trusts (PCTs) to provide training programmes and clinical governance for these GPs.

v Delivering a high quality service

Characteristics of a high quality service

For STIs:

- Most departments hold clinics at least four days per week and should have dedicated premises. Patients suspecting an acute STI should be seen on the day they present to a clinic, or on the next occasion the clinic is open.[17] This principle has been undermined by the huge increase in workload, much of which is related to sexual health advice-seeking and screening which forms an important part of the prevention and public health role of the specialty. A 48-hour access target is endorsed by the HCSC and will require considerable investment to establish.[3]

- Clinics should be in good quality, easily accessible premises. There should be a relaxed atmosphere to assist confidential discussion of sexually related conditions. Interviewing rooms should be sound attenuated and examination rooms should afford privacy.[18]

- Management includes taking a general and sexual history, physical examination and the collection of all appropriate specimens for a full STI screen. Patients should be offered a chaperone, in line with the General Medical Council (GMC) guidance.[19]

- Clinical examination is supported by immediate staining and microscopy of samples, and patients are given results before leaving. This requires fresh stains, swabs and other supplies, up-to-date and well-maintained equipment such as microscopes, and facilities for the storage and swift transfer of samples so that they arrive in the laboratories in optimal condition for processing.

- Patients often have more than one infection at one time. Sexually transmitted infections may be asymptomatic so patients are offered screening for other common conditions.

- Provision of free treatment for STIs is a legal requirement so treatments are usually stored and dispensed in the clinic.[20]

- Patients with STIs are advised on the need to notify sexual partners at risk of infection, and are offered counselling on sexual health in general. They are offered leaflets to support verbal information. They are also offered free condoms. Most clinics provide general contraceptive advice, some provide emergency and routine contraception methods, and all collaborate closely with related services.

- Follow-up appointments are required to assess resolution of symptoms and compliance with medication, undertake tests of cure, ensure partners have been notified, and for further sexual health advice if required.

- Medical staff are supported by receptionists, nurses and health advisers.

- Enhanced confidentiality for all patients who attend a clinic is set out in statute to shield their identity as well as diagnosis, and must be guaranteed by all members of clinic staff and any other person who becomes aware of their attendance.[20,21] A more recent trust directive extends this across primary and secondary care.[22]

- All patients presenting to GUM clinics are offered screening for HIV infection. This involves a discussion about the tests and the infection, which is time-consuming. This is especially important for individuals with high-risk behaviour.

- The contracting process should ensure that this guidance is followed.[23-25]

For HIV infection:

- Standards for NHS HIV services recommend the establishment of clinical networks as many smaller clinics cannot meet these standards alone.[11]

- At the first visit a full history is taken, physical examination performed, and an STI screen is offered if not previously done.

- Baseline investigations include viral load and CD4 lymphocyte subset, and investigations for co-existent or previous infection including tuberculosis if indicated. At this visit the patient may desire further counselling.

- Though treatment may not be indicated at this stage, services and facilities are described, including the provision of HAART and drugs for prophylaxis or treatment of complications. There may be a specialist pharmacist to assist.

- There are advantages in dietitians, physiotherapists and pharmacists taking part in all aspects of care, and patients should have access to community services and patient support groups.

- Patients require regular outpatient follow up with monitoring of immunological and virological parameters. When these investigations indicate the need, or symptoms develop, HAART will be introduced.

- When complications occur, patients require outpatient, day centre or inpatient care in dedicated beds staffed by specially trained nurses. Clinical teams of outpatient-based doctors may manage all the hospital care in outpatients, and the day centre will be managed primarily by nurses.

- Close cooperation and good communication between all those involved in the wards, outpatient clinics and the community is essential.

- Longer appointment times are required for HIV patients than those with STI.

- The contracting process should ensure that this guidance is followed.

Resources required for a high quality service

Specialised facilities

▪ modern tilting couches for the examination of female and disabled patients

▪ supplies and equipment for microscopy within the clinic

▪ facilities for collecting, storing and transporting samples to the laboratories

▪ equipment for the treatment of warts, which may include cryotherapy and electrosurgery, and access to laser therapy (some specialists undertake colposcopy)

▪ for HIV-infected cases, facilities such as arterial puncture for blood gases, lung function tests, negative-pressure rooms for obtaining induced sputum and for admission if pulmonary tuberculosis and other aerosol infections are present or suspected, and day care for treatment such as intermittent IV infusions.

Workforce requirements: clinical and support staff in STI clinics

Doctors Many consultants work in more than one hospital; they may be on call for emergencies at several hospitals. Time must be allowed for travel, and car parking space might be required. Some consultants undertake this work without any supporting medical staff. Those based at a single hospital with colleagues and good supporting staff have less onerous on-call commitments. Consultants are supported by non-consultant career grade doctors (NCCGs), clinical assistants, specialist registrars (SpRs) and SHOs.

▪ Doctors take patient history and undertake clinical examination of new patients except those seen by appropriately trained nurses operating within the nurse competency framework in sexual health.[26]

▪ They make diagnoses, prescribe and may dispense treatment.

▪ In smaller clinics they collect samples, undertake microscopy, advise on partner notification, undertake counselling and arrange follow-up appointments.

Nurses

▪ Nurses are trained to take samples for investigation and often undertake microscopy.

▪ They help with partner notification and counselling.

▪ They dispense prescribed treatment according to agreed written guidelines and Patient Group Directives (PGDs). This may include treatment of warts. Nurses can undertake an independent prescribers course.[27]

▪ Nurses must be familiar with the wide range of clinical and other problems that arise in HIV clinics and be trained to assist with or to undertake procedures such as obtaining induced sputum samples, intravenous infusions and biopsies. They need to know of, and liaise with, services in the hospital and community.

▪ Nurse practitioners undertake independent practice according to agreed written guidelines and PGDs.

Health advisers Health advisers are professionals unique to GUM. All clinics should have one or more health advisers on duty throughout all clinic sessions. They have four main roles:

▪ They advise patients on notifying partners at risk of infection. This involves identifying individuals and working with the patient to determine the best way to ensure partner attendance at a clinic. It may include talking to the partner on behalf of the patient.

■ They provide the main counselling service in clinics. All patients are anxious about attending a clinic, their diagnosis, treatment and sequelae. Patients whose behaviour has put them at risk of acquiring HIV infection may require much discussion before and after antibody testing. Ongoing support of HIV infected patients is often needed.

■ They ensure attendance of patients for review to assess response to treatment. This is a vital part of infection control, especially with the rising incidence of STIs and HIV infection.

■ They provide sexual health promotion through education for patients, partners and carers on STIs and HIV infection.

Receptionists These staff have a difficult role. They have the first contact with patients who are often anxious and occasionally aggressive. This pressure has escalated as waiting times to be seen have increased. For reasons of confidentiality and because patients may attend without appointments, clinics have their own dedicated healthcare records.

Secretaries Full secretarial support for consultants and other clinic professionals is essential. Secretaries ensure prompt, efficient correspondence on patients, support consultants in maintaining their diary and keep records up to date of educational materials, CPD, clinic adminstration, research projects, training and appraisal, personal appraisal and revalidation, audit, and specialist society, college and trust work. Secretaries often have to deal with anxious patients, ensure liaison between consultants, primary and secondary care colleagues, other clinical professionals and other agencies.

Clinic manager Larger clinics require a clinic manager to ensure the efficient and responsive running of the department. Roles include management of clinic staff, records and computer systems, ensuring adherence to trust and health service directives and regulations, ensuring effective communication systems both within and outside the department, and training for non-clinical staff.

Other staff These include clinical psychologists, psychosexual counsellors, pharmacists and dietitians.

vi   Quality standards and measures of the quality of specialist services

Consultants review the notes of patients to monitor quality of care and ensure that accurate diagnoses are entered on returns. (Workload and epidemiological returns are made to trusts, districts, regions and to the Public Health Laboratory Service (PHLS) on behalf of the DH.)

Genitourinary medicine clinics undertake internal and multidisciplinary audits which are an important part of training. Most regions have a well-developed system of regional audits which are reported to the regional offices of the National Health Service Executive (NHSE).

A national audit group has been established to develop audit tools. The first national audit on management of gonorrhoea has been undertaken. Specialty specific standards have been developed and are recommended as an integral part of the revalidation process.

The British Clinical Co-operative Group (BCCG), a special interest group, has conducted regular national surveys for over 50 years and published the results of clinic practices.

Specialist society guidelines

Specialist guidelines for all sexually transmitted infections (excluding HIV) were first published in 1999.[28] The updated and expanded guidelines include other areas of practice (eg care of adolescents and sexual assault patients) and are available online.[29] Guidelines for comprehensive management and treatment advice for HIV are published by the British HIV Association (BHIVA).[30]

National Institute for Clinical Excellence (NICE) guidelines

Currently there are no guidelines applicable to STIs/HIV. The HCSC report has recommended that NICE produce guidelines on HIV therapies.

Clinical governance

Clinical governance is overseen by the specialty society, the BASHH, through their clinical governance committee.[31]

CLINICAL WORK AND/OR LABORATORY WORK OF CONSULTANTS IN GENITOURINARY MEDICINE

Contributions made to acute medicine

Few GUM physicians participate in the general medical take but they do provide a consultation service, including out-of-hours provision.

Direct clinical care

Depending on the profile of their workload and specialist interests, consultants will undertake 7.5 direct patient care programmed activities (PAs) divided between outpatient GUM/HIV and inpatient HIV/AIDS work. Many consultants have outpatient clinics on more than one site. The antenatal screening programme for HIV infection is resulting in many new cases of HIV infection in pregnancy being detected. This is greatly adding to the unplanned direct patient clinical care for many consultants.

Inpatient work

This largely concerns HIV-infected patients. Admissions are mainly emergencies related to opportunistic disease or complications of HAART. Patients may be admitted for procedures such as endoscopy or insertion of a permanent IV line.

Ward rounds vary according to the numbers of patients involved and the supporting staff available. Many district general hospitals (DGHs) have only one or two inpatients at any one time. Consultants in DGHs may be single handed with minimal supporting staff. They may see the patients daily and manage most or all of the care themselves. Alternatively, inpatient care may be shared with colleagues in other disciplines, such as infection or thoracic medicine, with shared junior staff.

Larger units have several GUM consultants, some of whom specialise in the management of HIV disease, with either dedicated or shared junior staff. Regular ward rounds, preferably with the full team of junior medical staff, specialist nurses, pharmacists, physiotherapists, dietitians and others, provide an opportunity for clinical teaching.

Consultants in GUM swiftly see referrals from other wards, for example when HIV-infected patients are admitted to other services.

Outpatient work

STI clinics Most departments hold clinics at least four days per week. In a four-hour session consultants should allow three and a half hours for their own patients and half an hour for consultation, teaching and training. Clinical teaching forms a major part of the workload in teaching and non-teaching hospitals. Fewer patients will be seen when teaching but numbers vary according to the casemix and the supporting staff. Adequate time must be allowed to practise to a satisfactory standard, especially important for single-handed consultants.

Purchasers and trusts may require late evening, early morning or weekend clinics which must be staffed in the same manner as other sessions and by agreement in keeping with the 2003 consultant contract.[32]

HIV clinics Consultants seeing HIV-infected patients require the support of junior medical staff in training plus receptionists, nurses and health advisers. Ideally, where dedicated HIV clinics are held other healthcare professionals should be available including pharmacists, dietitians and clinical psychologists.

Other specialist clinics Consultants may undertake other clinics depending on casemix and local requirements. Many offer consultant specialist clinics such as psychosexual problems, erectile dysfunction, and clinical problem clinics such as pelvic pain. These require nursing support. Some services provide multidisciplinary clinics, such as those for genital skin or vulval disorders, staffed by a GUM physician, dermatologist and gynaecologist who see the patients together. These clinics provide opportunities for teaching and training.

Specialised investigative and therapeutic procedure clinics

Investigative clinics For some years GUM provided colposcopy but with the increasing pressures of other work this service is being reduced. Colposcopy is needed for vulval and HIV clinics.

Therapeutic procedure clinics Genital warts are common and persistent. They can be treated in dedicated sessions or during dedicated time. Trained nurses working to agreed written protocols and PGDs may provide treatment. One person using one room can treat four to six patients per hour.

Specialised services within the specialty

Referral from another provider is not required. The specialty emphasises ease of access, confidentiality of identity and diagnosis, clinical diagnosis supported by microscopy, systems for swift transfer of samples to supporting laboratories, and free treatment. In addition, sexual health counselling including contraception and provision of free condoms, discussion of HIV antibody testing, partner notification, management of erectile dysfunction, joint management of genital dermatoses and vulval disorders and, in some services, colposcopy are available. Most services provide HIV infection outpatient care and many provide the medical element of full HIV care.

Education on therapy and adherence are essential elements of specialised support for patients. Intermittent intravenous infusions and inhalation therapy are provided as required.

Specialist advice on call

All services provide a consultant on call. This includes advice on HIV post-exposure prophylaxis following needlestick injuries or sexual exposure, support for A&E departments, inpatients, and sometimes problems in the community. With the aid of junior staff some emergencies may be managed over the telephone or using other telemedicine modes. Some single-handed consultants still have one in one rotas at more than one hospital.

A single-handed consultant should only manage occasional inpatients. A team of five consultants can manage 10–20 inpatients with rotations for on-call and day-to-day consultant supervision but many consultants with a significant HIV patient cohort have rotas of less than one in five.

Other specialist activity including activities beyond the local services

Many services have set up outreach clinics, but problems associated with confidentiality, and the need for examination facilities, microscopy and readily available investigative support need to be overcome. Some specialists deliver care in primary healthcare settings and in prisons.

Clinically related administration

Correspondence with primary care and other medical colleagues is routine. Writing reports for social services, Disability Living Allowance and asylum seekers, and writing medico-legal reports is a significant workload.

Work to maintain and improve the quality of care

Leadership role and development of the service

The NSSHH has emphasised the need to set standards for more community-based care. Any service development must take into account the individual and the impact on public health. As a consequence, the increased awareness and case-finding anticipated will increase patient attendance at clinics. Adequate resources are the main requirement for improved patient care, as identified in the HCSC report.

The principal aim is for patients suspecting new STIs to be seen either on the day they present or on the next occasion the clinic is open.[3,17] It is to be determined whether this is best provided by open access or a flexible appointment system. Evening and weekend working would depend on adequate resources and agreement under the new contract.[32] Staff skillmix and multidisciplinary working requires more consideration but an overall increase in workforce is necessary to increase capacity. Discussion within the specialty and with purchasers and the DH is needed to introduce these improvements and to evaluate them.

Clinics for those with special needs, for example young persons, gay men, commercial sex workers (CSWs) and ethnic groups, are to be encouraged.

Improved laboratory diagnosis including the wide introduction of sensitive methods for detecting microrganisms, such as Nucleic Acid Amplification Tests (NAATs), and improved antimicrobial sensitivity testing are required. NAATs are more expensive than current methods but the technology is available to undertake tests for multiple organisms on single samples at little more than the cost of individual single investigations. Another improvement will be salivary antibody detection instead of serological testing. Implicit in these developments is the need to produce timely reports, entailing cooperation within trusts between laboratories and clinics, and more widely between the HPA and trusts, and may benefit from discussion between the Royal College of Physicians and the Royal College of Pathologists.

Improved computer systems within clinics are required in order to implement the standard dataset under review by the NHS Information Centre. Currently only aggregate data are collected. Clinical networking will also require better systems. Improvement will involve work with industry; the College GUM joint specialty committee can provide an impetus, but the BASHH will probably need to facilitate these changes.

Treatment of HIV infection needs antiretrovirals with enhanced potency and simpler dosing regimens with better side-effect profiles. Many clinics are currently working with the Medical Research Council (MRC) and industry in developing improved therapies.

Services should have agreed written guidance for all aspects of management. This will improve and maintain quality and maximise risk avoidance and risk management.

The specialty is working on a document which outlines the application of clinical governance in GUM. This will be made available to the College when it is finished and will be posted on the BASHH website.

ACADEMIC MEDICINE

There is a dearth of academic posts in the specialty.

Clinical contribution to NHS

Academic genitourinary physicians undertake similar clinical NHS duties to NHS consultants according to agreed job plans.

Teaching

Most teaching is still carried out by NHS consultants in outpatient clinics and on undergraduate and postgraduate courses. The paucity of teaching time in GUM in most undergraduate courses is of concern. More full-time academic posts would greatly enhance the capacity for teaching.

Research

The establishment of special interest groups in GUM by the BASHH is an important boost to the research agenda of the specialty. More academic posts are needed to ensure their success. In HIV medicine, academic posts have been critical to clinical and basic research, especially through the MRC. Specific funds have been identified by the MRC to implement and evaluate the NSSHH.

Other academic duties

These include participating in specialty development and helping to deliver the NSSHH.

WORKFORCE REQUIREMENTS FOR GENITOURINARY MEDICINE

For all the foregoing reasons it is essential that there is an urgent review of manpower in the specialty.

Current workforce numbers

There are a total of 267 WTE consultants in the UK (England 242, Wales 8, Northern Ireland 1, Scotland 16). Whole time equivalents are a better measurement, particularly in GUM where a large number of the current and future workforce are females who may be working part-time. 33% of consultants and 66% of SpRs are female; 20% are single handed. There has been less consultant expansion than in most other medical specialities, despite attendances at GUM clinics more than doubling. Expansion of consultants was 3.5% (actual, not WTE) between 2001 and 2002, and 36% over the previous nine years.

Number of consultant programmed activities (PAs) required to provide a specialist service to a population of 250,000

These figures assume 50% of consultations will be undertaken by consultants. Patients will also be seen by other staff, including doctors in training, staff grade, associate specialists, clinical assistants, and nurse practitioners who will see many patients but require consultant supervision.

15,000 new and follow-up consultations per 250,000 population per year

42 consultant weeks per year (8 weeks annual leave/bank holidays, 2 weeks CPD)

6 clinics

20 minutes per appointment

10–12 patients seen per clinic

2,500–3,000 consultations per year per consultant

National consultant workforce requirements

Whilst the manpower calculations have been made to reflect the ideal goal of consultant-delivered quality service it may not be realistic to expect the consultant expansion this would need in the foreseeable future. The specialty is commited to modernisation of practice and other ways of delivery of the service will be vigorously pursued.

The proposed number is three WTE consultants per 250,000. This would mean an increase of 162% across the UK, with 434 WTE consultants over the next few years. On data available almost one in three of female consultants in GUM work part-time. Of present NTN holders 66% are female and 12% are training part-time.

CONSULTANT WORK PROGRAMME/SPECIMEN JOB PLAN

Activity	Workload	Programmed activities (PAs)
Direct clinical care		
Outpatient clinics/clinical supervision	10–12 patients	**5–6**
Ward work including day care		**0.5**
On call		**0.5**
Patient-related administration		**1.0**
Total number of direct clinical care PAs		**7.5 on average**
Supporting professional activities (SPA)		
Work to maintain and improve the quality of healthcare	Education and training, appraisal, departmental management and service development, audit and clinical governance, CPD and revalidation, research	**2.5 on average**
Other NHS responsibilities	eg medical director/clinical director/lead consultant in specialty/clinical tutor	**Local agreement with trust**
External duties	eg work for deaneries/Royal Colleges/specialist societies/Department of Health or other government bodies etc	**Local agreement with trust**

References

1. Department of Health. *National strategy for sexual health and HIV.* London: The Stationery Office, 2001. www.doh.gov.uk/nshs/bettersexualhealth.pdf

2. Department of Health. *National strategy for sexual health and HIV. Implementation action plan.* London: The Stationery Office, 2001. www.doh.gov.uk/sexualhealthandhiv/pdfs/commissioning toolkit.pdf

3. House of Commons Health Committee. *Report on sexual health.* London: The Stationery Office, 2003. www.publications.parliament.uk/pa/cm/cmhealth.htm#reports

4. Health Protection Agency. *Epidemiological data – sexually transmitted infections.* www.hpa.org.uk/infections/ topics_az/hiv_and_sti/epidemiology /sti_data.htm

5. Health Protection Agency. *Regional and national distribution of primary and secondary syphilis in GUM clinics by sex: UK 1996–2002.* July 2004. www.hpa.org.uk/infections/topics_az/hiv_and_sti/sti-syphilis/epidemiology/ sti_table_a.htm

6. Fleming DT, Wasserheit JN. From epidemiological synergy to public health policy and practice: the contribution of other sexually transmitted diseases to sexual transmission of HIV infection. *Sex Transm Inf* 1999;**75**:3–17.

7. Moss GB, Overbaugh J, Welch M *et al.* Human immunodeficiency virus DNA in urethral secretions in men: association with gonococcal urethritis and CD4 depletion. *J Infect Dis* 1995;**172**:1469–74.

8. Rogers PA, Sinka KJ, Molesworth AM *et al.* Survival after diagnosis of AIDS among adults resident in the United Kingdom in the era of multiple therapies. *Commun Dis Public Health* 2000;**3**:188–94.

9. Evans DTP. Comparative sources of positive female chlamydia diagnoses and places of treatment of chlamydia in Leicester 1997–1999 inclusive. A changing trend? *Int J STD & AIDS* 2001;**12**:62.

10. Department of Health. *Report of CMOs advisory group on Chlamydia trachomatis.* London: DH, 1998.

11. Medical Foundation for AIDS and Sexual Health. *Recommended Standards for NHS HIV Services.* London: MedFASH, 2003.

12. Malcolm SE, Ng JJ, Rosen RK, Stone VE. An examination of HIV/AIDS patients who have excellent adherence to HAART. *AIDS Care* 2003;**15**:251–261.

13. www.bashh.org/directory.htm

14. Robinson AJ, Rogstad K; Genitourinary medicine modernization group. Modernization in GUM/HIV services: what does it mean? *Int J STD AIDS* 2003;**14**(2):89–98 (Erratum in *Int J STD AIDS* 2003;**14**(4):292).

15. Department of Health. *Implementing a scheme for general practitioners with special interests,* April 2002. www.doh.gov.uk/pricare/gp-specialinterests

16. General practitioners with special interests. *A step-by-step guide to setting up a general practitioner with a special interest* (GpwSI) service, April 2003. www.gpwsi.org

17. Department of Health. *The 'Monks Report'.* Report of the working party to examine work loads in genitourinary medicine. London: DH, 1988.

18. Department of Health. *Health building note 12, Supplement 1: Genitourinary medicine clinics.* Department of Health, Welsh Office. Department of Health (NI), 1990.

19. General Medical Council Standards Committee. *Intimate examinations.* December 2001. www.gmc-uk.org/ standards/intimate.htm

20. Ministry of Health. *The Public Health (Venereal Diseases) Regulations 1916.* London: Ministry of Health, 1916.

21. Department of Health and Social Security. *The National Health Service (Venereal Diseases) Regulations 1974.* London: DHSS, 1974.

22. The NHS Trusts and Primary Care Trusts (Sexually Transmitted Diseases) Directions 2000. The National Health Service Act 1977.

23. Association for Genitourinary Medicine. *Guidelines for a GU medicine service specification.* AGUM, 1995.

24. Association for Genitourinary Medicine. *Service standards in genitourinary medicine; advisory document for purchaser/clinical governance leads.* AGUM, 2000.

25. Association for Genitourinary Medicine. *Considerations for core service specification.* AGUM, 2000.

26. Association for Genitourinary Medicine. *Nurse competency framework in sexual health.* www.agum.org.uk

27. Department of Health. *Extension of independent nurse prescribing within the NHS in England: a guide for implementation,* February 2004. www.doh.gov.uk/nurseprescribing/index.htm

28. Radcliffe K, Ahmad-Jushuf I, Cowan F *et al.* UK national guidelines on sexually transmitted infections and closely allied conditions. *Sex Transm Infect* 1999;**75**:Supplement 1.

29. www.bashh.org/guidelines/ceguidelines.htm

30. British HIV Association (BHIVA). *Guidelines for the treatment of HIV-infected adults with antiretroviral therapy,* July 2003. www.bhiva.org

31. www.bashh.org/committees/cgc/

32. British Medical Association. Main documentation for the consultant contract in England. www.bma.org.uk/ap.nsf/ Content/_HubCCSCcontractdocument.

Geriatric medicine

i   Description of the specialty and clinical needs of patients

The essence of geriatric medicine is to assess and treat the medical and rehabilitative needs of older people. This is achieved through comprehensive geriatric assessment. The evidence base demonstrates that outcomes for older people with multiple pathologies and functional problems are improved if they are managed by an interdisciplinary team led by a consultant geriatrician.

The core work of a geriatric medical service may take place in a number of different inpatient areas including the A&E department, surgical wards and specialised elderly medical wards. The emergency treatment of older people within the general hospital is frequently followed by intensive rehabilitation, both in the general hospital and in less acute settings such as community hospitals and sometimes in the patient's own home. Intermediate care is a potentially important development in which geriatric medical services should have an integral role in planning and delivering care for older people in the community. For a small number of heavily dependent patients with ongoing requirements for specialist review there will be a need for NHS-funded long-term care.

Comprehensive geriatric services have an important role in the community, including outpatients, community rehabilitation teams, and in day hospitals. In partnership with social services and the local primary care teams, geriatric medical services can support older people who require specialist supervision of their medical condition and improvement or maintenance of their physical function in their own home.

Geriatricians can also provide subspecialty services for orthogeriatrics, movement disorders, falls and osteoporosis, and stroke (of which the last three may be services for patients of any age). These areas, together with continence, delirium, palliative care and old-age psychiatry, form the basis of expertise within a comprehensive service for older people.

ii   Organisation of the service and patterns of referral

Primary, secondary and tertiary levels

To provide integrated holistic care for older people, geriatric medical services should cross the boundary of primary and secondary care. Care pathways should embrace the increasing physical and psychological needs of normal ageing together with crises associated with acute illness. Tertiary referrals in the specialty are uncommon. Key to the provision of health services for older people is a partnership across the whole health and social care framework in a locality.

The assessment of an acutely ill older person should occur as soon as possible using appropriate imaging and diagnostic facilities. Organisation of community and hospital services for older people should be geared towards this aim, which should usually be performed in a district general hospital (DGH). There is no evidence that any one pattern of service organisation (integrated with general medicine, age related or needs related) is superior, though the format chosen will vary according to the size and facilities in each hospital. Patients admitted urgently to geriatric medical services might be referred directly by their GPs through medical admissions units, or from other acute areas such as surgical or psychiatric facilities.

Rehabilitation aims to optimise or maintain physical function and well being, and should commence as soon as the patient's acute illness has stabilised. Although this will usually take place in hospital, rehabilitation may take place away from the main hospital site in the proposed forms of intermediate care. The needs of vulnerable, frail, older patients are often complex and require careful assessment and evaluation, usually necessitating close working with social services and collaboration with formal and informal care networks.

Day hospitals can provide comprehensive geriatric assessment and rehabilitation of older people in the community, and may play a part in intermediate care services. These facilities can also contribute to the delivery of the subspecialties of geriatric medicine (eg falls, movement disorders and stroke care). However, the role of the day hospital will depend on the availability of nursing, paramedical and medical staff, and other local resources.

With care in the community the numbers of NHS continuing care beds have been reduced, and the previously expanded numbers of private nursing and residential beds are also falling. Geriatricians continue to have a vital role and duty to provide care for older people in these institutions in liaison and formal collaboration with GPs (some of whom will have a special responsibility for the care of older people).

Relationship with other services/agencies

Multidisciplinary working necessitates close liaison with many complementary services (Box 1) as well as the mainstream specialties in a DGH.

Box 1: Medical and paramedical services supporting the assessment and rehabilitation of older people.

Activities of daily living
Occupational therapy

Care management
Social work services

Communication
Speech and language therapy
Audiology
Hearing therapy
Ophthalmology
Optician services
Dental Services

Elimination
Continence adviser
Stoma therapist
Urological/gynaecological services
Urodynamic assessment
Personal laundry services

Nutrition
Dietetic advice
Enteral and parenteral feeding services including percutaneous endoscopic gastrostomy (PEG)
Dental services
Videofluoroscopy

Mental state
Psychiatry of old age
Clinical psychology

Mobility
Physiotherapy
Wheelchair and aid supplies
Orthotics
Podiatry
Orthopaedic services
Chiropody

Palliative care
Specialist pain relief
Hospice support

---

iii Working with patients: patient-centred care

Patient choice and involving patients in decisions about their treatment

Geriatricians are committed to rooting out ageism in the delivery of medical care and recognise that competent, informed adults have an established right to refuse medical procedures, sometimes in advance. Respect for patient autonomy is at the centre of practice, particularly when dealing with advance directives and issues relating to nutrition in advanced old age. Medico-legal issues such as power of attorney, Court of Protection and testamentary capacity are important in geriatric medical practice together with seeking patients' views on cardiopulmonary resuscitation, assisted ventilation, artificial feeding, and other interventions.

Patients with chronic conditions and the role of the carer

Geriatricians recognise the importance of involving informal carers in decisions about complex treatment in old age and consider a patient's quality of life and disability-free life expectancy as important goals of treatment rather than absolute longevity. Patient and carer support groups have a role in the management of chronic conditions in older life, particularly with conditions such as stroke, Parkinson's disease and dementia. In addition, patient and carers views form an important part of the clinical governance process in hospital departments of geriatric medicine, either individually or within focus groups established as part of implementation of the National Service Framework (NSF) for Older People.

Older people should be treated as individuals at all times and offered choice in treatment, discussion and planning of future care. Services need to be made easily accessible, regardless of the end provider, through involving older people and their carers in service planning, for example:

■ integrating commissioning arrangements between NHS trusts, local authorities and primary care groups or trusts

■ using a single assessment process

■ integrating community services to ensure rapid and flexible access to equipment

■ ensuring a single point of access to services

■ providing services that are inclusive not exclusive (eg not excluding patients with dementia).

Older people may expect from specialist services:

■ to be involved in decisions made about their health and future care

■ adequate numbers of appropriately trained staff

■ clear and sensitively expressed explanations of their medical condition/illness and the treatment options available, unless their ill health prevents this, in writing if required

■ that information will be shared with relatives, friends and carers if they wish

■ that relatives, friends or other advocates may give and receive information on their behalf if the patient has difficulty in understanding or communicating and gives consent

■ practical advice on appropriate support services and information to enable them to adapt to illness and disability

■ written detailed information on local health and social services, voluntary organisations and benefits

■ support to be available for their family and close friends

- access to their health records and the security of knowing that everyone in the NHS is under a legal obligation to keep records confidential
- health premises to be accessible to people with disability
- appropriate and punctual transport arrangements.

All specialist elderly units should have policies for:

- discharge of patients
- communication with GPs and other members of the primary healthcare team
- the provision of drugs on discharge from hospital
- written patient information about life in hospital and the choices to be made, discharge plans and the timescales involved, follow up and care arrangements in the community.

Opportunities for education and access to information

Information should be readily available on:

- a healthy lifestyle
- the dangers of smoking and excessive alcohol consumption
- healthy eating and the problems of obesity
- the benefits and importance of regular exercise
- home safety and advice on how to avoid personal accidents
- social support and welfare benefit rights
- bereavement counselling
- benefits of vaccinations
- high blood pressure causes and corrections.

Promoting health and self-care

Local health economies should actively develop programmes to promote disability prevention:

- Specialist elderly services should develop a culture of health promotion alongside disease management and rehabilitation.
- Geriatricians should discuss health promotion and preventative healthcare programmes, which should be regarded as a legitimate subspecialty, with primary care groups. This could involve more formal links with nursing homes.
- Health promotion posters and literature should be readily available in patient contact areas.

iv   Interspecialty and interdisciplinary liaison

Consultants in geriatric medicine pioneered the concept of interdisciplinary team working to ensure that medical illness and functional capacity in older people was assessed and treated. It is the essence of good practice in acute assessment and rehabilitation settings for the consultant to lead at least one interdisciplinary case conference per week. These may be less frequent in long-term care. Other career grades, including staff grade, associate specialists and general practitioners with a special interest (GPSI) have a role in delivering a comprehensive service in the community and in hospital.

v Delivering a high quality service

Characteristics of a high quality service for older people

- adequate access to acute teams specialising in needs of older people (at the main hospital site) with interdisciplinary team support, including acute stroke unit and wards specialising in management of older people with fractures
- locally agreed policies for admission and referral made available to older people
- access to specialist rehabilitation wards for stroke, orthogeriatric problems and general rehabilitation with interdisciplinary team support
- access to comprehensive assessment and rehabilitation in the community, which could be via a day hospital, including rapid access facilities and opportunities for intermediate care support
- access to outpatient clinics for older people with specialist clinics for falls, cerebrovascular disease, continence, Parkinson's disease and orthogeriatric problems
- community rehabilitation teams and crisis intervention based on an interdisciplinary model with specialist medical involvement
- education, training and support programmes for non-specialist wards and clinicians not specialising in care of older people
- pathways of care for stroke, falls, osteoporosis, delirium, Parkinson's disease and fractured neck of femur
- active partnership working between health and social services, considering the views of older people and carers, to develop services and to ensure appropriate joint learning and training for all groups of staff
- a programme of health promotion and preventative healthcare
- a system of quality assurance facilitating clinical governance and ensuring the highest possible standards of healthcare for older people.

Resources required for a high quality service

- laboratory and imaging investigation facilities and specialised neuroimaging, Doppler scanning and swallowing assessment facilities
- good gymnasium for early rehabilitation and areas to perform adequate assessment of activities of daily living such as occupational therapy bathrooms and kitchens
- appropriate numbers of skilled healthcare and social workers within the interdisciplinary team caring for an older person.

vi Quality standards and measures of the quality of specialist services

- The British Geriatrics Society (BGS) (**www.bgs.org.uk**) has guidelines, policy statements, and statements of good practice in the care of older people.
- The Health Advisory Service in England (**www.healthadvisoryservice.org**) and NHS Quality Improvement Scotland (**www.show.scot.nhs.uk**) utilise quality indicators when assessing services for older people.
- The NSF for Older People (**www.doh.gov.uk/nsf/olderpeople.htm**) has set out standards and targets for rooting out age discrimination, person-centred care, intermediate care, general

hospital care, stroke, falls, mental health in older people and promoting an active healthy life. Standard 5, relating to stroke care, is based upon implementation of the intercollegiate *National clinical guidelines for stroke* (**www.rcplondon.ac.uk/pubs/books/stroke/**) which are regularly updated.[1]

The work of consultant geriatricians and their teams is not covered directly by National Institute for Clinical Excellence (NICE) guidance, with the exception of the guidance for pressure ulcer prevention. However, the delivery of high quality care for older people is a priority of visits by the Healthcare Commission (**www.healthcarecommission.org.uk**).

Examples of clinical quality indicators

▪ discharge communications received by the primary healthcare team in less than 48 hours

▪ patient and carer satisfaction with discharge (using a standardised assessment instrument)

▪ delay to discharge due to equipment delays

▪ number of patients readmitted to hospital or institutional care shortly after discharge.

Patients under the care of an individual consultant geriatrician entering long-term institutional care from an inpatient setting should have documented evidence of a formal multidisciplinary assessment with consultant involvement prior to placement. This should be measured by an annual audit of a 10% sample of all institutional placements from any individual hospital.

Patients seen as outpatients or day patients by an individual consultant or member of his or her team should have at least one recorded assessment of both their mental and functional status in the case records. Where clinically relevant (but not invariably) this will involve the use of a standard measurement scale (eg Abbreviated Mental Test or Barthel Index) or equivalent. This should be measured annually by random audit of 20 sets of case notes by a third party.

Inpatients or outpatients with atrial fibrillation under an individual consultant should have had an assessment of whether or not they should receive long-term thromboprophylaxis. The decision and its rationale will be recorded in the case records. (This is an example of an accepted evidence-based prescribing indicator. Other accepted indicators might be utilised.) This should be measured by audit of 20 sets of notes annually by random sample, identified by prescription of digoxin. Rotational substitution of an alternative evidence-based indicator or range of indicators would be anticipated on an annual basis.

CLINICAL WORK AND/OR LABORATORY WORK OF CONSULTANTS IN GERIATRIC MEDICINE

Contributions made to acute medicine

In many areas, consultant geriatricians participate in the acute unselected take for adults of all ages, which may involve as many as 89% of all geriatricians. In this situation their commitment to emergency medicine may be to the detriment of their ability to deliver specialised services for older people. Alternatively, geriatricians may work alongside organ-based physicians in delivering cover for emergency medicine in situations where they can preferentially care for older people on an age-related or needs-related basis. In all situations, geriatricians must ensure an appropriate balance between their emergency role and other duties, particularly in supervising rehabilitation and delivering subspecialty services such as falls, stroke care or orthogeriatrics. Most physicians performing acute take duties should not have to take personal responsibility for more than 25 acute admissions per day.

Direct clinical care

The work of individual geriatricians differs widely in content and load across the United Kingdom. This reflects variations in local supporting services, specialist activity, geographical sites to be covered and involvement in the acute emergency intake.

Most consultants in geriatric medicine maintain specific sessional commitment to the inpatient core areas of acute assessment and rehabilitation. Additionally, they will have some community responsibilities through outpatient, day hospital and outreach facilities. In well-staffed departments the responsibility for the common subspecialisms of geriatric medicine (see section i) will be divided between consultants. In smaller departments the availability of these subspecialty services will depend on local circumstances and the interests of individual consultants.

Local requirements and personal interests have led many geriatricians to incorporate organ subspecialisms into their work. Such specialisms include diabetes mellitus, clinical pharmacology, gastroenterology and heart failure.

The relationship between geriatric medicine and the community will often mean that some services are provided away from the main hospital site. The development of intermediate, or post-acute care outside hospital, will necessitate increasing cooperation with primary care.

Inpatient work

Acute inpatient care   Depending on casemix, the number of beds and support staffing, a consultant would expect to perform at least two assessment ward rounds per week. A consultant should not normally be expected to care for more than 20 acutely ill assessment patients at any one time. It is anticipated that each consultant might receive between 5–10 acutely ill new specialty patients per week.

Rehabilitation   A consultant with supporting medical staff should be expected to care for no more than 20 rehabilitation patients at any one time, with 200–300 discharges per year. A consultant would normally be expected to complete at least one rehabilitation ward round each week per 20 patients.

Community care   Depending upon the local model of intermediate care, and commissioners' priorities, departments of geriatric medicine should expect to have a significant role in the community, including domiciliary assessments, reviewing patients in care homes (NHS and private sector), assessing patients who require long-term care, and delivering intermediate care. These duties of community geriatricians may be undertaken in partnership with social services, by GPSIs in older people, and perhaps nurse/therapist consultants.

Continuing care   In some areas of England and Wales this work is much less frequent than in the past. When undertaken, a consultant geriatrician should have direct responsibility for no more than 30 continuing care beds and would normally be expected to review the needs of these patients at least once every two weeks.

Referral work including interspecialty and interdisciplinary liaison   A consultant would expect to deal with 5–10 referrals per week.

Case conferences, speaking to carers and discharge planning   This may be included in ward rounds but additional time should be allowed for these activities in circumstances of a heavy inpatient load

Outpatient work

General geriatric medicine and general internal medicine outpatient clinics   The number of patients seen will depend on the time taken to evaluate a complex new patient (45–60 minutes) or a review patient (10–20 minutes) and local resources. For example, when there is no support from a registrar, staff grade or other physician, two to four new patients can be seen plus 7–10 review patients.

Specialised clinics   These may include clinics for stroke and transient ischaemic attack, movement disorders (eg Parkinson's disease), cognitive dysfunction (memory), metabolic bone (osteoporosis), continence and falls. The numbers of patients seen is as above for general and geriatric medicine clinics.

Day hospitals   A high-turnover day hospital might expect to see 600 new patients a year in a 30-placed unit. Each consultant should have no more than 12–15 patients each at any one time. The consultant should hold interdisciplinary case conferences every one to two weeks.

Services beyond the base hospital   These may include clinics at other hospitals, outreach clinics, domiciliary work and hospice work.

Work to maintain and improve the quality of care

This work encompasses duties in clinical governance, professional self-regulation, continuing professional development (CPD), and education and training of others. For many consultants at various times in their careers it may include research, serving in management and providing specialist advice at local, regional and national levels.

The BGS has produced detailed guidance on clinical governance and the amount of time that will be required to fulfil these requirements. Generally, a lead clinician in clinical governance would need one session of programmed activity (PA) whilst participation would need approximately 0.25 PA. This does not include any time required for revalidation, CPD or participation in appraisal, which are mandatory activities for all consultants.

Leadership role and development of the service

Departments of geriatric medicine are expected to take an active role in the development of services for older people in primary and secondary care. This is particularly important in the development of intermediate care and work to meet the targets of the NSF for Older People. Such work for designated individuals should be recognised in the job-planning process alongside management duties such as running the department, the responsibility for the delivery of teaching, clinical governance and the research agenda for a group of geriatricians.

ACADEMIC MEDICINE

Academic geriatricians usually make a significant contribution to the NHS service for older people but have fewer clinical sessions to allow for university commitments which include teaching and research. Consultant geriatricians teach not only undergraduate medical students but also other disciplines. Many NHS geriatricians teach and undertake research where there is no academic department. All academic and NHS geriatricians have a responsibility for the postgraduate training of higher specialist trainees in geriatric medicine that culminates in the award of a Certificate of Completion of Specialist Training (CCST).

WORKFORCE REQUIREMENTS FOR GERIATRIC MEDICINE

There were 1,037 (999 WTE) consultants in geriatric medicine in the UK in 2002, which represents one WTE per 55,000 of the population. Compared with 761 in 1997, this represents an average annual increase of 55 (or approximately 7%) and a 25% expansion since 1993.

The BGS has recommended that to care for the population aged over 75 years there should be one WTE geriatrician per 50,000 of the population (one WTE for 4000 people >75 years). However, this calculation may underestimate future requirements, for example:

■ Geriatricians are increasingly involved in unselected acute medicine (30% of consultants in 1995 rising to 88.6% in 2002). Previously estimated to equate to one WTE per 35,000 of the population, this 'non-geriatric' work may account for 7.8 hours (approximately two PAs) per week. Therefore, where geriatricians participate in the acute medical take, 20% more consultants (one per 250,000 population) would be required if current work in the specialty is to be maintained, making an estimate of one WTE consultant per 40,000 population.

■ The 2002 College Census has indicated that consultant geriatricians currently exceed the European Working Time Directive maximum of 48 hours a week by 7.8 hours.[2] As a consequence, the Federation of Royal Colleges has estimated that an additional 210 consultant geriatricians are required, which represents a 20% increase and an additional one WTE per 250,000 of the population.

■ Many subspecialty and community developments are associated with modernisation and new care pathways. These include implementation of the NSF for Older People, developing existing subspecialty services such as care for stroke and falls, and new activities including intermediate care, complex assessment and community-based work, particularly in nursing and residential homes.

The arguments presented above suggest that the projection of 1,368 consultants by 2009 (for England and Wales) may have to be re-calculated. For the present, 7.05 WTE per 250,000 population is suggested, equivalent to 1,371 for England and 81 for Wales making a total of 1,643 WTE for the UK.

CONSULTANT WORK PROGRAMME/SPECIMEN JOB PLAN

Typical job plan for a consultant geriatrician participating in the acute emergency take

Activity	Workload	Programmed activities (PAs)
Direct clinical care		
Acute ward rounds (including interdisciplinary meetings and interviewing relatives)	20–25 patients	2
Rehabilitation ward rounds (including interdisciplinary meetings and interviewing relatives)	20 patients	1
Intra-hospital liaison/ domiciliary visits		0.5
General/geriatric medicine clinic	3 new and 7–10 review patients	1
Specialist clinic, day hospital, other subspecialty work		1
Post-take ward round		1
Patient-related administration		1
Total number of direct clinical care PAs		**7.5 on average**
Supporting professional activities (SPA)		
Work to maintain and improve the quality of healthcare	Education and training, appraisal, departmental management and service development, audit and clinical governance, CPD and revalidation, research	**2.5 on average**
Other NHS responsibilities	eg medical director/clinical director/lead consultant in specialty/clinical tutor	**Local agreement with trust**
External duties	eg work for deaneries/Royal Colleges/specialist societies/Department of Health or other government bodies etc	**Local agreement with trust**

References

1. Royal College of Physicians. *National clinical guidelines for stroke 2nd edition.* London: RCP, 2004. www.rcplondon. ac.uk/pubs/books/stroke

2. The Federation of the Royal Colleges of Physicians of the United Kingdom. *Census of consultant physicians in the UK, 2002. Data and commentary.* London: The Federation of the Royal Colleges of Physicians of the United Kingdom, 2002.

Haematology

i   Description of the specialty and clinical needs of patients

Haematology encompasses the diagnosis and clinical management of a wide spectrum of blood disorders. Haematologists undergo general professional training in medicine followed by specialist training in all aspects of clinical and laboratory haematology. Most develop further expertise in one or more subspecialties including:

- haemato-oncology: acute and chronic leukaemias, lymphoma, multiple myeloma
- haemostasis/thrombosis: inherited and acquired bleeding and thrombotic disorders
- management of haemoglobinopathies
- transfusion medicine: blood transfusion services, therapeutic apheresis
- paediatric haematology.

In addition to their clinical role, haematologists provide the professional direction in the haematology/transfusion laboratory and provide advice on the interpretation of a wide range of tests with an emergency and on-call service 24 hours a day, 365 days a year, for GPs and hospital clinicians. Specialist units in surgery, medicine, paediatrics and obstetrics in a general hospital all depend upon this haematological service. The incidence of haematological disease is increasing. An indication of the numbers of patients to be seen annually is given in Table 1.

Table 1. The increasing incidence of malignant haematological disease

Disease	Incidence, England & Wales	Per million population	Per 500,000	Per 250,000
Acute leukaemia	2,400	48	24	12
Chronic myelogenous leukaemia	500	10	5	2–3
Chronic lymphocytic leukaemia	4,000	80	40	20
Non-Hodgkin's lymphoma 'high grade'	2,000	40	20	10
Non-Hodgkin's lymphoma 'low grade'	5,000	100	50	25
Hodgkin's lymphoma	1,200	24	12	6
Myeloma	3,000	60	30	15
Myelodysplasia/myeloproliferative diseases/other	2,000	40	20	10

ii   Organisation of the service and patterns of referral

Primary, secondary and tertiary levels

The haematology laboratory supports primary care by providing a range of tests which may reveal different types of anaemia, bleeding or clotting disorders, or evidence of blood cell cancers.

The haematologist provides advisory and interpretative services to back up the laboratory results and is an essential link in the referral of patients with suspected haematological disease. Following diagnosis in the laboratory the clinical haematology service is responsible for ensuring that the patient is seen in a haemtology clinic within an appropriate time, which may need to be within hours or within a few weeks of diagnosis. Close liaison with primary care is essential for best practice in all cases. The haematologist should ensure that patients with non-haematological disease are referred appropriately to other clinicians where necessary.

Secondary care of patients with haematological disorders varies in complexity. The British Committee for Standards in Haematology has defined four levels of care for haematological malignancies.[1] All general hospitals will be expected to provide care at levels 1 or 2 (detailed below), whilst levels 3 and 4 are considered to be tertiary care. These guidelines are due for revision, in particular for level 2 care, in order to differentiate between the facilities required for haematological patients when neutropenic and those with solid tumours when the neutropenic state is shorter and much less intense.

Level 1 care is for patients with general haematological disorders including a number of haematological malignancies. Among them are patients with slowly developing malignant diseases in a stable phase and patients with malignant disease requiring chemotherapy that is unlikely to produce prolonged neutropenia. The dual role of the haematologist – combining laboratory and clinical work – requires that those hospitals offering a level 1 service have a minimum of two consultant haematologists.

Level 2 care provides facilities for patients with haematological malignancy who require more intensive chemotherapy regimens. Dedicated inpatient haematological teams with their own junior staff at senior house officer (SHO) level and higher, specially trained nurses and facilities for the management of prolonged neutropenia are essential. Such units should have a minimum of three consultant haematologists and close collaboration with medical oncology if a medical oncology unit exists.

Level 3 care requires facilities for delivering autologous stem cell therapy following very intensive chemotherapy. Units offering level 3 care need additional facilities for patient management, including stem cell harvesting and more extensive isolation facilities.

Level 4 care applies to units offering tertiary referral services. These units would provide care for patients in need of, for example, allogeneic stem cell transplantation, specialist services in haemostasis and thrombosis, and paediatric haematology services.

Although these levels of care were defined to describe facilities for management of haematological malignancies, it is appropriate to apply them to other specialised areas of haematological practice. Thus, units may offer specialist services to cover one or more other aspects of haematology, for example haemoglobinopathy, congenital and acquired bleeding disorders, or transfusion practice.

Clinical networks and community arrangements

Many disorders of the blood are protracted and some, such as inherited disorders, are lifelong. Some require prolonged intensive treatment, while others pursue a relapsing and remitting course or stable phases punctuated by acute emergencies. Such a spectrum of disorders requires integrated care within a network system whereby the patient is managed jointly between primary care and the local hospital, with tertiary referral centres aware of the patients and their conditions and ready to give advice and help as necessary. The very nature of these diseases has engendered a culture of networking amongst haematologists, of which good examples are the organisation of haemophilia services and the inclusive nature of the Medical Research Council (MRC) leukaemia trials groups (now known as National Cancer Research Institute (NCRI) trials). More formal arrangements are being established, particularly in haemato-oncology where cancer network groups are now in operation. Similar informal networks exist for the management of patients with a haemorrhagic disorder, particularly for inherited bleeding disorders and for families with thrombophilia.

Relationship with other services/agencies

Terminal care entails particularly close collaboration between haematologists and other services. In this situation the hospital-based Macmillan nurse often provides a key link between secondary care and hospice or community services.

Robust networks or collaborations should be in place for anticoagulant control. Whether this service is based mainly in the community or in the local hospital varies according to local arrangements, but scrupulous quality control and immediate access for patients with problems linked to anticoagulation are essential. In many cases a small team of anticoagulant specialist nurses, working in conjunction with consultant haematologists, supervise the control of such patients in both the community and hospital settings.

iii Working with patients: patient-centred care

Patient choice and involving patients in decisions about their treatment

Patients with a haematological disorder, particularly those with lifelong chronic disorders or malignancy, should receive a detailed explanation of the disorder, the treatment options, their likely success rate and associated side effects. In many instances this is provided in conjunction with a haematology specialist nurse, and this crucial role has been highlighted in the recent guidance from the National Institute for Clinical Excellence (NICE).[2] Easily understood written information about a haematological disorder and the drugs to be used should be given to patients. Written informed consent is increasingly sought for those receiving complex treatments such as chemotherapy and monoclonal antibody therapy. Haematologists are also closely involved with their patients in decision making about drug therapy for malignant conditions, where both the benefit to the patient and the expected toxicity must be carefully balanced. Patients in the final phase of their illness will have treatment options carefully explained, alongside discussions with their family, when treatment with drugs and blood product support is no longer helpful.

A recommendation of treatment with a blood product can be unacceptable to groups of patients with certain religious beliefs, for example Jehovah's Witness patients. The haematologist will respect this belief and follow local guidelines to manage the situation

Opportunities for education and promoting self-care

Patient education plays a crucial role in the safe management of the haematology patient. With assistance from specialist haematology nurses, education enables the patient to recognise symptoms, such as fever and bleeding, which need urgent attention or early self-referral.

Some haematological disorders lend themselves to care at home, where the patient, carer or visiting home nurse can administer therapy. Examples include home treatment with factor VIII in haemophilia, administration of heparin by injection, and home chemotherapy delivery. Increasingly, patients on oral anticoagulant therapy are able to self-test at home.

Access to information, patient support groups and the role of the expert patient

Abundant written information is available to patients, produced by organisations such as CancerBACUP (**www.cancerbacup.org.uk**), the Leukaemia Research Fund (**www.lrf.org.uk**) and the Haemophilia Society (**www.haemophilia.org.uk**).

There are active support groups for many haematological disorders throughout the UK. These meet locally or may have helpful websites for patient information. Examples include the Leukaemia Care Society (**www.leukaemiacare.org**), the UK Myeloma Forum (**www.myeloma.org.uk**), the Ideopathic Thrombocytopenic Purpura (ITP) Support Association (**www.itpsupport.org.uk**), the Aplastic Anaemia Trust (**www.theAAT.org.uk**), and the Haemophilia society. Most large groups have excellent local networks, for example Macmillan Cancer nurses.

Haematologists recognise the expert patient and often involve a patient representative in the preparation of national guidelines for haematological care.

iv   Interspecialty and interdisciplinary liaison

Multidisciplinary team working

Multidisciplinary team (MDT) meetings are an established part of the work of the haematologist and the members of the haematology team. Haematological cancer team meetings may involve several haematologists, consultants in radiotherapy and oncology, consultant radiologists and histopathologists. Similar meetings are held to discuss patients with severe bleeding disorders and patients with haematological problems associated with pregnancy. These meetings are an important setting in which to agree and document the diagnostic and therapeutic decisions made for haematology patients. Regular meetings with biomedical and clinical scientists working within the discipline also take place.

Working with other specialists

Haematologists work in joint clinics with radiation oncologists or obstetricians and paediatricians to effect shared care. Close liaison between specialists is necessary in the care of complex problems in patients with haematological disease. In the field of haemostasis, joint care is needed for surgical interventions throughout a patient's life. For patients with complex malignant haematological diseases, the haematologist may consult a nephrologist, respiratory physician, palliative care physician and medical microbiologist.

The regular meetings and function of the hospital transfusion committee and hospital transfusion team are a requirement of all hospitals where blood is transfused. This remit is fully described in the document *Better blood transfusion*.[3]

v   **Delivering a high quality service**

Resources required for a high quality service

Specialised facilities

Some indication of the specialised facilities required is given below, dependent on the nature of service offered. For hospitals caring for patients with haematological cancers, facilities should be organised as set out in the document *Improving outcomes in haematological cancers.*[2]

Outpatients   Facilities should be close to the haematology laboratory for rapid turnaround of blood samples. Where this is not possible, patient-testing equipment should be located nearby or a rapid sample transportation service available. Sensitive information and patient education should be delivered to patients and their families in an appropriate environment. In some hospitals, outpatient facilities are combined with day care facilities

Day care   Haematology day care areas are crucial to the delivery of blood products, the majority of chemotherapy, and infusional treatments (bisphosphonates, IV iron, immunoglobulin, coagulation factors and monoclonal antibodies). The development of good facilities has greatly relieved pressure on inpatient beds and is more acceptable to patients. Sufficient staff numbers are needed to cover the frequent phone calls received from patients undergoing specialist treatment and to offer a 'walk in' service. The area should have full resuscitation equipment and staff trained regularly to use it. Separate day care areas facilitate therapeutic apheresis and cytopheresis in more specialist units.

Inpatients   All hospitals looking after haematology patients should have some single room accommodation available for the care of immunosuppressed or neutropenic patients. Their complexity and number will vary with the size of the hospital and the level of care offered between levels 1 and 4, as defined above. Above level 1, inpatient beds should be grouped together.

Minimum requirements are rooms with full toilet and shower/bath, with adequate space for IV pumps and X-ray equipment. At level 3 and 4 of care, filtered air and positive pressure rooms are needed. In units offering care at levels 2 and above, haematology patients should be cared for on a dedicated ward with adequate haematology nurses.[2] Each shift should have nurses capable of accessing IV and specialist IV lines (eg Hickmann or other catheters). Hospitals delivering intrathecal chemotherapy will have a designated clinical area in which this is performed.[4]

Workforce requirements: clinical and support staff

The haematology team of a typical large district hospital would offer level 2 care for patients with haematological disease and would comprise the following members:

▪   consultant haematologists

▪   clinical nurse specialists: haemato-oncology nurses responsible for the safe delivery of IV chemotherapy, patient education and IV access; anticoagulant nurses to assist in the running of anticoagulant services, including community dosing and the outpatient management of venous thromboembolic disease (Clinical Leaders of Thrombosis (CLOT) nurses); transfusion nurses (or equivalent scientific grade) (Specialist practitioners of transfusion (SPOT) nurses)

▪   haemophilia nurses (units with a specialist interest in haemostasis)

▪   haematology pharmacist

▪   data manager.

The team should have close links with other health professionals, depending on its subspecialty, including:

- palliative care team
- IV access team
- psychiatric team to provide psychological support, bereavement counselling
- pain control team
- patient support groups and appropriate charities
- dietitian.

vi Quality standards and measures of the quality of specialist services

Specialist society guidelines

Haematology is a highly complex and rapidly changing field of medicine and it can be difficult for individual haematologists to keep abreast of all relevant developments in order to make appropriate decisions. To meet this need the British Society for Haematology (BSH) established a specialist subcommittee, the British Committee for Standards in Haematology (BCSH), to provide robust evidence-based guidance in all areas of haematology. The BCSH was established in 1964 and has published over 100 guidelines on aspects of haematology since 1984. The guidelines are now produced through a well-defined process designed to fully assess available evidence and involve all relevant stakeholders; the draft guidelines are reviewed by a wide spectrum of UK haematologists. They have been disseminated by publication in peer-reviewed journals and, more recently, on the BCSH website (**www.bcshguidelines.com**) which currently receives over 30,000 page hits per month.

Other important guidelines include those for haemophilia produced by the UK Haemophilia Centre Doctors' Organisation (UKHCDO), part of the Haemophilia Alliance (**www.haemo philiaalliance.org.uk/docs/who.htm**).

National Institute for Clinical Excellence (NICE) guidelines

In recent years NICE has appraised several new therapies available for the treatment of some leukaemia and lymphoma, specifically the drugs fludarabine, rituximab and imatinib. However, these guides relate to only a small fraction of the overall workload of haematologists, unlike the BCSH guidance discussed above.

NICE has also issued guidance on the organisation of healthcare for patients with haematological cancer, which will almost certainly highlight resource deficiencies to be addressed as clinical governance issues by individual trusts.[2]

Clinical governance

A consultant haematologist contributes actively to trust clinical governance arrangements by assuring the quality of the results issued from the laboratory, including participation in national quality assurance schemes, and by ensuring the laboratory meets the quality standards set by Clinical Pathology Accreditation (CPA). This forms part of their personal professional development and that of the other team members. The production of policies for use of the laboratory and the management of patients, and participation in audit of these policies, also contributes to effective clinical governance. Correct membership and function of the hospital transfusion team is crucial for safe transfusion practice.

CLINICAL WORK AND/OR LABORATORY WORK OF CONSULTANTS IN HAEMATOLOGY

Contributions made to acute medicine

Although not usually directly involved, the haematologist is regularly consulted on emergency problems arising in acute medical take patients, particularly with regard to anticoagulant therapy. However, emergency admissions in all specialties may result in urgent haematology consultations.

Direct clinical care

Table 2. Recommended maximum clinical workload for consultant haematologists[5]

Activity		Annual numbers of patients
Inpatients		250
Outpatients	New	250
	Return	1,500
Day cases/ward attenders		1,500
Ward consults		100

Inpatient work

There is considerable variation in the type of work carried out by a consultant haematologist, depending on the specialisation and size of the hospital. For a typical district general hospital (DGH) serving a population of 250,000 patients, there should be a minimum of two programmed activities (PAs) for ward rounds and ward referrals per week per consultant. All consultant haematologists, irrespective of specialty, will have significant numbers of patients with complex medical problems in whom the clinical condition can change significantly within a few hours. Time should be designated for MDTs. Haematology patients should be reviewed at the same level of intensity at weekends.

Day case work

A significant amount of haematological activity takes place in a day case ward. Patients receiving transfusions or chemotherapy will be seen by a member of the haematology team on each visit. Depending on the expertise of the supporting members of the team the consultant haematologist may not need to review these patients daily but will be responsible for ensuring appropriate guidelines on management are followed. These patient reviews may be made by junior medical staff or haematology clinical nurse specialists.

If patients are managed only in a day case area and do not attend other outpatient clinics, consultant haematologists will personally review the patients at regular intervals and will be available at all times to support the team members.

Outpatient work

Recommended outpatient activity is given in the above table. There is considerable variation in practice, however, depending on the expertise and number of supporting team members and on the complexity of case review. Some new referrals need not be seen in a haematology clinic but a letter should be sent to the referring doctor with a helpful management plan.

Specialist investigative and therapeutic procedures

Bone marrow aspirates and trephine biopsies will be undertaken to confirm diagnosis on a large number of haematology patients (approximately 150–250 per year). Medical staff usually perform these but nurses are increasingly being trained in the procedure. The haematologist will produce the laboratory report of marrow aspirates whilst specialist haemato-oncological pathologists may report the trephines in some hospitals.

Therapeutic procedures may include the insertion of central or Hickman lines for chemotherapy. Intrathecal chemotherapy is given by specifically designated haematologists under strictly controlled conditions (see above).

Specialist on-call arrangements

Haematologists provide an on-call service for both their laboratory work and for patients under their care. This should not exceed a one-in-three rota for care that requires daily patient review by a haematologist. Highly specialised advice by telephone may demand a greater intensity of rota and is often essential in transplant and haemostasis centres.

Other specialist activity including activities beyond the local services

Blood transfusion One consultant member of the haematology team should have specific responsibility for the transfusion service. Appropriate consultant time should be designated for the safe delivery of this service.[3] The consultant should be a member of the hospital transfusion team together with a transfusion practitioner and the head of blood bank. This team is responsible for meeting the standards outlined in *Better blood transfusion* and is responsible for considerable audit and educational activity and for ensuring that appropriate policies and guidelines are in place.

Specialist outpatient clinics These may be held weekly or less frequently and are supported by relevant MDTs. Joint consultant specialist clinics may be held with consultants in obstetrics, orthopaedics, paediatrics, clinical oncology and others.

Anticoagulant services The consultant haematologist is usually the lead clinician for anticoagulant services in a hospital.[6] He/she is responsible for ensuring that appropriate guidelines for management of anticoagulation are in place and that individuals who dose patients are competent. These individuals may include nurses, clinical pharmacists and biomedical scientists (BMS) in the anticoagulation team. Computerised dosing schedules can facilitate the delivery of the anticoagulant service at hospital clinics. Some patients may be managed remotely, with arrangements made for taking samples from patients in the community, and dosed either by their own GP or by the hospital anticoagulant team. Increasingly, patients can be managed in primary care and in their own home.

Anticoagulant patient numbers and service workload is usually collated separately from other haematology workload and varies considerably. A typical DGH would expect to manage 1,500–2,000 patients per year (18,000–24,000 dose interventions per year). Consultant haematologists are frequently consulted about patients with anticoagulant-related problems both in the hospital and in the community. Advice is sought prior to surgery or other therapeutic procedures.

Hospital and primary care liaison activity   Consultant haematologists are regularly consulted about the management of patients in all specialties. Many of these consultations may be dealt with on the telephone but frequently the consultant needs to see the patient. GPs appreciate close contact with the haematology consultants; 30–50% of the laboratory work typically comes from primary care and telephone consultations are frequent.

Clinically related administration

Keeping accurate records of all patients is vital to ensure continuity of care between colleagues, including those in primary care, and must be timely due to the significant changes in a patient's status that may develop in haematological conditions.

The consultant haematologist should actively participate in the organisation and planning of outpatient and day case facilities, and contribute to the management of ward areas to ensure adequate facilities and staffing.

Roles in the laboratory   Abnormal GP and hospital blood films and the authorisation of other results are reviewed daily and shared between members of the consultant haematology team. This frequently leads to urgent referrals from primary care or intra-hospital referrals and contributes to the unpredictable workload of the consultant haematologist. Depending on their specialist interest the consultant will have a variable input to the day-to-day running of the laboratory or a section within it. Some haematologists may undertake research within the routine laboratory and supervise BMS staff directly.

Clinical and laboratory networks   MDT and other specialist meetings are held to develop clinical networks for the management of patients with malignant disorders and for patients with certain haemostatic disorders, often in other hospitals within the network. The development of pathology laboratory networks may also mean that the consultant haematologist is responsible for an area of laboratory work across different locations, which will involve added travel time. The configuration of pathology services is now under review following the publication of *Modernising pathology services* and will clearly change with increased collaborative working.[7] No one model is favoured and many work patterns are being piloted. Those adopted will be dependent on local circumstances. This work is being overseen by the Department of Health Pathology Modernisation Oversight Group which will help publicise and support best practice.

Work to maintain and improve the quality of care

This work encompasses duties in clinical governance, professional self-regulation, continuing professional development (CPD) and education and training of others. For many consultants at various times in their careers it may include research, serving in management and providing specialist advice at local, regional and national levels.

This work requires additional designated PAs. As a general guide, time must be allocated for continuing medical education (CME) (one PA); teaching (one PA); administration and management (one PA); with further PAs for those consultants with a lead managerial role or significant research commitment.

Active participation in audit projects of clinical outcomes and processes contributes to the maintenance of high quality care. Haematologists will also participate in local, regional and national educational meetings.

Leadership role and development of the service

The head of service must have strong leadership skills in order to coordinate the roles of members of the haematology team and to ensure that adequate resources for the haematology department are obtained through the business planning processes. All consultant haematologists participate in both national trials of patient management and clinical audits assessing the effectiveness of their service. Broad awareness of developments on both the national and local agenda are essential to ensure that the haematology department is able to provide the most effective up-to-date service. A consultant haematologist is responsible for the production and implementation of local guidelines, taking into account national haematology guidance produced by NICE or the BCSH.

Education and training

All haematologists participate in the teaching and training of nurses, biomedical scientists and clinical scientists, and postgraduate medical staff in all specialties. A majority of hospitals, whether they are teaching centres or DGHs, now also have undergraduate medical students.

Mentoring and appraisal of medical staff and other professional staff

The senior consultant with management responsibility will undertake appraisal of consultants. Doctors undertake the record of in-training assessment (RITA) of specialist registrars (SpRs) and SHOs. Haematologists with a significant role in the laboratory may also participate in the appraisal and assessment of senior BMS.

Continuing medical education

Consultant haematologists are expected to participate in the Royal College of Pathologists scheme for CPD and would be expected to attend local, regional and national meetings.

Research – clinical studies and basic science

Haematology departments in large teaching centres will have an active research programme, which may be either laboratory or clinically based. All hospitals participate in clinical trials in accordance with the trust's research governance arrangements. Consultants with a large research/academic commitment are considered below (see Academic medicine section).

Local management duties

One member of the consultant team will usually be appointed head of service or equivalent. This consultant will be responsible for setting the strategic direction of the service and for the delivery of a high quality, effective service for patients. Haematologists will take part in trust-wide management activities and play a key role in leading the development of the service. Participation in business planning and governance activities is necessary because of the dual responsibility for services within medicine and pathology. This may be shared between two individuals in a centre with a large clinical workload or be the responsibility of one member of the team of haematologists in a DGH. Consultant haematologists work closely with BMS to ensure that staff members are competent and that appropriate guidelines and procedures are in place.

Regional and national work

Due to the increasingly specialist nature of some areas of haematology, participation in regional and national organisations is common. The modernisation agenda and emphasis on patient choice will contribute to the significant duty of haematologists to ensure that the laboratory service and patient care are delivered safely and effectively. All haematologists contribute to the development of evidence-based guidelines through the BCSH.

ACADEMIC MEDICINE

Although academic medicine is in crisis with a number of vacant professorial posts and the loss of almost one-third of clinical lecturer posts, the Research Assessment Exercise (www.rae.ac.uk) has shown that haematology remains one of the more academic specialties. More than 40% of trainees take time out during higher specialist training to follow a research project, many proceeding to a higher degree. Approximately 10% of the consultant workforce are in academic posts funded by the Higher Education Funding Council for England (HEFCE), which means that many with research training will take NHS consultant posts. This research expertise is reflected in the enthusiastic support for national studies of the NCRI and the British National Lymphoma Investigation Group (BNLIG), and the work presented at the annual scientific meeting of the BSH.

The 2003 consultant contract identifies five PAs for academic work and one to two for supporting professional activity, which will certainly have an impact on the time that clinical academics will be able to devote to direct clinical care. The impact of this on numbers and work patterns will become clear over the next year or two.

The input of clinical scientists in the subspecialty areas of haematology must be recognised. The Clinical Science Forum of the BSH has identified over 100 clinical scientists working primarily in areas such as molecular cytogenetics, thrombosis, blood transfusion, immunophenotyping and bone marrow transplantation. The BSH, in conjunction with the Royal College of Pathologists (RCPath), has developed a training scheme for grade A scientists. They will be able to join the College by examination and this will enhance the flow into the specialty.

WORKFORCE REQUIREMENTS FOR HAEMATOLOGY

Current workforce numbers

There are 800 haematology consultants in the UK/Northern Ireland (720 WTE).

Whilst consultant numbers have increased by 50% over the last seven years, the 2002 Census showed that haematologists are working between three and 11 PAs above the standard working week.[8] This figure confirms that of the Clinical Benchmarking Company, who found that the median excess of sessions across the UK was 6.5.[9]

Consultant PAs required to provide a specialist service to a population of 250,000

The Intercollegiate Committee on Haematology, in association with the BSH, published the document *Haematology consultant manpower in the 21st century* which provides a template for calculating workforce by trust.[5] The document recommends a minimum of two consultant haematologists in each acute trust offering laboratory and clinical services. Using a combination of laboratory workload and finished consultant episodes (FCEs), the formula can be used to calculate the requisite number of consultant haematologists per unit with increasing activity and complexity of care. In practice, most acute DGHs serving a population of 250,000 should have 3.7 WTE consultant haematologists. The total target figure for WTE consultants in the UK will be approximately 862 which will be achieved over the next five to seven years.

The PAs for a population of 250,000 is given in the suggested job plan.

National consultant workforce requirements

Several recent initiatives (European Working Time Directive, *Better blood transfusion*, the European directive on haemo-vigilance, and the NHS Cancer Plan) will impact on workforce requirements within haematology.[3,10,11] For example, the NHS Cancer Plan estimated that at least 149 additional posts are needed. Implementation of the demands of *Better blood transfusion* and the European Directive on Haemo-Vigilance will require an additional 30–40 consultants.

Early retirement is having an increasing effect. Over 20% of the consultant workforce is now aged over 55 and a survey by the RCPath in 2003 indicated that 22 consultants were planning to take early retirement, whereas the same cohort surveyed the previous year indicated only seven planning to retire early. This is a current increase of yearly retirements by a factor of three. In addition, 30% of haematologists and over 50% of trainees are female, some of whom will wish to work part-time. We consider that each consultant haematologist is the equivalent of 0. 94 WTE when making workforce calculations (see Table 3).

Table 3. Summary of workforce requirements

For Cancer Plan	Approx. 149 posts
Implementation of *Better blood transfusion* and European Directive on Haemo-Vigilance	Approx. 30–40 posts
Implementation of European Working Time Directive (in order to create legal rotas)	Approx. 100 posts
Current shortfall in staffing (identified to avoid single-handed practices)	Approx. 110 posts
Total	Approx. 380 posts

Tertiary units, such as those offering allogeneic transplantation (level 4 services), specialist coagulation services and academic units require a minimum of five consultants. These numbers depend upon the specialties on offer within the hospital and the subspecialties within the department.

The impact of these initiatives will certainly lead to some shifting of cancer care to cancer centres but will also emphasise patient pathways and the quality of care in cancer units, where less-intensive care will be administered. This, in addition to continued provision of general haematological support, is unlikely to mean any significant reduction in staffing from the current level but will entail more networking and patients moving between centres. There will need to be more provision of high technology diagnostic services and haemato-morphology. It is clear that cross-cover will be required for the smaller units to create legal rotas and this will lead to more inter-trust networking.

The specialty will need to look at alternative methods of service provision, entailing an increase in clinical nurse specialists and other support staff, and the efficient and appropriate use of non-consultant career grade (NCCG) posts. Haematology is a leading specialty in the use of clinical nurse specialists and non-training junior grades. In areas such as thrombosis and haemostasis, support staff including BMS and pharmacists are providing a clinical service. The potential for changing skillmix will become apparent as the implications of the improving outcomes guidance (IOG) on haematological cancer, *Better blood transfusion* and the National Service Frameworks (NSFs) in Cardiovascular Disease and Stroke are worked through, but it is anticipated that the input of other staff will increase as it has already in haemophilia care and, to a lesser extent, haemoglobinopathy management.

Job planning to implement the 2003 consultant contract is underway. Each job plan should assign at least three PAs for work done to maintain and improve the quality of care (see below). The job plans for clinical academics will be even more defined. Universities will insist on an identifiable academic component and will not continue to support the clinical service to the degree that has occurred historically. There are at least 80 academic posts identified in the UK and their reduced clinical input will clearly have an impact on service delivery.

Annual consultant workforce requirement

Over the last five to seven years, between 30 and 40 consultant haematologist posts have been appointed each year. Approximately one-third are retirement posts and two-thirds are newly created posts. The number of Certificates of Completion of Specialist Training (CCST) awarded each year has previously matched the number of appointments. The increasing number of consultants taking early retirement over the last two to three years has meant that the majority of those awarded the CCST are needed to fill retirement posts, with little additional capacity for new appointments. In practice, however, many new posts have been appointed, leaving the established replacement posts vacant. The number of vacancies has increased steadily and is now approaching 6% of the workforce.

On current CCST numbers haematology will not be able to maintain the previous level of expansion and will not be able to achieve the numbers envisaged to maintain and enhance the level of practice. More trainees have been sought through the Workforce Advisory Group, which has realised the extent of the problem in the specialty. This has led to more favourable recognition but will not translate rapidly into increased consultant numbers. Expansion will depend on more networking and imaginative development of skillmix until the new numbers begin to come through.

CONSULTANT WORK PROGRAMME/SPECIMEN JOB PLAN

Activity	Workload	Programmed activities (PAs)
Direct clinical care		
Diagnostic laboratory work		2–3
Ward rounds/ward referrals/ MDT meetings		2
Outpatient clinics		2–3
Marrows and other specialist procedures		0–0.5
Lead haematologist lab		0–1
Lead haematologist transfusion		0–1
Lead haematologist anticoagulation		0–1
On-call and weekend work	This should not exceed a 1:3 rota	
Total number of direct clinical care PAs		**7.5 on average**
Supporting professional activities (SPA)		
Work to maintain and improve the quality of healthcare	Education and training, appraisal, departmental management and service development, audit and clinical governance, CPD and revalidation, research	**2.5 on average**
Other NHS responsibilities	eg medical director/clinical director/lead consultant in specialty/clinical tutor	**Local agreement with trust**
External duties	eg work for deaneries/Royal Colleges/specialist societies/Department of Health or other government bodies etc	**Local agreement with trust**

NOTES

1. Consultants with a significant academic workload will have separate PAs identified for NHS and/or university components.

2. Consultant job plans must take into account the European Working Time Directive.

References

1. British Committee for Standards in Haematology. Guidelines on the provision of facilities for the care of adult patients with haematological malignancies. *Clin Lab Haematology* 1995;**17**:1–10.

2. National Institute for Clinical Excellence. *Improving outcomes in haematological cancers.* London: NICE, 2003. www.nice.org.uk

3. Department of Health. *Better blood transfusion: appropriate use of blood. HSC 2002/009.* London: DH, 2002.

4. Department of Health. *Updated national guidance of the safe administration of intrathecal chemotherapy, HSC 2003/010.* London: DH, 2003.

5. Intercollegiate Committee on Haematology and British Society for Haematology. *Haematology consultant manpower in the 21st Century.* British Society for Haematology: London, 2001.

6. British Committee for Standards in Haematology. Guidelines on oral anticoagulation: third edition. *Br J Haematol* 1998;**101**:374–387.

7. Department of Health. *Modernising pathology services.* London: DH, 2004.

8. The Federation of the Royal Colleges of Physicians of the United Kingdom. *Census of Consultant Physicians in the UK, 2002. Data and commentary.* London: The Federation of the Royal Colleges of the United Kingdom, 2002.

9. Clinical Benchmarking Company Ltd. Annual Reports (1996/7); (1997/8); (1998/9).

10. European Blood Safety Regulations: 2002/93/EC and 2004/33/EC.

11. Department of Health. *The NHS cancer plan: a plan for investment, a plan for reform.* London: DH, 2001. www.doh.gov.uk/cancer/cancer plan.htm

Immunology

i Description of the specialty and clinical needs of patients

The clinical practice of immunology, as defined by the World Health Organisation (WHO), encompasses clinical and laboratory activity dealing with the study, diagnosis and management of patients with diseases resulting from disordered immunological mechanisms, and conditions in which immunological manipulations form an important part of therapy.[1] In the UK, the practice of immunology largely conforms to this WHO definition with immunologists providing combined clinical and laboratory services for patients with immunodeficiency, autoimmune disease, systemic vasculitis and allergy.

Patients with immunologically mediated diseases comprise a diverse group who present to a variety of medical specialties. Within this group, patients with primary immunodeficiency disorders (PID) have particular clinical needs given the relative rarity of their chronic conditions and the attendant diagnostic delay, with the need for complex therapy and lifelong immunological follow up. Such patients require access to a specialist clinical immunology service for optimal care. Patients with autoimmune disease, systemic vasculitis and serious allergy require access to the relevant organ-based specialty working in partnership with a high quality immunology laboratory to ensure prompt diagnosis and optimal management of their condition.

Allergy has recently been recognised as a specialty in its own right. Historically, in view of the immunological principles underlying allergic disease and the patchy development of allergy services, many immunologists established, and continue to provide, a significant allergy service including desensitisation therapy. There are insufficient specialist allergists in the NHS at present.

ii Organisation of the service and patterns of referral

Clinical immunology has evolved over the past two decades from a laboratory base to a combined clinical and laboratory specialty. A typical immunology service is based in a teaching hospital and led by a consultant immunologist, and comprises a mixture of clinical and laboratory staff. The clinical team will include specialist registrars (SpRs) in immunology and immunology nurse specialists, while the laboratory team is comprised of biomedical and clinical scientists.

The advent of laboratory accreditation has led many district general hospitals (DGHs) to seek formal consultant immunology input into their diagnostic immunology services. In many instances laboratory duties are combined with clinical work. In some parts of the country, this arrangement has enabled the development of a clinical network linking the regional immunology service to surrounding DGHs, thus ensuring wider delivery of clinical immunology services.

The majority of referrals to immunologists involve patients with suspected immune deficiency, severe allergy, systemic autoimmune disease and vasculitis. Referrals emanate from colleagues in both hospital and primary care.

iii   Working with patients: patient-centred care

Patient choice and involving patients in decisions about their care

Patients with immunodeficiency disorders have a lifelong need for specialist immunological care. As their primary physician, immunologists work in close partnership with colleagues from other disciplines to ensure that their patient's complex multisystem complications are managed optimally across disciplines.

Access to information, patient support groups and the role of the expert patient

The Primary Immunodeficiency Association (PIA) and other patient groups provide a vital source of educational and pastoral support for patients. Both adult and paediatric immunologists serve on the medical advisory panel of the PIA and play an important educational and advisory role in raising awareness of immunodeficiencies among the wider medical profession and policy makers. Immunologists are also actively involved in patient education by making regular presentations to regional and national patient meetings and contributing to patient newsletters.

The concept of the expert patient is particularly apposite to patients with primary immuno-deficiency who have a lifetime's experience of the problems associated with defective immunity. The active solicitation of patients' views on the quality of the clinical service afforded to immuno-deficient patients is a requirement for accreditation of immunodeficiency services by the United Kingdom Primary Immunodeficiency Network (UKPIN), a multidisciplinary organisation comprising clinicians, nurses and scientists. Regular meetings between UKPIN and the PIA patient body about matters of mutual interest – ranging from the supply of therapeutic immunoglobulin, relative risk of variant Creutzfeld-Jakob disease from blood products and research into PID – ensure that patients' views are well represented in both medical and industrial forums.

iv   Interspecialty and interdisciplinary liaison

Immunologists work as members of multidisciplinary teams (MDTs) that include nurse specialists. Nurse specialists in immunology play a leading role in all aspects of immunoglobulin infusion, from supervision of hospital clinics to the training and supervision of patients who undertake self-infusion of immunoglobulin as part of the home therapy programme. In many centres, immunology nurse specialists undertake skin testing for allergy and train patients with life-threatening allergic disease in the use of self-injectable adrenaline. Some immunology nurse specialists have completed the extended prescribing course for nurses and have gone on to set up autonomous clinics for the diagnosis and management of allergic diseases.

Several other complementary services including radiology and cellular pathology are essential for the efficient delivery of a good immunology service. Multidisciplinary meetings provide education and improved liaison for patient care. A comprehensive diagnostic immunology laboratory underpins the diagnosis of all immunological disease.

Considering the propensity of antibody deficient patients to develop complications involving multiple organ systems, immunologists must liaise closely with colleagues in a range of specialties including respiratory medicine, ear nose and throat (ENT) surgery, haematology, ophthalmology and gastroenterology. Access to specialist microbiology and virology laboratories is vital for the early detection and optimal management of the infectious complications of immunodeficiency.

v **Delivering a high quality service**

A high quality clinical immunology service will be well staffed (medical, scientific, nursing and secretarial), well resourced and consultant led. It must be supported by an accredited immunology laboratory providing a full repertoire of investigations encompassing immunochemistry, auto-immunity, allergy, and cellular and molecular immunology.

vi **Quality standards and measures of the quality of specialist services**

The Department of Health (DH) has recently published specialist definitions for clinical immunology (definition number 16) and laboratory immunology (included in definition number 25 pertaining to specialised pathology services), which provide a benchmark for the practice of immunology.[2,3] The quality of the laboratory immunology service has been underpinned by Clinical Pathology Accreditation UK (CPA) since 1993. Enrolment with CPA was made a mandatory requirement by the DH for all laboratory disciplines including immunology in 2003.

The process of accreditation of clinical immunology services for immunodeficiency through a system of peer review by UKPIN is actively underway. Participation in both clinical and laboratory accreditation ensures that immunology services comply with current standards of clinical governance. UKPIN fulfils an important educational role in the development of guidelines on the diagnosis and management of immunodeficiencies (**www.pinguidelines.org.uk**). The Network also develops the immunodeficiency register and works closely with governmental agencies involved in the provision of therapeutic agents for patient care.

CLINICAL WORK AND/OR LABORATORY WORK OF CONSULTANTS IN IMMUNOLOGY

Contributions made to acute medicine

Most immunologists do not participate in the on-take rota for unselected medical emergencies.

Direct clinical care

The clinical work of consultant immunologists is largely outpatient based, with the following broad work patterns:

- Immunologists are solely responsible for patients with primary immunodeficiencies (antibody deficiency, combined T and B cell deficiency, complement deficiency and phagocytic defects).
- Stem cell transplantation is increasingly being considered for young adults and children with primary immune deficiencies. The long-term follow up of these patients is an expanding area of work for immunologists.
- In centres without dedicated allergists, consultant immunologists are responsible for patients with severe allergic disease (food allergy, drug allergy, venom allergy, anaphylaxis).
- In most centres, consultant immunologists perform joint clinics with paediatricians to care for children with immunodeficiencies and allergy.
- Many immunologists have an interest in connective tissue disease and perform joint clinics with rheumatologists for patients with autoimmune rheumatic disease and systemic vasculitis.

■ Immunoglobulin infusion clinics for patients with antibody deficiency form an integral part of the clinical workload of consultant immunologists. A recent audit of primary antibody deficiency in the UK and discussions within the specialty suggest that a single consultant should be responsible for a maximum of 50 patients with antibody deficiency in order to deliver optimum care.[4] With the increasing recognition of intravenous immunoglobulin as a therapeutic immunomodulator, these infusion clinics have expanded in some centres to include non-antibody deficient patients, for example inflammatory neuropathies.

Outpatient work, including day cases

■ primary immunodeficiency clinics

■ severe allergic disease clinics

■ combined clinics with paediatricians for children with immunodeficiency and allergy

■ combined clinics with rheumatologists

■ immunoglobulin infusion clinics for antibody replacement and therapeutic immunomodulation.

The complexity of clinical referrals requires that assessment of patients at the first consultation is given sufficient time, which limits the number of patients that can be seen in a single outpatient session. A consultant immunologist working alone will typically see 5–10 patients (new and follow up) in a single session, depending on the complexity of the patients' problems. A consultant should be responsible for a maximum of 50 patients with antibody deficiency in order to deliver optimum care.[4]

Laboratory immunology

Consultant immunologists are responsible for directing diagnostic immunology services and perform a wide range of duties including clinical liaison, interpretation and validation of results, quality assurance, assay development, and supervision of biomedical and clinical scientists and SpRs. Some consultants perform a limited amount of 'hands on' laboratory work.

In view of the work pressures on immunologists, CPA guidelines stipulate that a single consultant immunologist should not support more than two laboratories outside their base hospital at any one time and the weekly off-site commitment to these should not be more than two programmed activities (PAs) (including travelling time).

The nature of on-call duties in immunology only rarely warrants the out-of-hours attendance of consultant immunologists. However, it is essential that an on-call specialist immunology service is available for discussion of clinical problems and emergency laboratory investigations. The frequency of on-call duties for consultant immunologists will be determined by the number of colleagues in a centre. Where possible, an on-call rota with a frequency of one in two or one in three is recommended although it is recognised that single-handed consultants will have difficulty with this arrangement. In such cases, the possibility of forming a consortium with colleagues in adjacent regions to provide an acceptable level of cover should be explored.

Work to maintain and improve the quality of care

Leadership role and development of the service

Immunologists are proactive in embracing service developments and developing initiatives that deliver improved patient care. Training patients to use home immunoglobulin therapy via intravenous or subcutaneous routes is evidence of this. Home intravenous immunoglobulin (IVIg) therapy, initially developed for patients with primary antibody deficiency, has now been extended in some centres to patients with autoimmune neuropathies in whom it is used for maintenance immunomodulatory therapy.

In the laboratory, immunologists take a lead role in the assessment of new diagnostic tests for immunological diseases, followed, if appropriate, by their introduction into routine clinical practice.

Education and training, clinical governance and management duties

Immunologists are actively involved in a range of duties which are essential to the maintenance of high standards of clinical practice. These include education and training of SpRs, laboratory scientists and nurses; continuing medical education (CME); clinical governance; local management; and national work for the Royal Colleges of Physicians and Pathologists and specialist immunological societies (the British Society of Immunology (BSI), the British Society for Allergy and Clinical Immunology (BSACI) and UKPIN). With the development of a competency-based curriculum in immunology, it is envisaged that a consultant will need to devote one weekly PA to teaching and training activities.

Research – clinical studies and basic science

The direct relevance of immunology to much of clinical medicine and its strong scientific foundations provides ample opportunities for clinical studies of new immunomodulatory therapies, the recognition of new diseases (as shown by recent descriptions of new forms of severe combined immunodeficiency and type I cytokine deficiency) and translational research. Despite their heavy NHS commitments, many immunologists are actively involved in clinical and laboratory studies at national and international levels.

ACADEMIC MEDICINE

The few full-time academic immunologists make a proportionately greater contribution to research whilst shouldering a significant clinical workload for the NHS, as detailed in the preceding paragraphs. With the disappearance of many university immunology departments and recent medical school expansion, consultant immunologists have major undergraduate and postgraduate teaching commitments.

WORKFORCE REQUIREMENTS FOR IMMUNOLOGY

Currently, 49 consultant immunologists serve the entire population of England and Wales.

Limited data are available on the workload of immunologists, who are based mainly in teaching hospitals. Increasing awareness of immunological diseases, coupled with the need to provide specialist advice and direction to immunology laboratories, including those in larger DGHs, has placed a traditionally understaffed specialty with many single-handed consultants under great strain.

An estimate of the number of consultant immunologists required in England and Wales is based upon the recent workload survey undertaken by the Royal College of Pathologists, the College Census and extensive consultation within the specialty.[5,6] The RCPath survey showed that immunologists worked a median of 57 hours a week (14.4 PAs) while the Census showed that an individual immunologist worked 23.8 hours in excess of his or her contractual obligation performing the various activities detailed above.

Workforce requirements have been calculated on the basis that most immunologists are based in teaching hospitals, and the population served by existing consultant immunologists is 38.9 million.

Since there is insufficient data on immunology workload at a DGH level, it is not possible to calculate workforce requirements for a population of 250,000. Instead, the projected estimates are based on the assumption that each consultant will not be expected to exceed his or her contractual obligation of 10 PAs and no consultant will have to practise single-handedly (currently 19% of consultant immunologists work single-handed).

On this basis, it is estimated that 114 WTE consultants in immunology are required to serve the population of England and Wales (53.4 million). This translates into one consultant immunologist per 513,400 of the population compared to the existing provision of one per 1.1 million of the population. This is 0.49 WTE for 250,000 population, which is an expansion of 128%. This estimate is approximately in line with the DH's own recent estimate of consultant requirements in immunology. Consultant numbers will need to expand by 5.5% per annum over the next 10 years to achieve this figure.

CONSULTANT WORK PROGRAMME/SPECIMEN JOB PLAN

Activity	Workload	Programmed activities (PAs)
Direct clinical care		
Outpatient clinics	5–10 patients per clinic	**3–4**
New patients	3–4 patients per clinic	
Follow-up patients	6–8 patients per clinic	
IVIg infusion	6–10 patients per clinic	
Ward consultation and telephone advice		**0.5**
Allergy, including desensitisation immunotherapy		**1**
Laboratory work		
Clinical liaison, interpretation of results		
Quality assurance		
Assay development		
Hands on laboratory work		
Supervision of DGH immunology laboratories		
Total laboratory work		**3–4**
Total number of direct clinical care PAs		**7.5 on average**
Supporting professional activities (SPA)		
Work to maintain and improve the quality of healthcare	Education and training, appraisal, departmental management and service development, audit and clinical governance, CPD and revalidation, research	**2.5 on average**
Other NHS responsibilities	eg medical director/clinical director/lead consultant in specialty/clinical tutor	**Local agreement with trust**
External duties	eg work for deaneries/Royal Colleges/specialist societies/Department of Health or other government bodies etc	**Local agreement with trust**

References

1. Lambert et al. Clinical immunology: guidelines for its organisation, training and certification: relationships with allergology and other medical disciplines – a WHO/IUIS/IAACI report. *Clin Exp Immunol* 1993;**93**:484–91.

2. Department of Health. *Specialised services national definitions set 2nd edition: Specialised clinical immunology services (all ages) – definition no. 16*, December 2002.
    www.dh.gov.uk/PolicyAndGuidance/HealthAndSocialCareTopics/ SpecialisedServicesDefinition/fs/en

3. Department of Health. *Specialised services national definition set: Specialised pathology services (all ages) – definition no. 25*, December 2002.
    www.dh.gov.uk/PolicyAndGuidance/HealthAndSocialCareTopics/SpecialisedServices Definition/fs/en

4. Spickett GP, Ashew T, Chapel HM. Development of primary antibody deficiency by consultant immunologists in the UK: a paradigm for other rare diseases. *Qual Health Care* 1995;**4**:263–8.

5. Royal College of Pathologists. *Medical and scientific staffing of the National Health Service pathology departments.* London: RCPath, 1999.

6. The Federation of the Royal Colleges of Physicians of the United Kingdom. *Census of consultant physicians in the UK, 2002. Data and commentary.* London: The Federation of the Royal Colleges of Physicians of the United Kingdom, 2002.

Infectious diseases (including tropical medicine)

i Description of the specialty and clinical needs of patients

With the advent of antibiotics and vaccination programmes in the 1950s and 1960s, the interest in, and significance of, infectious disease began to wane. However, in the last few decades, increased awareness about new infections and re-emerging diseases have put the focus back onto infectious diseases (ID) as a specialty. Although the concept of a fever hospital, common in the early twentieth century, is clearly outdated there are now modern ID units in many British teaching hospitals.

Many patients with acute infections have multisystem problems and require the resources of a modern general hospital. New infections such as HIV have challenged modern medicine and it is widely recognised that global travel has made us all vulnerable to infections from other parts of the world. The recent outbreaks of severe acute respiratory system (SARS) and avian influenza have demonstrated this in a dramatic manner, while imported diseases like malaria and dengue fever pose continued threats. Advances in medicine have increased the number of immunosuppressed patients at risk from opportunist infections such as invasive fungal infection, while the complexity of modern hospital care has increased the risk of nosocomial infections such as methicillin-resistant *Staphylococcus aureus* (MRSA) and *Clostridium difficile*.

The discovery of new pathogens and better insight into host-pathogen interactions have increased the need for academic ID research. Increasingly, ID units have an academic base with networks of multidisciplinary groups within host universities. The focus is on understanding basic mechanisms in infection and immunity in order to inform improvements in the prevention and treatment of infections. Some ID doctors specialise in tropical medicine, usually in an academic setting, and many will have spent time abroad in training and to carry out research. They will act as a resource for others, particularly if they are based in one of the five currently recognised tropical centres in the UK.

Recent reports, including the House of Lords Select Committee report on antibiotic resistance, *Fighting infection*, and those from the Chief Medical Officer, *Getting ahead of the curve* and *Winning ways*, demonstrate the importance that parliament and the Department of Health (DH) place on combating and controlling infections.[1,2,3]

ii Organisation of the service and patterns of referral

The majority of ID units are based in academic departments of medicine in teaching hospitals, though some are in larger district general hospitals (DGHs). Most units are ward based with appropriate isolation beds, although one or two departments are mainly consultation based with few specialty inpatient beds. A few centres have paediatric ID units, which operate largely on a consultation basis. The typical, ward-based adult ID physician is responsible for 500–600 finished consultant episodes (FCE) per year, plus about 1,200 outpatients visits and numerous hospital consultations, although this figure will vary depending on the way the department functions.

Referrals for admissions come primarily directly from GPs but also from emergency departments. There are frequent transfers from other specialties in the hospital and often from outlying DGHs where there is often no ID expertise. A broad range of conditions are dealt with, from community-acquired infections such as gastroenteritis or pneumonia, imported fevers such as malaria and typhoid, to complex problems such as fever of unknown origin or infections in immunocompromised hosts such as those with AIDS. Many ID departments also provide travel medicine advice to patients in the form of specific travel clinics or telephone advice lines, to which patients often self-refer.

Infectious diseases physicians work closely with colleagues in medical microbiology and in public health. They aim to improve management of infection not only in hospitals but also in the wider community. This is reflected in an increasing trend to provide joint training for young doctors in ID and microbiology and in plans to develop joint training in public health medicine. Infectious disease physicians also work with local drug-dependency services because of the increase in blood-borne viruses such as HIV, hepatitis C and hepatitis B. For similar reasons, there are often links to local prisons and to refugee centres. These specific issues mandate close working relationships with social services departments.

iii Working with patients: patient-centred care

The onset of the HIV/AIDS pandemic in the 1980s produced a group of very vocal and articulate AIDS activists who have raised the level of patient involvement in their own care. Infectious disease physicians engaged with this movement early on and have tried to involve patients in decision-making in many aspects of inpatient and outpatient care, not only around the subject of HIV. Most ID units deal with tropical and imported diseases and see patients from a wide variety of geographic, ethnic and cultural backgrounds. This requires a willingness to address a range of patient-related issues and to involve patients, families, religious leaders and community supporters to achieve the best outcomes for often disadvantaged immigrants and refugees. These interactions also create opportunities for ID units to provide education in disease prevention, early recognition of problems and appropriate ways to access healthcare. The diverse background of the patient groups means there is a high demand for interpreters for those whose English is poor, which adds significantly to the time required for the individual consultation.

Although a large proportion of the work of ID units is concerned with emergency admissions and management of acute infections, all units help to manage chronic conditions. Most commonly, this involves the care of people with chronic blood-borne virus infections like HIV and hepatitis B and C. However, patients with tuberculosis (TB) or more chronic bacterial infections, such as osteomyelitis or infection of prosthetic joints or blood vessels, also require long-term care and follow up. Many ID units have taken on the role of assessing and managing people with chronic fatigue syndrome. Dealing with patients with chronic conditions leads ID physicians to engage with carers, community support groups and patient-advocacy groups. Information about various infections and treatments is available in wards and clinics, sometimes in collaboration with patient support groups, such as the Terence Higgins Trust for HIV, or with patient representatives.

iv Interspecialty and interdisciplinary liaison

Infectious diseases doctors work closely with physicians in the more traditional organ-based specialties. They collaborate with hepatologists in the joint management of hepatitis C, with respiratory physicians to manage TB and with genitourinary physicians to manage HIV. Surgical colleagues liaise concerning the infective complications of surgery and the surgical interventions necessary for the management of infection, such as the drainage of pus. There is increasingly important work with radiology to diagnose and manage complex infections.

Control of infection within hospitals and in the community requires close links with laboratory microbiology and with public health doctors. With improvement in the outlook for people with HIV, ID physicians now work with obstetricians, neonatologists and paediatricians to improve the antenatal care of infected women and to prevent HIV infection of newborn children.

Patients with infections, whether acute or chronic, often have complex needs, which can only be addressed through effective multidisciplinary team (MDT) working. Specially trained ID nurses can improve patient care and infection control. Patients need the help of occupational therapists and physiotherapists, particularly for rehabilitation after serious infections. Dietitians and social workers are also important contributors to the teams. More recently specialist pharmacists, either specialising in HIV or in antimicrobials, have joined MDTs and improved standards of prescribing for what are often very expensive drugs, and have improved patient education. This has been particularly important in helping HIV-infected patients adhere to long, complex antiretroviral drug regimens.

v   Delivering a high quality service

Characteristics of a high quality service

The aim of developing and maintaining a high quality service is central to the practice of an ID physician. Because the ID physician is not restricted by organ or dependent on performing procedures, it is the quality of specialist opinion and management that defines them. The ID physician must be open-minded and responsive to change. They must stay abreast of the literature in a rapidly-changing field where new pathogens and diagnostic possibilities are continually being recognised. The ID physician must be able to recognise infection emergencies such as meningococcaemia, be alert to rare diagnoses such as SARS or Lassa fever and be attuned to the possibility of outbreaks that may affect the community. Effective MDTs and cross-specialty liaison are key to this.

Resources required for a high quality service

Although not procedure-driven, ID physicians nevertheless require resources and specialist facilities in order to deliver a high quality service.

- Each unit should have an adequate number of single patient rooms to prevent cross infection and to prevent vulnerable, immunocompromised patients from nosocomial infection.

- Now that multi-drug resistant TB (MDRTB) and diseases like SARS are real threats, it is important to have facilities for appropriate respiratory isolation of infected patients. Units should have single rooms with negative pressure ventilation (and appropriate monitoring and alarms) to minimise the risk of respiratory droplet spread of infection. Effective protective masks and clothing should be worn by staff when necessary.

- There should be easy access to intensive care support.

- Nationally, one or two units will need to maintain additional specialist equipment, such as a Trexler isolator (eg for Lassa fever). All units will need equipment for the safe isolation and transfer of such patients to such special isolation units.

- ID units need sufficient trained physicians, physicians in training and specialist-trained nurses to provide optimal care for infected patients.

Infectious diseases physicians are also required to take a lead in implementing the DH smallpox plan and will be key personnel in providing leadership, training, clinical diagnosis and management of this and other potential illnesses which may result from deliberate release of biological agents.

vi Quality standards and measures of the quality of specialist services

Specialist society guidelines

Unlike many specialties, ID is not centred on one organ or one disease and has to deal with a vast array of possible infections and conditions. Each individual infection may present relatively few patients to an individual ID unit, making the derivation of quality standards more difficult. Nevertheless, specialist societies have developed, and are developing, guidelines for some of the more common infections.

■ The British Infection Society is leading on this and is piloting a peer-review scheme to ensure external quality assurance of ID units (**www.britishinfectionsociety.org**).

■ The British HIV Association updates guidelines for HIV management and conducts audits on different aspects of HIV care (**www.bhiva.org**).

■ Infectious diseases physicians also refer to appropriate guidelines developed by the Infectious Diseases Society of America (**www.idsociety.org**) and, for TB and pneumonia, the British Thoracic Society (**www.brit-thoracic.org.uk**).

National Institute for Clinical Excellence (NICE) guidelines

NICE has developed some guidance related to infections, such as hepatitis C and infection control, and others will follow in the future (**www.nice.org.uk**).

Clinical governance

All ID units are involved locally and nationally in promoting good clinical governance. Consultants undergo annual appraisal and there are annual reviews of doctors in training. The specialist advisory committee of the College has a rolling programme of inspection for ID training programmes in the UK. Infectious disease physicians take an active role in teaching and training medical students, medical trainees and allied clinical staff. They also maintain active continuing professional development (CPD), monitored by the College.

CLINICAL WORK AND/OR LABORATORY WORK OF CONSULTANTS IN INFECTIOUS DISEASES

Contributions made to acute medicine

A large proportion of admissions to ID units come directly from the community as acute admissions. In addition, about half of the ID specialists in the UK take part in the acute medical service, taking in unselected admissions in addition to their specialist work. Diseases may often present mimicking infections and ID doctors must be able to recognise these and liaise with general physicians appropriately. Experience of general medicine is an important part of ID training.

Direct clinical care

Inpatient work

Most ID units have inpatients for whom the ID consultant is directly responsible (between 15–25 patients). This involves providing on-call cover 24 hours a day, 7 days a week. On-call rotas are usually one in three or one in four for nights and weekends but, because the number of consultants is limited, it may be as arduous as one in two in some units. New admissions are seen within 24 hours and ward rounds are consultant led. An important additional inpatient activity is seeing referrals in the hospital from other specialties – in many cases this entails unsolicited consultations, often with the medical microbiologist, on patients with positive blood cultures. Infectious disease consultants with general medical duties also take part in separate rotas with other physicians in general medicine for the acute unselected medical take.

Outpatient work

The ID consultant will provide one to three specialist clinics per week and may also do a general medical clinic. Clinics will usually involve a mixture of new and review patients, including ward discharge follow-ups (six new patients or 15 review patients or a combination). There may be specialist clinics in HIV, viral hepatitis, TB, travel medicine and chronic fatigue syndrome.

Specialist procedures

Infectious diseases is not a procedure-driven specialty but some ID units provide additional specialist services. Increasingly, outpatient intravenous antibiotic services are run from ID units whereby patients (referred from a wide variety of hospital departments) can receive specialist treatment either in the clinic or in their own homes. Previously they may have required admission to hospital or a more prolonged hospital stay. Vaccination services may be offered to protect current patients from hepatitis infections or for prevention of travel-related diseases.

Other specialist activity

Some ID specialists may run outreach clinics at DGHs, hospices (eg for AIDS), prisons or refugee centres. Most ID consultants provide telephone advice for GPs, consultants at DGHs and within their own hospital.

Work to maintain and improve quality of care

This work involves clinical governance, keeping up to date through CPD, taking part in professional self-regulation, peer review and teaching and training others. Most ID consultants are involved in research, either through basic science academic activity, collaboration with scientists, or by involvement in clinical trials such as the Medical Research Council (MRC) trials in HIV infection. At some stage in their careers, consultants will be involved in local trust management activity and many will be involved with planning and development at a national level through specialist societies and the College.

ACADEMIC MEDICINE

More than half of ID consultants and about 80% of those involved with tropical medicine hold contracts with a university. In most instances, line management is through the medical school but consultants will have honorary NHS contracts and will devote some of their time to NHS work. Clinical duties will be limited by their academic commitments but they will be expected to participate in inpatient and outpatient care in some manner and to be included in on-call rotas for the specialty. They will have a vital role in educating medical and other students about infection. Universities, Royal Colleges and the General Medical Council will have to consider how those who are conducting research in the tropics can keep up with changes in the NHS and be eligible for revalidation.

MEDICAL WORKFORCE REQUIREMENTS FOR INFECTIOUS DISEASES

Current workforce numbers

There are about 110 consultants in England and Wales with a certificate of completion of specialist training (CCST) in ID and/or tropical medicine, approximating to one ID consultant per 550,000 of the population. It should be noted, however, that some of these are engaged primarily in research and others are based primarily in the tropics. The situation is somewhat better in Scotland where there are 20 consultants, giving a ratio of one per 270,000 of the population.

Comparisons can be made with Scandanavian countries such as Sweden and Norway where there is one ID specialist for around 50,000 patients. Holland and Australia, which have health systems more closely comparable to that in the UK, have approximately one specialist in ID per 200,000 of the population (see appendix 1 for European comparisons). In order to reach similar levels of provision in England and Wales, ID consultant numbers would need to double over the next 10 years.

National consultant workforce requirements

The College and the British Medical Association (BMA) recommend that there should be two to three whole time equivalent (WTE) infection specialists per 300,000 population (average DGH unit size), at least one of whom should be an ID consultant (others might be consultants in medical microbiology or public health). This equates to 0.83 WTE per 250,000, which would require an increase of 172% resulting in 193 WTE across the UK in the next few years. More specialists will need to be trained to reach acceptable levels for optimum patient care, particularly as some will have academic commitments and others will be involved in acute medicine commitments. There is still one well-established medical school in the UK with no ID specialists and most of the newly established medical schools have no clear plans to develop ID as an academic specialty. This, in turn, further limits the number of training slots available to provide future ID specialists.

CONSULTANT WORK PROGRAMME/SPECIMEN JOB PLAN

Infectious diseases (may include on call for general internal medicine)

Activity	Workload	Programmed activities (PAs)
Direct clinical care		
Inpatients (including on call)		3–4
Outpatients		2–4
Consultations		1–2
Work away from base		0–1
Total number of direct clinical care PAs		**7.5 on average**
Supporting professional activities (SPA)		
Work to maintain and improve the quality of healthcare	Education and training, appraisal, departmental management and service development, audit and clinical governance, CPD and revalidation, research	**2.5 on average**
Other NHS responsibilities	eg medical director/clinical director/lead consultant in specialty/clinical tutor	**Local agreement with trust**
External duties	eg work for deaneries/Royal Colleges/specialist societies/Department of Health or other government bodies etc	**Local agreement with trust**

Infectious diseases plus medical microbiology

Activity	Workload	Programmed activities (PAs)
Direct clinical care		
Inpatients (including on call)		1–2
Outpatients		1–2
Consultations		1–3
Work away from base		0
Microbiology lab		2–3
Total number of direct clinical care PAs		**7.5 on average**
Supporting professional activities (SPA)		
Work to maintain and improve the quality of healthcare	Education and training, appraisal, departmental management and service development, audit and clinical governance, CPD and revalidation, research	**2.5 on average**
Other NHS responsibilities	eg medical director/clinical director/lead consultant in specialty/clinical tutor	**Local agreement with trust**
External duties	eg work for deaneries/Royal Colleges/specialist societies/Department of Health or other government bodies etc	**Local agreement with trust**

Appendix 1: Comparison of European countries and infectious diseases specialists*

Numbers of infectious diseases specialists (including adult and paediatric) per million population [no data available from countries not shown in table]

Country	Population (million) approx.	ID specialists per million population
England, Wales and Northern Ireland	53.6	<5
Belgium	10	<5
Greece	10.3	<5
Germany	82	<5
Republic of Ireland	3.6	<5
Scotland	5.1	<5
Netherlands	15.8	5–10
Denmark	5.3	5–10
Portugal	10	5–10
Finland	5.2	10–20
Norway	4.5	10–20
Slovakia	5.4	10–20
Slovenia	2	10–20
Switzerland	7.3	10–20
Iceland	0.3	20–40
Croatia	4.8	20–40
Sweden	8.8	20–40
Turkey	68	20–40
Italy	58	40–60

*Figures are estimates from the Union of European Medical Specialists (UEMS).

Numbers of infection specialists (including adult and paediatric infectious diseases and microbiology) per million population*

Country	Population (million) approx.	'Infection specialists' (ID + microbiology) per million population
England, Wales and Northern Ireland	53.6	5–10
Greece	10.3	5–10
Republic of Ireland	3.6	5–10
Belgium	10	10–20
Germany	82	10–20
Netherlands	15.8	10–20
Scotland	5.1	10–20
Denmark	5.3	10–20
Portugal	10	10–20
Finland	5.2	20–40
Turkey	68	20–40
Slovakia	5.4	20–40
Iceland	0.3	40–60
Norway	4.5	40–60
Croatia	4.8	40–60
Sweden	8.8	40–60
Italy	58	40–60
Switzerland	7.3	No data
Slovenia	2	No data

*Figures are estimates from the Union of European Medical Specialists (UEMS).

References

1. House of Lords. *Fighting infection.* Report of the select committee on science and technology. London: The Stationery Office, 2003.

2. Department of Health. *Getting ahead of the curve: a strategy for combating infectious diseases (including other aspects of health protection).* A report from the Chief Medical Officer. London: DH, 2002. www.doh.gov.uk/cmo/idstrategy

3. Department of Health. *Winning ways: working together to reduced healthcare associated infection in England and Wales* A report from the Chief Medical Officer. London: DH, 2003.

Medical oncology

i Description of the specialty and clinical needs of patients

Medical oncologists are physicians trained in the diagnosis, assessment and treatment of patients with cancer in order to provide the best possible outcome, whether that is cure, or palliation and prolongation of good quality life. They provide counselling for patients and their families on cancer genetics, screening and preventative measures.

Medical oncologists are trained in the integration of systemic therapies such as chemotherapy, endocrine therapy, biological therapy and immunotherapy with the other modalities of treatment provided by the multidisciplinary team (MDT). They are trained in the highly developed communication skills required to fully involve patients in treatment decisions.

Their role is to assist in establishing the complete diagnosis and staging of the patient, to discuss and agree treatment options with the patient, and to supervise their treatment and any complications of the cancer or its treatment that may arise. They specialise in the introduction of new treatments through research trials and their application through audit.

ii Organisation of the service and patterns of referral

Primary, secondary and tertiary levels

Primary care The patient's GP usually initiates the referral for diagnosis and should remain integral to the continuing support and treatment of the cancer patient in the community. To this end, communication between the hospital-based medical oncology service and the GP is crucial so that the GP can provide appropriate supportive and anti-cancer medication, and assist in the management of toxicity, symptom control and terminal care.

Secondary and tertiary care Medical oncologists are linked to a tertiary cancer centre and a secondary cancer unit within a regional cancer network to a varying degree depending upon local arrangements.

Medical oncology forms part of a MDT with surgeons, specialist physicians, clinical oncologists, radiologists, pathologists, clinical nurse specialists, research practitioners and other professions allied to medicine (PAMs).

Clinical networks and community arrangements

Medical oncologists are expected to subspecialise in one to three tumour sites and to participate in the appropriate site-specific MDT and network tumour board to promote access to best quality cancer care throughout the unit/centre/network. They lead the development of systemic therapy standards of care according to nationally and locally agreed guidelines.

Following initial assessment it is common for patients to be cross-referred to the most expert and appropriate subspecialty tumour team according to diagnosis.

Relationship with other services/agencies

Medical oncology works closely with local support services both in the hospital and community, including physiotherapy, occupational therapy, social work, district nursing and hospice teams. Integration with palliative care services is vital in the provision of appropriate care.

Complementary services

Many patients will seek complementary therapies that help them exercise mind over body and the medical oncologist can provide guidance and enable them to integrate these with their allopathic treatment.

iii   Working with patients: patient-centred care

Patient choice and involving patients in decisions about their treatment

Medical oncology works with patients to provide a holistic approach to care that recognises their right to information, autonomy, support and guidance that is sensitive to their cultural background and appropriate to their knowledge and beliefs.

At all stages of care, information should be easily comprehensible to the patient and, if necessary, supported by appropriate interpreters and advocates. Options and consequences should be clearly described to the patient, who should be invited to participate in making treatment choices to the degree that they wish. Verbal information should be complemented with written material or other records that can be taken away by the patient.

Opportunity for education and patient support groups

Local self-help groups can improve patient education, and medical oncology provides staff education within the specialist oncology team, the general hospital and the community services that provide much of the patient care. Patients receiving palliative treatment need extra education and support to cope with their chronic condition. They need access to information not only within the hospital setting but also from local and national groups such as CancerBACUP.

iv   Interspecialty and interdisciplinary liaison

Working with other specialists

The majority of referrals to medical oncology come from specialist surgeons or physicians who have made a diagnosis or who wish to seek advice about a potential diagnosis.

The NHS Cancer Plan and, in particular, the two-week wait initiative requires that all suspected cancer patients referred urgently by their GP or consultant should be seen by an appropriate cancer specialist within two weeks.[1] By 2005, definitive treatment as agreed by the MDT should begin within four weeks of referral.

Multidisciplinary team working

All newly diagnosed patients should be discussed in the relevant MDT meeting and a recommended treatment plan agreed according to tumour-site guidelines and protocols. Continuing liaison between members of the MDT is necessary to refine and develop patients' treatment.

v   **Delivering a high quality service**

Characteristics of a high quality service

A high quality service can be judged by the criteria of patient satisfaction, adherence to national and network guidelines and accreditation standards, and the achievement of outcomes that are audited and compared with national cancer care standards and published reports.

Medical oncology works through the network tumour boards to lead the development of evidence-based treatment protocols and the integration of clinical research trials into patient care. Medical oncology usually leads the development of systemic therapy guidelines and the review of their application through the drugs and therapeutics boards of networks and trusts.

Collection of accurate information is vital to the practice of medical oncology in order to inform all the above developments. It is expected that the local databases currently used will be amalgamated into a national cancer dataset. With its tradition of research, medical oncology is well placed to lead the organisation of data collection and the audit of outcomes.

Contribution to the national collaborative studies of the National Cancer Research Network (NCRN) is expected of all medical oncology units together with more specialised translational research in those based in academic centres.

Resources required for a high quality service

Specialised facilities

■   outpatient clinics with appropriate support staff to act as patient advocates and chaperone clinical examination

■   joint or parallel tumour site-specific clinics with other clinicians in the MDT for common cancers

■   dedicated day care treatment ward with trained oncology nurses and medical supervision

■   pharmacy chemotherapy preparation suite with trained oncology pharmacists

■   inpatient beds on a dedicated oncology ward supported by an adequate number of trained oncology nurses and appropriate support staff

■   single rooms for the management of infection

■   on-site access to acute medical and surgical specialties and intensive care unit beds

■   emergency diagnostic services in pathology and radiology

■   IT support to access patient records, pathology and radiology reports and to enable computerised prescription of chemotherapy to minimise error.

Workforce requirements – clinical and support staff

The consultant medical oncologist can only function fully when supported by a MDT.

■   *Trainee medical staff* assist in patient care and outpatient clinics.

■   *Clinical nurse specialists* coordinate treatment, investigation and information and they should be available for all the common tumour sites. Their role includes counselling patients about their diagnosis and explaining treatment options and their consequences. They are the point of contact for patients and relatives to discuss issues relating to diagnosis or treatment and for emotional support.

- *Research nurses* recruit and treat patients in clinical trials. They should be present in all units within the NCRN to assist with assessment of patient eligibility for specific trials; counselling and explanation of treatment options and trial procedures in conjunction with the written patient information sheet; coordination of trial-related investigations and clinic visits; assessment of patients in trials and collection of case report forms.

- *Data managers* collect diagnostic information on all patient treatment and outcomes; complete case record forms; assist in preparing data records for external monitoring; and, together with research nurses, maintain trial conduct and data collection according to the principles of good clinical practice.

- *Oncology pharmacists and nurses* prepare, check, and administer treatment. They prepare chemotherapy in appropriate facilities, check all prescriptions and advise on drug interactions, protocol deviations and safety.

- *Secretaries and clerical staff* provide and file results of investigations and records of letters and MDT meetings.

vi Quality standards and measures of the quality of specialist services.

The NHS Cancer Plan published by the Department of Health (DH) sets down a broad framework of standards related to the diagnosis and treatment of cancer.[1] It describes the integration of cancer care and the importance of multidisciplinary working.

National cancer care standards are based on the NHS Cancer Plan and the *Improving outcomes guidance* and provide an extensive framework for measuring the quality of the care process for cancer centres and cancer units.[1,2] There is already a peer-review accreditation system coordinated by the Commission for Healthcare Audit and Inspection (CHAI) to monitor performance against these standards.

National Institute for Clinical Excellence (NICE) guidelines

The production of the series of *Improving outcomes guidance* is now coordinated by NICE.[2] They are generally site-specific, and provide guidance on the appropriate service framework for each disease or group of diseases. They define multidisciplinary standards of care for each stage of the care pathway.

NICE also produce health technology appraisals for oncology, which usually concern the appropriate use of new and existing anti-cancer drugs.

Specialist society guidelines

Publication of original research and meta-analyses in oncology journals provides outcome measures against which treatment of specific patient groups can be compared.

Medical oncology has developed specialty-specific standards of good medical practice which can be used for auditing medical oncologists. The Joint Collegiate Council for Oncology also provides standards of care against which the quality of a chemotherapy service can be assessed.

Standards for training accreditation are produced by the College, the Joint Council for Higher Medical Training (JCHMT) and the postgraduate medical and dental education deans. Standards for research governance derive from the Medical Research Council (MRC) and the European Union clinical trials directive.[3,4]

CLINICAL WORK OF CONSULTANTS IN MEDICAL ONCOLOGY

Contributions made to acute medicine

Very few medical oncology consultants now practise acute general medicine. Future training and subspecialisation requirements make this likely to cease entirely in the near future. Clinical governance requirements mean it is unlikely that a medical oncologist will maintain sufficient expertise in both acute general medicine and oncology.

All medical oncologists, however, are expected to treat critically ill patients with oncological emergencies such as neutropenic sepsis. They must maintain a general level of competence in internal medicine in order to coordinate the provision of cancer treatment with the frequent co-morbidities of an often elderly population, and to recognise when to refer for specialist assistance.

Direct clinical care

The medical oncologist is the leader and coordinator of an extended team of professionals who aim to provide optimum cancer care for the patient and to define the appropriate objectives for diagnosis, cure, palliation and terminal care.

Most cancer patients receive their care in the outpatient setting of clinics and day care wards, supported by sufficient inpatient facilities for intensive diagnosis, treatment and management of complications.

Consultant job plans in medical oncology are currently evolving with the 2003 contract but, in general, a full-time equivalent would comprise 7.5 programmed activities (PAs) of direct clinical care with each four-hour outpatient clinic likely to require one to two hours subsequent patient administration activity (to a maximum of four outpatient clinics and two administration PAs per week).

Other direct care activities to be included are MDT meetings, a minimum of one inpatient ward round per week, and clinical management responsibilities of lead clinician, clinical director, training director or rotation organiser. The number of ward rounds will vary according to the frequency of acute illness in the patients and the composition of the clinical team.

The remaining 2.5 PAs comprise the supporting professional activities of teaching and training, audit and clinical governance, continuing professional development (CPD), research participation in NCRN trials, and translational research in academic centres. Specialist skills may be developed through a wide variety of activities from, for example, intensive high-dose chemotherapy to palliative care.

Clinically related administration will vary with the type of patients seen, the complexity of treatment and the availability of appropriate support staff. Most outpatient clinics will entail one to two hours of direct clinical care administration for the organisation and prescription of patient treatment.

Work to maintain and improve the quality of care

Leadership role and development of the service

Coordination of cancer patient care through regular MDT meetings has improved patient access to oncological care and the timeliness of delivery. Medical oncology continues to develop MDTs for all tumour sites.

Cancer medicine and systemic therapy are undergoing rapid change with the development of multiple diagnostic tools and treatment modalities. The assessment and introduction of this new technology has, for the most part, been led by medical oncology with emphasis on audit and research.

Medical oncology has typically assumed responsibility for the coordination and continuing care of patients with complex cancer treatment and needs to ensure that the care pathways deliver timely and appropriate treatment.

Medical oncology promotes awareness of the principles of good cancer care throughout the extended medical community through hospital-based teaching and educational activities in primary care. It also generates improved patient awareness of how to access and attain good quality care through careful dissemination of information and local self-help groups.

In addition, medical oncologists frequently take on extra leadership roles as clinical director, medical director, director of clinical trials units, lead clinician for cancer networks and as advisers for a variety of organisations such as the Association of Cancer Physicians (the medical oncology specialist society), the Royal College of Physicians, the Joint Collegiate Council for Oncology, the DH, cancer charities and ethics committees.

Clinical governance

With its tradition of audit and research, medical oncology is strongly orientated towards maintaining clinical effectiveness through the application of staff appraisal, CPD, audit and the acceptance of responsibility for clinical governance.

Other specialist activity beyond local services

Most medical oncologists will be based in a cancer centre and provide a number of direct clinical care PAs in a peripheral cancer unit within their network. For some, the principal site of activity and hence inpatient admitting rights and responsibilities is within a district general hospital (DGH) cancer unit and they will visit their cancer centre for a limited number of PAs relating to audit, research and CPD. The activities at the secondary site may include MDT meetings and a range of outpatient consultation and treatment services but should not involve sole responsibility for inpatient care.

If the secondary site is a cancer unit then arrangements must be made for local consultant cover (for example a haematologist or a general physician) with appropriate protocols for the care of oncological emergencies.

ACADEMIC MEDICINE

Academic medical oncologists should expect a reduced clinical commitment of six PAs per week for direct clinical care and, consequently, four or more PAs for teaching and research.

Those who retain clinical activities will be expected to participate in local clinical teams and duty rotas and to lead their particular field of research activity within a cancer centre and the wider cancer network.

Additional academic duties may include teaching both undergraduates and postgraduates, examining and inspecting at other institutions, and participation in national societies and research committees.

The training and supervision of specialist registrars (SpRs) in medical oncology is becoming more detailed and time consuming. A new competency-based curriculum has been developed in which the formal assessment of competence in practical procedures and the assessment of knowledge, skills and attitudes of the aspiring medical oncologist will fall to the existing consultant body. Assessment tools are being developed which will include mini clinical examination (mini-CEX), 360-degree appraisal and direct observation of clinical procedures. Many of these assessments are designed to be conducted in the course of a normal outpatient clinic or ward round. Consultant medical oncologists who are regularly involved in supervision of trainees will see fewer patients in a fixed four-hour period in the clinic or the wards than previously.

Academic medical oncology continues to be influential in the design of national and international clinical trials, the development of new therapies, the exploration of new translational ideas and the conduct of basic laboratory research.

WORKFORCE REQUIREMENTS FOR MEDICAL ONCOLOGY

In 2000, the College recommended a figure of 1.25 WTE medical oncologists per 200,000–250,000 population. This requires about 250 WTE, equating to a total of approximately 300 medical oncologists in the UK. In November 2000, there were 138 medical oncologists in the UK, this figure rising to 196 in January 2004. There is, therefore, still a substantial shortfall against the figure recommended in 2000. An increase of 53% is required urgently to reach the figure of 300 medical oncologists. However, treatment options for patients with common cancers have increased substantially in the past three years leading to a significantly greater workload for medical oncologists. Therefore, it is likely that the current workforce requirement for medical oncology in the UK is actually a minimum of 400 posts, which represents an increase of 120%.

CONSULTANT WORK PROGRAMME/SPECIMEN JOB PLAN

The workload of a medical oncologist, measured by the number of new patient referrals seen per year, should be approximately 200. This takes into consideration the continuing care required by most patients over repeated episodes of treatment and the intensive monitoring required for chemotherapy treatment. This figure will depend upon the subspeciality interest and casemix of the consultant's practice.

Academic medical oncologists with a reduced direct clinical care commitment and a correspondingly greater teaching and research requirement should see approximately 100–150 new patients per year. However, due to the lack of specialist oncologists in much of the UK, the current workload of the majority of medical oncologists will exceed these figures.

An on-call rota of oncology specialists should provide 24-hour emergency cover, if necessary in conjunction with colleagues from haematology or clinical oncology to ensure sufficient numbers for a rota, which should not exceed one in five.

The volume of on-call work will depend on the patient practice of the oncologist, the intensity of treatment, and the trainee staff cover. It varies from telephone advice with the occasional requirement for attendance (category B), to frequently required urgent attendance on, for example, transplant units or where only limited general medical senior house officer (SHO) cover is available (category A). Further alterations in rotas may be required by the introduction of the European Working Time Directive.

Activity	Workload	Programmed activities (PAs)
Direct clinical care	Clinical research is an integral part of all clinical PAs for a medical oncologist	
Outpatient clinic	3–4 new patient consultations per week: approx 1 hour each. Routine follow-up of well patients: 10–15 minutes consultation. Management of patients with relapsed or metastatic disease: approximately 30 minutes.	**3–4**
Day care ward work	May form part of a mixed outpatient clinic. Patient assessment and chemotherapy prescribing: approximately 30 minutes	**1–2**
Clinical administration		**2**
Inpatient ward rounds	Number of patients will vary depending on nature of practice 5 –20 would be typical	**1–2**
MDT meetings	Frequency and duration will vary according to size of MDT sessions, up to 4 hours is not uncommon	**1–2**
Total number of direct clinical care PAs		**7.5 on average**
Supporting professional activities (SPA)		
Work to maintain and improve the quality of healthcare	Education and training, clinical trials and research, appraisal, departmental management and service development, audit and clinical governance, CPD and revalidation	**2.5 on average**
Other NHS responsibilities	eg medical director/clinical director/lead consultant in specialty/clinical tutor	**Local agreement with trust**
External duties	eg work for deaneries/Royal Colleges/specialist societies/Department of Health or other government bodies etc	**Local agreement with trust**

Note: Medical oncologists, particularly in academic centres, may work with other consultant medical oncologists as part of a team sharing the outpatient and inpatient care of a group of patients. In this case, responsibilities may vary weekly or monthly, for which an annualised job plan is required.

References

1. Department of Health. *The NHS cancer plan: a plan for investment, a plan for reform.* London: DH, 2000.

2. National Institute for Clinical Excellence. *Improving outcomes guidance.* www.nice.org.uk/page.aspx?o=guidelines. completed.

3. Medical Research Council. *Guidelines for good clinical practice in clinical trials.* London: MRC, 1998.

4. Directive 2001/20/EC of the European Parliament and of the Council of the European Union. *Official Journal of the European Communities* 2001;L121:34–44. www.europa.eu.int/eur-lex/en/search/search_lif.html

Neurology

i   Description of the specialty and clinical needs of patients

Neurology is the branch of medicine dealing with disorders of the nervous system, including the brain, spinal cord, peripheral nerves and muscle. These can be conditions managed almost entirely in the community (epilepsy and migraine), acute neurological emergencies (stroke and meningitis) or chronic disabling conditions (dementia, multiple sclerosis and Parkinson's disease).

Specialist care is provided by consultant neurologists, increasingly in collaboration with specialist nurses, members of the professions allied to medicine, and other physicians and surgeons including primary care physicians. Neurologists provide a clinical lead in these teams and promote the cause of their patients.

Many neurologists have other roles in undergraduate and postgraduate education or research and clinical governance, and they may be involved in service planning for people with neurological disorders.

Academic neurologists are appointed by universities, the Medical Research Council (MRC) and occasionally by other agencies. They promote research and teaching of university students in addition to providing patient care and teaching other health professionals. They have an important responsibility in the planning and implementation of neurology teaching to both undergraduates and postgraduates and may have more general university responsibilities. They are likely to have fewer clinical responsibilities than is usual for other neurologists.

Patients referred to neurologists may have straightforward disorders or highly complex and unusual conditions. Sixteen common diseases account for 75% of all new outpatient referrals – the investigation and management of which have become more complex in the light of new medical and surgical treatments. The remaining 25% of patients have more unusual disorders, which may require expert assessment, sophisticated investigation and elaborate treatment. Without exception, patients need prompt, effective and competent diagnosis and treatment.

The model of care for neurological services in the future will be laid out in the National Service Framework (NSF) for Long-Term Conditions.

ii   Organisation of the service and patterns of referral

Primary, secondary and tertiary levels

All patients with significant neurological symptoms need a diagnosis and prompt appropriate treatment. This can be achieved by rapid access to a local high quality neurological service which is part of a clinical neuroscience network. The network should include a group of local neurological services functioning in local hospitals and the community which are linked with neurology and neuroscience centres, share common protocols and guidelines, and use specialist services that may be based only in some parts of the network.

Neurology and neurosurgery centres   Neurology and neurosurgery centres are crucial to the provision of high quality care and are staffed by neurologists, neurosurgeons, clinical neurophysiologists, neuroradiologists, neuropathologists, neuropsychologists and other specialist staff. All relevant modern investigative equipment should be available. Where all the neuroscience specialties are based at such centres an appropriate environment is created for the management of both the more common disorders and rarer complex conditions that often require input from more than one professional. All neurologists should be attached to a neurology and neurosurgery centre to ensure that patients have equitable access to high quality facilities for care, including other specialist opinions on rare disorders, and to ensure high quality continuing professional development (CPD).

Neurology centres   Neurologists work together in neurology centres to provide a general and special interest neurological service with clinical neurophysiology, neuroradiology and neurorehabilitation services, but without inpatient neurosurgery facilities. It is anticipated that the number of these centres will increase.

Most acute hospitals have neurological outpatient departments but the extent of neurology consultant involvement in the management of inpatients at district general hospitals (DGHs) varies greatly depending on local circumstances. In many cases support is limited to advising the local admitting physician. With the increasing number of neurologists and a potential reduction in the involvement of general physicians in the care of those with neurological diseases, there is a trend towards the establishment of local neurological beds. An on-call service with adequate support services, facilities, beds, and senior and junior staffing has been introduced for the admission of neurological emergencies.

Some general neurology services are being devolved to community level where general practitioners with a special interest (GPSI) in neurology and nurse specialists take a lead in the diagnosis and management of patients. Neurologists will be involved in this development, providing training and supervising staff.

Clinical networks and community arrangements

Neurology is included in the national specialist services definitions set, and primary care trust (PCT) consortia should commission services.[1] Increasingly, neurological services are being organised and commissioned on a network basis to ensure equity of access and to meet national targets. This may change if practice-based commissioning is developed.

Relationship with other services/agencies

Closer links between the community rehabilitation teams, the local hospital and the regional neuroscience or neurology centre should provide seamless care so that rigid boundaries are removed from every level of the service. Neurologists should be part of the multidisciplinary teams (MDTs) providing care for all patients with chronic neurological diseases. These teams include specialist and general nurses, physiotherapists, speech and language therapists, occupational therapists, dietitians and social care workers. Within each district, a neurologist should work with the MDT for patient care in each major chronic neurological condition. Rapid access to these therapy services in the community is essential.

Complementary services

Neurologists do not routinely provide complementary services, though many of their patients use them for pain relief and the treatment of mechanical disorders of the spine.

iii   Working with patients: patient-centred care

Patient choice and involving patients in decisions about their treatment

At every stage, neurologists keep patients informed and involved in planning their care. Following the initial outpatient consultation and investigation a diagnosis can usually be made and treatment plans discussed with the patient, their family and the GP. A minority will require ongoing care, for which a detailed plan should be made jointly with the patient, the GP and, where relevant, rehabilitation services and other local community services. People with neurological conditions should be able to access the most appropriate part of the service at all times. Where indicated clinically they should have easy access to services at the regional neuroscience or neurology centre.

Neurologists aim to take account of the wishes and aspirations of their patients and respect and work within their ethical and religious traditions wherever possible.

Opportunities for education and promoting self-care

At present, patient education is often undertaken by specialist nurses and others rather than neurologists, partly because of the scarcity of neurological services. Good quality information is widely available from the Association of British Neurologists (ABN) and patient groups. Neurological patients are encouraged to develop strategies for self-care. Those with chronic disorders such as multiple sclerosis are particularly adept at this.

Patients with chronic conditions

Long-term management and care strategies are required for the common chronic disabling neurological disorders such as stroke, dementia, epilepsy, Parkinson's disease and multiple sclerosis, and for many less prevalent conditions, including motor neurone disease and muscular dystrophy. Where relevant, a key worker should be appointed to assist in the patient's management, especially at the interfaces between health and social services, vocational re-entry and education.

Neurologists are often part of the team providing palliative care for their patients. Particular skills are required to provide care in the final phase of chronic, deteriorating conditions. In some, such as motor neurone disease, input is appropriate from the point of diagnosis. Patients, carers and family need to be kept fully informed about the prognosis and the range of services available, whether in a hospice, nursing home or their own home. It is essential to coordinate pain control, and emotional and psychological care. Neurological teams should support carers and family with practical issues after death and offer bereavement counselling. All of this requires a new approach to train neurological palliative care staff and volunteers and to support the emotional well being of these staff.

Access to information, patient support groups and the role of the expert patient

Patients should have access to high quality information about their neurological condition, investigations and treatment. People with neurological conditions, carers and local branches of neurological charities, together with a wide range of healthcare workers, all contribute to discussions about how neurological services can best be delivered and promoted in each district.

Increasingly, neurological patients are experts in their condition and can expect to be part of the MDT as expert patients. This patient expertise must be recognised by non-neurological hospital staff, for instance in the control of medication during a routine surgical admission.

Availability of clinical records/results

Since many neurological conditions are lifelong, patient records should be universally available to all treating agencies. This may become increasingly possible by electronic means.

iv   Interspecialty and interdisciplinary liaison

Multidisciplinary team working

The key to improving neurology services locally is a closer working partnership of neurologists and other neurological staff with primary care and social services, to offer a coordinated, comprehensive care package incorporating all relevant aspects of the local health system. This should include care and support in the interval between referral and the appointment with a neurologist.

Working with other specialists

People with chronic neurological conditions need to be under the direct care of a designated specialist who is skilled, available and who has access to the appropriate resources. This may be a neurologist or an elderly care physician, psychogeriatrician, clinical geneticist or consultant in rehabilitation medicine. Joint care may be appropriate so long as clinical responsibility is defined clearly. Care may be given by a neurological nurse specialist or other paramedical specialist with appropriate competencies but there must be direct access to an appropriate neurological specialist. More nurses are needed with a special interest in the major common neurological diseases (epilepsy, stroke, dementia, multiple sclerosis, Parkinson's disease and motor neurone disease). More nurses with broader expertise in neurological conditions are also needed. If such nurses are well integrated in the regional neuroscience network they can play a major role in improving and hastening appropriate care and in liaison and communication. Advice and support from neurologically trained staff should be available to patients who have a chronic neurological problem such as Parkinson's disease and are admitted to other wards or units.

Working with GP specialists

Neurologically trained GPSIs should play a greater role at the interfaces between community, primary, secondary and tertiary care to improve clinical care, communication, information and access to services. Neurologists need to work closely with GPSIs, nurse specialists and other healthcare professionals to explore the most effective way to meet outpatient standards and to consider new ways of delivering services. The confidence and competence of GPs in handling common outpatient neurological problems should be enhanced if they work more closely with neurologists. Shared care protocols and guidelines are being developed to offer wider access to appropriate key investigations, including computed tomography (CT). The aim is to break down traditional divisions between primary, secondary and tertiary-based practice, to provide a seamless high quality neurological service based around local needs as part of the broader neurosciences network.

v   **Delivering a high quality service**

Characteristics of a high quality service

Neurologists want to ensure that people with neurological conditions have timely access to a high quality, comprehensive, coordinated, patient-centred and expert service, with equity of provision regardless of geography, age, race and gender. Neurologists need to explore the optimal sites for general neurology outpatient clinics with commissioners, including GPs. These may include community-based clinics in addition to local hospital outpatient departments. All emergency admissions with acute neurological problems to a local hospital should be placed under the care of consultant neurologists and their teams. These standards cannot be achieved without a significant increase in the number of neurologists and a change in the way neurologists work.

Short outpatient waiting times must be achieved. The NHS Plan requires that, by the end of 2005, patients referred by GPs must wait no longer than 12 weeks.[2] These waiting times must be considerably reduced so that routine patients can be seen within four weeks. Outpatients considered urgent by the referring clinician or neurologist should not wait more than a week. These goals may be achievable by having a neurology outpatient clinic in each district every weekday. A designated consultant neurologist in each district should be easily accessible on a daily basis (including weekends) to speak to GPs directly about urgent clinical concerns.

In addition to general follow-up neurology clinics, specialist clinics are being established at local hospitals for the common neurological conditions (multiple sclerosis, epilepsy, Parkinson's disease, stroke and dementia). These clinics need the support of doctors, allied health professionals, specialist nurses and other professionals. They will foster team-based working in order to provide patients with a full range of facilities. Patients with specific and unusually complex conditions should be reviewed in specialist multidisciplinary clinics where time is available to address their needs and those of their carers. Neurologists will need to access such clinics and will often be involved in their management.

Resources required for a high quality service

Specialised facilities

An increase in neurological beds to approximately 15 per 100,000 of the population is needed. Until these facilities are introduced all patients admitted to a local hospital with a major neurological problem should at least have immediate access to an expert neurological opinion and be assessed by a neurologist within 24 hours, or possibly via a telemedicine link. Neurosurgery and certain neurological emergencies require rapid access to the designated regional neuroscience centre, for which adequate numbers of neurocritical care beds are essential.

Neurological conditions should be investigated soon after consultation with a neurologist. Where possible, and where the patient desires it, a one-stop service should enable consultation and investigations on the same day. Adequate access to brain imaging is vital – emergency CT brain scanning in all local hospitals is needed 24 hours a day, seven days a week, and greater access to out-of-hours emergency magnetic resonance imaging (MRI) facilities is required. Emergency and routine scans should be reported by a neuroradiologist in person or by imaging link. Routine waiting times for CT or MRI should not exceed four weeks.

A clinical neurophysiology service is required by the local neurological service for electro-encephalogram (EEG) and electromyogram (EMG) investigations. The service should offer urgent appointments in local hospitals for emergency admissions, and routine appointments within four weeks for an EEG and eight weeks for an EMG. An adequate neuropsychology service is necessary and should be based locally.

Workforce requirements: clinical and support staff

The workforce must include sufficient trained neurologists to meet this service, together with an adequate number of trainees. Neurological teams will include neurologically trained nurses and allied healthcare professionals. This will need to be mirrored in the community with enhanced training for GPs and trained GPSIs. There is a need to increase the pool of neurophysiological measurement technicians, radiographers and psychologists who have the skills to investigate people with neurological disorders.

vi Quality standards and measures of the quality of specialist services

Specialist society guidelines

- *Acute neurological emergencies in adults.*[3] (**www.theabn.org/downloads/AcuteNeurology.pdf**)
- *Neurology in the United Kingdom: numbers of clinical neurologists and trainees.*[4] (**www.theabn.org/downloads/neurology numbers.pdf**)
- *Neurology in the United Kingdom: towards 2000 and beyond.*[5] (**www.theabn.org/downloads/2000 and beyond.pdf**)
- *Levelling up: Neurological Alliance 2002.*[6] (**www.neurologicalalliance.org.uk/docs/levelling_up/level.pdf**)
- *Academic neurology in the United Kingdom: threats, opportunities and recommendations for the future.*[7] (**www.theabn.org/downloads/CRAC-full-version-2003.pdf**)
- *Standards of care for people with neurological disorders.*[8] (**www.theabn.org/downloads/Jun%2004-standards4-GSV.pdf**)

National Institute for Clinical Excellence (NICE) guidelines

- Alzheimer's disease: donepezil, rivastigmine and galantamine (No. 19).[9] (**www.nice.org.uk/cat.asp?c=14400**)
- Motor neurone disease: riluzole (No. 20) (**www.nice.org.uk/cat.asp?c=14401**).[10]
- Multiple sclerosis: beta interferon and glatiramer acetate (No. 32).[11] (**www.nice.org.uk/cat.asp?c=27588**)
- Multiple sclerosis: management of multiple sclerosis in primary and secondary care.[12] (**www.nice.org.uk/cat.asp?c=27588**)
- Head injury: triage, assessment, investigation and early management of head injury in infants, children and adults.[13] (**www.nice.org.uk/cat.asp?c=56817**)
- Epilepsy: the diagnosis and care of children and adults with epilepsy.[14] (**www.nice.org.uk/cat.asp?c=229249**)

Clinical governance

Neurologists should not work in isolation and should either be attached to a specified neurology and neurosurgery centre, or be a member of a neurosciences network with a single contract of employment. Neurologists should have a base hospital at which the majority of their clinical work and other duties are undertaken. None should work at more than two trusts. Days split between two sites should be avoided whenever possible.

CLINICAL WORK AND/OR LABORATORY WORK OF CONSULTANTS IN NEUROLOGY

Contributions made to acute medicine

Most neurologists have no direct involvement with the acute medical take. Increasingly, however, they are involved in the acute care of people with neurological disorders as recommended in *Acute neurological emergencies in adults*.[3]

Direct clinical care

Direct clinical care involves work relating to the prevention, diagnosis or treatment of neurological illness, and emergency work carried out during, or arising from, on call, ward rounds, outpatient activities, clinical diagnostic work, other patient treatment, MDT meetings about direct patient care and related administration. This also includes the time spent supervising specialist nurses and non-consultant grade staff and trainees.

Inpatient work

Inpatient work may take the form of ward rounds, consulting on patients on other wards (ward liaison) and care of emergency admissions on the neurology unit or in intensive care. Job plans should assign one to three sessions for this purpose, including all relevant administration. Liaison with MDTs and other staff, discharge planning, writing discharge summaries and patient-related administration following ward liaison are also inpatient activities.

Outpatient work

The number of outpatient clinics will depend on other duties, in particular the amount of inpatient work. The ABN recommends that a job plan should not normally contain more than three outpatient sessions, including subspecialty clinics, in a week, each of which will normally be no more than a full (four-hour) programmed activity (PA).

When consultants are expected to spend time on more than one site, travel time must be included as working time within a programmed direct clinical care activity, either as additional paid time or by a corresponding reduction in clinical activity.

It is expected that the number of clinics per session per year would take account of other clinical duties (including ward work), teaching, holidays and study leave and lie between 38 and 44 clinics per session. Definitions of new and old patients can be found on the ABN website. Clinics should be reduced by 25% if trainees or students are to be supervised. The time to be allocated per neurological outpatient, as suggested by ABN, is:

- 30 minutes per new patient for a consultant appointment or 40 minutes for a specialist registrar (SpR)
- 15 minutes per follow-up patient for a consultant appointment or 20 minutes for a SpR.

Specialist investigative and therapeutic procedures

Most neurologists do not undertake investigative or therapeutic procedures, with the exception of activities such as botulinum toxin injection. This may change in the future with carotid stenting, the introduction of thrombolysis in acute stroke and the management of implanted devices in patients with movement disorders.

Specialist on call

On-call duties should not exceed one in three with appropriate remuneration in accordance with nationally agreed terms and conditions.

Other specialist activity

This would not normally form part of a neurologist job plan although some neurologists have regional or supra-regional clinical responsibilities.

Clinically related administration

The ABN recommends that a minimum of an additional 50% of time per clinic is included in direct clinical care for:

- responses to referrals (including the grading of letters) by telephone, email or other means
- administration relating to patients attending clinics, such as arranging and reviewing investigations, giving any further opinion, and arranging for copy and other letters to be sent to patients.

Work to maintain and improve the quality of care

Leadership role and development of the service

This is an integral component of the activity of many neurologists, especially those with clinical director roles. Provision must be made in the job plan for local clinical management, governance, unit meetings, audit and other meetings to support patient care and service development.

Education and training

This varies between university NHS trusts and 'non-teaching' trusts, but should be an identified component of the job plan where applicable. Allowance must be made for educational supervision, competence assessment and training needs for neurology trainees and others. The extent of this allowance will vary considerably depending on the role and seniority of a participating trainee, whether non-participating health professionals are present and whether undergraduate students needing teaching are present. A set period should be allocated in the weekly job plan for these activities.

Mentoring and appraisal of medical staff and other professional staff

Neurologists are involved extensively in mentoring and appraisal of junior medical staff and other team members.

Continuing medical education

Continuing medical education must be included in the job plan. A minimum of one PA or two half PAs for attending postgraduate educational meetings and for private study is recommended. On occasions, the meetings will involve the neurologist in teaching colleagues and neurological trainees. Provision and funding for 10 days study leave per annum for consultant neurologists is mandatory.

Clinical governance

All neurologists should be aware of the requirement for clinical governance.

Research – clinical studies and basic science

Consultants should understand research governance and be encouraged to continue research with up to one PA per week being made available where appropriate.

Local management duties

The following responsibilities, which are not usually undertaken by the generality of consultants, should be agreed between a consultant and the employer and cannot be absorbed within the time that would normally be set aside for supporting professional activities:

▪ medical director or director of public health

▪ clinical director or lead clinician

▪ Caldicott guardian

▪ clinical audit or governance lead

▪ undergraduate or postgraduate dean

▪ clinical tutor or regional education adviser.

Regional and national work

▪ trade union duties

▪ inspections for the Commission for Healthcare and Inspection (CHAI)

▪ external member of an advisory appointments committee

▪ assessments for the National Clinical Assessment Authority

▪ work for the Royal Colleges in the interests of the wider NHS, eg as examiner or member of a specialist advisory committee

▪ work for a government department

▪ specified work for the General Medical Council (GMC)

▪ work for the ABN.

ACADEMIC MEDICINE

Academic departments of neurology are based mainly at university medical schools and remain vital for the development of quality neurological services and for the training of undergraduates and postgraduates.

Clinical contribution to NHS

Academic departments are usually linked closely to neurology and neurosurgery centres. Such departments should be well integrated with local clinical services, and should support research and educational activities undertaken by NHS staff at all levels in the neuroscience network.

Teaching

Academic departments of clinical neurology should play a major role in the coordination and teaching of undergraduate basic neuroscience and clinical neurology.

Research

The future development of neurological services should benefit from health services research. Effective clinical networks increase opportunities for many forms of research, including randomised trials and observational epidemiology.

WORKFORCE REQUIREMENTS FOR NEUROLOGY

At present there is one neurologist per 140,000 population in England. To provide comprehensive neurological care, including the care of the acutely ill neurological patient, one whole time equivalent (WTE) consultant neurologist is required per 40,000 population.

Table 1. Current workforce

	Department of Health (September 2003)[15]	Department of Health – WTE
Consultants (England)	410	355
National training numbers (NTN) (UK stock)	190	166
Senior house officers (SHO) (UK)	149	144
Associate specialists (UK)	8	5
Staff grades (UK)	15	12
Hospital practitioners/clinical assistants (UK)	65	15

(Note: there are about 10 neurologists who are not members of the ABN, mostly in independent practice.)

Consultant workforce requirements to manage new referrals to neurology clinics

Assuming there are approximately 320,000 new referrals to neurology clinics per year, based on the figure of 79,972 in the second quarter of 2003, and assuming that neurologists have an average of three clinics per week with six new patients per clinic, then 423 WTE are required to meet outpatient demand in England. This equates to 2.16 WTE per 250,000 population or one neurologist to 115,000 population.

Increasing numbers of follow-up cases and the effects of the NSF in facilitating re-entry into the neurology service, suggest that current manpower projections may underestimate the true need.

Consultant workforce requirements to provide acute care for people with neurological disorders

There are a number of models of care that can be used. Previously, ABN guidelines have recommended one neurologist per 100,000 of the population, which requires approximately 600 WTE neurologists in the UK, with 2.5 WTE in each DGH.[4] Assuming that academic neurologists spend time in a DGH, the numbers would be made up of 560–570 NHS neurologists and 78 academic neurologists.

To provide a 24-hour service in every DGH requires five consultant neurologists per hospital (excluding academic neurologists who tend to be based at centres), making a total of 1,250.

Other neurologists are based primarily at neurology and neurosurgery centres. At least five are needed at each neurosurgery centre to deliver the basic 24-hour service. With approximately 35 such centres nationally, an additional 175 neurologists will be needed.

In summary, this model demands 1,250 NHS neurologists, 175 centre-based neurologists and 78 academic neurologists, which gives a total of approximately 1,400 nationally, or a population ratio of 1:43,000.

This model represents an excellent aspiration but it is not a realistic possibility as there are currently insufficient neurologists in training. Additional NTNs and recruitment from overseas may help but neurology faces recruitment difficulties in common with other specialties. In 2003, 23.5% of consultant posts were unfilled following advertisement. A more desirable and realistic target is 909 WTE across the UK by 2012 (3.9 WTE for 250,000 population).

Present numbers of SpRs are insufficient to generate the expansion required to deliver this service and neurologists will need to come from other health systems. However, even if this level of penetration of neurological services into the country was ever achieved, the workforce would still be between a half and a third of the number of neurologists currently found in almost every other European country. (In Europe, the population per neurologist is between 8,100 and 38,500, which contrasts to the current UK ratio of 177,000 population per neurologist.)

CONSULTANT WORK PROGRAMME/SPECIMEN JOB PLAN

Activity	Workload	Programmed activities (PAs)
Direct clinical care Inpatient work including ward rounds	10–15 patients	**2**
Ward liaison and emergencies		**1–2**
MDT including radiology meetings and other clinical administration		**1–2**
Outpatient work including travel	6 new patients	**3**
Total number of direct clinical care PAs		**7.5 on average**
Supporting professional activities (SPA) Work to maintain and improve the quality of healthcare	Education and training, appraisal, departmental management and service development, audit and clinical governance, CPD and revalidation, research	**2.5 on average**
Other NHS responsibilities	eg medical director/clinical director/lead consultant in specialty/clinical tutor	**Local agreement with trust**
External duties	eg work for deaneries/Royal Colleges/specialist societies/Department of Health or other government bodies etc	**Local agreement with trust**

References

1. Department of Health. *Specialised services national definition set: Specialised neurosciences services (adult) – definition no. 8*, December 2002. www.dh.gov.uk/PolicyAndGuidance/HealthAndSocialCareTopics/SpecialisedServices Definition/fs/en

2. Department of Health. *The NHS plan: a plan for investment, a plan for reform.* London: DH, 2000.

3. Association of British Neurologists. *Acute neurological emergencies in adults.* London: ABN, 2002. www.theabn.org/downloads/AcuteNeurology.pdf

4. *Neurology in the United Kingdom: numbers of clinical neurologists and trainees.* London: ABN, 1996. www.theabn.org/downloads/neurology numbers.pdf

5. *Neurology in the United Kingdom: towards 2000 and beyond.* London: ABN, 1997. www.theabn.org/downloads/2000 and beyond.pdf

6. Neurological Alliance. *Levelling up.* London: Neurological Alliance, 2002. www.neurologicalalliance.org.uk/ docs/levelling_up/level.pdf

7. Association of British Neurologists Clinical Research and Academic Committee. *Academic neurology in the United Kingdom: threats, opportunities and recommendations for the future.* London: ABN, 2003. www.theabn.org/ downloads/CRAC-full-version-2003.pdf

8. Association of British Neurologists. *Standards of care for people with neurological disorders.* London: ABN, 2003. www.theabn.org/downloads/Jun%2004-standards4-GSV.pdf

9. National Institute for Clinical Excellence. *Alzheimer's disease: donepezil, rivastigmine and galantamine (No. 19)*, January 2001. www.nice.org.uk/cat.asp?c=14400

10. National Institute for Clinical Excellence. *Motor neurone disease: riluzole (No. 20)*, January 2001. www.nice.org.uk/cat.asp?c=14401.

11. National Institute for Clinical Excellence. *Multiple sclerosis: beta interferon and glatiramer acetate (No. 32)*, February 2002. www.nice.org.uk/cat.asp?c=27588

12. National Institute for Clinical Excellence. *Multiple sclerosis: management of multiple sclerosis in primary and secondary care*, February 2002. www.nice.org.uk/cat.asp?c=27588

13. National Institute for Clinical Excellence. *Head injury: triage, assessment, investigation and early management of head injury in infants, children and adults*, June 2003. www.nice.org.uk/cat.asp?c=56817

14. National Institute for Clinical Excellence. *Epilepsy: the diagnosis and care of children and adults with epilepsy*, October 2004. www.nice.org.uk/cat.asp?c=229249

15. www.publications.doh.gov.uk/stats/d_results.htm

Nuclear medicine

i   Description of the specialty and clinical needs of patients

Nuclear medicine comprises all applications of radioactive materials in diagnosis, therapy and research, with the exception of the use of sealed radiation sources in therapy. Nuclear medicine deals with a wide range of pathology across all age ranges, but specific clinical practice involves major input in oncology, cardiology, nephro-urology, orthopaedics, rheumatology and neuropsychiatry.

The pursuit of this field requires a highly specialised team, of which a well-trained nuclear medicine physician is a central component. In contrast to Europe, Canada, USA and Australia, the specialty in the UK has lagged behind in terms of recognition and funding.

The range and complexity of diagnostic investigations has increased considerably in recent years, reflecting both continuing radiopharmaceutical development and the wider availability of tomographic cameras. Through the use of receptor-specific ligands, monoclonal antibodies and small peptides, there are now tracers available for tissue recognition at molecular level.

Advances in drug radio-labelling and delivery systems have led to a parallel expansion in unsealed source therapy, extending the range of conditions that can be treated by this approach. This, together with the expanding role of nuclear cardiology studies in coronary heart disease, the rising importance of positron emission tomography (PET) in cancer staging and follow up, and the delivery of sentinel node imaging in patients with breast cancer and melanoma, will have a major impact upon future workload patterns.

In research, single photon emission computed tomography (SPECT) and PET are now seen as essential tools in new pharmaceutical evaluation, if not discovery. Gene therapy is being monitored with labelled vectors with first applications emerging in cardiology. The field is involved in the development of new ligands for specific syndromes, such as movement disorders, schizophrenia, Alzheimer's disease, the unstable plaque in CAD and thromboembolic disease, and in specific functional biology signals such as apoptosis, hypoxia and neo-angiogenesis.

ii   Organisation of the service and patterns of referral

Nuclear medicine services are hospital based. Provision varies according to the size and casemix of the population served and reflects the degree of centralisation of nuclear medicine services within individual hospitals. Service delivery varies between hospitals of different types.[1] Small departments undertaking a limited range of diagnostic investigations follow an outpatient clinic model and are often organised within departments of radiology. Larger centres offering a comprehensive range of both imaging and non-imaging diagnostic procedures and unsealed source therapy require day care and dedicated inpatient facilities. Often both types of department offer the bone densitometry service and occasionally specialist bone clinics for osteoporosis management.

In most centres, nuclear medicine studies are performed in one department within the hospital, but the service is delivered in one of two ways. There may be specialist nuclear medicine practitioners, either physicians or radiologists, covering the full range of procedures, or individual practitioners may be responsible for specific clinical aspects aligned to their main specialty. Examples of the latter would be several system-specific radiologists, a cardiologist for nuclear cardiology or an endocrinologist for thyroid therapy, all with further training in radionuclide procedures. The way in which the service is delivered in individual hospitals reflects how it has developed historically depending on funding, local expertise and the interests of individual practitioners.

Currently, not all hospitals have on-site nuclear medicine facilities, but access to these services is required in most hospitals. Surveys indicate that some trusts are performing only a small number of non-imaging nuclear medicine procedures annually, raising questions of service quality.[1] Taken with predicted manpower shortages, an urgent review of nuclear medicine service delivery in the UK was undertaken by the Intercollegiate Standing Committee in 2003.[2] A 'hub-and-spoke' model was proposed, based upon the existing specialist nuclear medicine departments and the cancer centre framework. It was recommended that priority be given to ensuring nuclear medicine specialist support for all UK cancer networks. Central (hub) functions would include protocol development and the full range of imaging and non-imaging tests and unsealed source therapy for benign and malignant disease, and would likely be provided from the cancer centre and/or from the major specialist departments. Smaller departments (spokes) would undertake radionuclide imaging and therapy for benign disease, where appropriate.

Clinical networks and relationships with other services

Some areas have already developed a form of the 'hub-and-spoke' model of provision, comprising a large department, often within a teaching hospital, linked to a number of local district general hospitals (DGHs). Specialist services and inpatient facilities are provided in the central unit, and consultants undertake sessions in central and outreach hospitals. Even where there is no formal arrangement, most areas have a large department where nuclear medicine consultants with particular expertise provide advice and receive tertiary referrals from other centres for specific procedures such as PET, specialist tumour imaging or therapeutic procedures. There is inevitably a close working relationship with the complementary radiology services.

iii   Working with patients: patient-centred care

Patient information is vital in delivering good care, and detailed written information is required, especially for patients undergoing radioactive therapy procedures. This information is continually reviewed and revised, both locally and nationally. The joint specialty committee is currently pursuing ways of providing a central information resource for patients.

It is not always easy to organise patients' appointments according to their choice due to the nature of some of the investigations and radioisotope availability. Some departments have developed initiatives to do this whenever possible, particularly in cases where post-therapy restrictions on daily activities are required.

Direct booking of appointments is also problematic because Ionising Radiation (Medical Exposure) Regulations (IRMER) require all investigations to be justified by the practitioner. Under this legislation, 'practitioner' has a specific meaning and in nuclear medicine it must be the doctor holding a certificate granted under the Medicines (Administration of Radioactive Substances) Regulations. Authorisation by others against justification criteria set by the practitioner is allowed, but the large number of people potentially involved in direct booking makes training for this impractical.

Patients are not currently sent the reports of their scans directly. These reports sometimes contain unexpected information which provides only part of the clinical picture and needs to be put into context by the referring clinician, especially where malignancy is diagnosed. It is felt to be inappropriate for patients to receive nuclear medicine results in isolation and without reference to the clinician managing their case. Where the nuclear medicine physician is managing the case, for example in radionuclide therapy, they will be in a position to discuss the issues with the patient directly.

iv   Interspecialty and interdisciplinary liaison

Non-medical personnel are essential to routine nuclear medicine service provision. Staffing arrangements vary between departments but may include:

- physicists and other clinical scientists
- medical technical officers
- radiographers
- radiopharmacists
- specialist nuclear medicine nurses, including nurse practitioners
- medical laboratory scientific officers.

Play specialists and cardiac technicians may contribute to the specialist services in centres with a high paediatric or cardiac casemix. There is a legal requirement for a medical physics expert and a radiation protection adviser.

Local circumstances, particularly the level of overall clinical support within departments, dictate regular clinical commitments to some specialist areas such as nuclear cardiology, endocrinology and paediatrics. Most nuclear medicine specialists undertake radionuclide therapy and may be the lead clinicians in joint clinics, for example in the management of benign and malignant thyroid disease.

Nuclear medicine can provide specialist services in support of almost every other specialty so the specialists liaise with a wide range of other colleagues. In most centres, there is a particularly close liaison with radiology, oncology, cardiology, neurology, nephrology, urology, orthopaedics and endocrinology. Participation in cross-specialty meetings is valuable for cost-effective service provision. The growing importance of the multidisciplinary team (MDT) meetings in the delivery of cancer care has enhanced this role, allowing the development of cross-specialty liaison within the framework of joint clinics for the management of complex malignancy.

v   Delivering a high quality service

Characteristics of a high quality service

A high quality service involves significant teamwork. It produces accurate results in a timescale appropriate to the patient's need. It should have sufficient scientific support to allow development in response to new evidence. The definition of explicit service standards provides a framework for improving patient care.

It is a legal requirement that all procedures are carried out in accordance with written procedures and protocols, and these are usually derived from the British Nuclear Medicine Society (BNMS) or European guidelines.[2,3]

The delivery of nuclear medicine services in departments where there is no sessional commitment to nuclear medicine is decreasing. However, where this still exists, or where departments undertake very few studies, there are implications for service quality and clinical governance. The situation is compounded in some centres by dividing a limited number of nuclear medicine cases between a large number of consultants, thereby diluting individual experience.

Single-handed specialists working independently cannot easily fulfil the requirements of clinical governance. A minimum of 0.4 whole-time consultant overlap within single-handed practices is encouraged to avoid clinical isolation. This may be achieved by single-handed practitioners rotating to another unit as part of their weekly commitment, or by another practitioner rotating in to the unit when it is more appropriate to the caseload.

The potential of telemedicine links with larger centres is being explored as a means of sharing experience and opinions between departments, and to allow a wider audit of performance than currently possible. The introduction of a national picture archiving and communication system (PACS) may also help in this objective, though not all PACSs deal well with nuclear medicine datasets. However, the use of telemedicine and distance reporting should not be seen as a substitute for local clinical involvement in the long term, as issuing reports, whilst extremely important, is only part of the role of the nuclear medicine specialist.

Resources required for a high quality service

Outpatient investigations   The following specialist facilities are required:

- two dedicated patient waiting areas, one for radioactive and one for non-active patients and accompanying persons
- separate radiopharmaceutical administration areas
- dedicated toilet facilities
- examination rooms and quiet counselling room for pregnant and breast-feeding mothers, appropriate to the casemix
- secure radiopharmaceutical storage area
- image analysis area
- data reporting room
- educational and library area
- separate paediatric waiting/play area where appropriate
- room for cardiac stressing where appropriate – this may be a shared facility with cardiology
- appropriate imaging equipment for the casemix, maintained to a quality defined in published literature
- radiation protection measures to comply with all relevant legislation.

Inpatient work   Inpatient unsealed source therapy must take place in a dedicated facility complying with all statutory requirements for radiation protection and waste disposal, staffed by appropriately trained nurses and physics personnel. Therapy rooms should have individual shower and toilet facilities.

There is a current shortfall in provision of inpatient unsealed source therapy beds in the UK. Published survey data of 20 European countries highlights wide variations in access to isolation facilities.[3] In 1999, 1,520 isolation beds were available for a population of 478 million, giving a mean European provision of one bed per 314,500 population. At the same time the UK provided one bed per 667,000, which was inadequate to meet the existing workload pressures within acceptable waiting times. The situation is currently being reviewed, but a substantial increase in bed provision is still required urgently to match predicted demand for unsealed source treatment. The proposed expansion of nuclear medicine services within cancer centres has not occurred, but this would provide opportunities for closer cross-specialty liaison. The shared use of purpose-built shielded facilities should be encouraged to ensure cost-effective room occupancy.

For departments offering therapy, there must be arrangements to support close collaboration with relevant MDTs.

vi Quality standards and measures of the quality of specialist services

Specialist society guidelines

Generic quality guidelines for the provision of radionuclide imaging services have been developed in the UK by the BNMS.[4] These cover aspects of clinical effectiveness, safety and timeliness, and include explicit recommendations on appropriate facilities, equipment, staffing, administration, referral prioritisation, performance and reporting of investigations. The British Cardiac Society (BCS), the British Nuclear Cardiology Society and the BNMS have also produced joint guidelines for recommending, performing, interpreting and reporting myocardial perfusion studies.[5] The College has produced guidelines on the role of radioactive iodine in the management of benign thyroid disease and thyroid cancer.[6,7]

The training standards for doctors working in nuclear medicine and in the related subspecialty of radionuclide radiology have been specified in the appropriate Colleges' curriculum documents.[8,9] The Institute of Physics in Engineering and Medicine (IPEM) training scheme ensures appropriate training and experience for clinical scientists. The BNMS are also developing guidelines for the training and experience required for extension of roles by non-medical healthcare professionals. The guidelines offer a structure for the contracting process and for peer review through the BNMS organisational audit programme.

National Institute for Clinical Excellence (NICE) guidelines

Reports from NICE on the management of specific diseases, for example thyroid and lung cancer, have referred to the appropriate use of nuclear medicine services in specific circumstances. In addition, the NICE technology appraisal of myocardial perfusion scintigraphy has identified some guidelines for its appropriate use.[10]

CLINICAL AND LABORATORY WORK OF CONSULTANTS IN NUCLEAR MEDICINE

Contributions made to acute medicine

A majority of nuclear medicine consultants have no direct clinical commitment to acute medicine. This is especially true of the more recently trained physicians. There are, however, a few who have had dual training and still contribute to the acute on-call service as well as supporting the routine clinics in either general internal medicine (GIM) or another specialty such as respiratory medicine or endocrinology. There is one training post in the UK specifically for those who wish to continue this role. However, the specialty does provide diagnostic services to acute physicians and faces increasing demands for rapid access to tests and reports. This is particularly true with the 'one-stop shops' for outpatients and acute medical assessment units. It is a pressure to which the specialty is trying to respond.

Direct clinical care

Nuclear medicine specialists are responsible for the selection, supervision and reporting of diagnostic investigations, administration of unsealed source therapy and provision of appropriate follow up. Subspecialist areas include nuclear cardiology, oncology, metabolic bone disease, thyroid disease (both benign and malignant) and paediatrics.

The workload of nuclear medicine specialists covers a broad spectrum, ranging from reporting non-imaging studies to complex tomographic imaging and radionuclide therapy. Workload estimates must balance the time required for procedures grouped by type and allow for variations between consultants. The workload capacity of a consultant will also be affected by the degree of support available from nurses, physicists, technical and clerical staff, reflecting the ability for delegation. Therefore, the number of patients that can be dealt with by a consultant will vary according to the casemix of the department and the role of any individual working within it. Procedures have been considered in categories according to their complexity. The times listed below are approximations reached by consensus between consultants working in departments of different types.[11] It is assumed that figures will allow a balance to be achieved between straightforward reports and those procedures requiring more detailed assessment or patient care.

Table 1. Time allocation for procedures grouped by type

Procedure	Time required	
	Non-training environment (time in minutes)	Training environment (time in minutes)
Routine non-imaging studies, planar imaging and bone densitometry	10	13
Tomographic imaging	15	20
Complex procedures and image co-registration studies	30	40
Positron emission tomography (PET)	40	50
Stressing prior to cardiac imaging, including prior assessment and advice on drug therapy	25	30
Outpatient thyroid therapy: new patient	45	60
Outpatient thyroid therapy: follow up	15	20
Inpatient therapy and other outpatient therapies:	Variable according to length of patient stay and amount of care shared with other specialties. On average, allow 40 minutes for pre-treatment visit, one hour on day of administration and 15 minutes per day per patient on subsequent days or follow-up visits	

The number of cases that may be dealt with in each clinical programmed activity (PA) session can be calculated from the above figures according to the departmental and individual's casemix. The time taken to complete procedures includes time spent on:

- clinical vetting and discussion of referrals (justification of requests is a legal requirement), planning the procedure and consulting with the patient
- reviewing data to confirm that procedures are of a satisfactory technical standard which may involve further discussion with other professional staff or with individual patients
- reporting clinical data and reviewing clinical notes or other imaging
- checking the written report.

Where work is mixed during a PA, the clinical component can be apportioned pro-rata. It is emphasised that the workload estimates listed relate to uninterrupted clinical activity, both with and without the additional time taken with a trainee. No account has been taken of other interruptions that might reduce efficiency. Efficiency will suffer if clinical sessions cannot be protected. This is more likely to be an issue in small departments where a single consultant may be less able to delegate routine queries to other staff.

In devising work programmes, consideration should be given to the concept of fixed commitments. These include procedures undertaken on a regular basis, such as outpatient clinics, special procedures, teaching and MDT meetings. Administrative work, teaching and training, and some reporting activities could be considered flexible commitments. Further adjustments are suggested where individual consultants are also responsible for administering radiopharmaceuticals and are required to monitor or oversee work delegated to others.

It should be remembered that the reporting of studies and supervision of trainees in a department has to continue during a colleague's annual or professional leave, as the studies will continue to be performed by technical staff to maintain the diagnostic service. This prospective cover should be allocated time within the PAs in the job plan. In some weeks this may completely replace the supporting professional activities, which will then be done in the allocated extra clinical time for the rest of the year. The exact allocation will depend on normal workload intensity and local circumstances, but is likely to be one PA or more per week. A further time commitment will be required for paediatric imaging and training. Additional time for training will vary according to the stage of training and personal competence and experience of the trainee concerned. The figures in the table above should be considered an average guide.

On-call duties

Most nuclear medicine departments are not able to provide an on-call nuclear medicine service. Most agree that a service should be available for urgent cases at weekends and bank holidays, which requires access to out-of-hours radiopharmacy and technical support. With the increasing expectation of services being available 24 hours in order to encourage efficient use of inpatient beds and equipment, it is possible that there will be pressure to extend the hours of availability, if not to provide a full on-call service. This will place a significant burden on the specialist as most departments have only a few trained clinicians and would result in rotas with a potential frequency of one in two. Centres undertaking inpatient therapy have to provide some form of on-call availability.

Dual-accredited physicians should expect to be included in the rota for general medical duties, including acute medical take.

Work to maintain and improve the quality of care

This work encompasses duties in clinical governance, professional self-regulation, continuing professional development (CPD) and education and training of others. For many consultants at various times in their careers it may include research, serving in management and providing specialist advice at local, regional and national levels.

Leadership role and development of the service

Nuclear medicine has developed rapidly over the last twenty years with the development of new equipment and new pharmaceuticals. The nuclear medicine physician has a significant part to play in leading these developments, and in bridging the gap between clinical colleagues and patients, and the scientists developing new procedures. Clinicians should expect to modify current protocols to improve standards and to gain the expertise to introduce new techniques when evidence of their efficacy becomes available. The development of nuclear cardiology, PET and radio-immunotherapy are examples of recent advances.

Education, training and workforce development

Nuclear medicine is a multidisciplinary specialty. In addition to undergraduate teaching and postgraduate teaching of nuclear medicine trainees and specialist registrars (SpRs) in other specialties (eg cardiology and radiology), nuclear medicine consultants will have substantial training commitments to non-medical staff including physicists, radiographers, technicians and specialist nurses. The small number of specialists trained in nuclear medicine means that a disproportionate amount of education and training will fall to these consultants when compared with many other clinical specialties.

This training often has to occur alongside clinical work, and those involved would require a time allowance, likely to be an average of at least three hours per week.

The physician should also take an active role in collaborating with groups, including patient representatives, to improve the written information available to patients. This can be a time-consuming iterative process; how much time will depend on how much support is available from other healthcare professionals.

Continuing medical education, clinical audit and clinical governance

Consultants are expected to spend at least 50 hours per annum on continuing medical education (CME). Formal participation in interdisciplinary meetings is a requirement for good clinical practice, and additional time should be allowed for informal clinical consultation. The nuclear medicine consultant is often a named core member of the group at cancer MDT meetings. Clinical audit will often be undertaken at regional or national level. Provision may be required for some consultants to take a lead role in clinical governance.

Research

Nuclear medicine techniques are used extensively in medical research.

Local management duties

Nuclear medicine consultants have unique legal responsibilities with respect to the Administration of Radioactive Substances Advisory Committee (ARSAC) certification for diagnostic, therapy and research procedures. This, and their expertise in radiation protection of the patient, often demands their participation on radiation protection and research ethics committees, over and above the more common management duties of all consultants.

Regional and national work

The small number of nuclear medicine consultants nationally results in an unusually strong commitment to external duties relating to educational and professional issues. Depending on frequency, this may be included as a weekly PA, but agreement on how leave for external duties will be handled should be included in the job plan.

The time commitment to supporting activities has been extrapolated from a published model.[1] As this aspect of workload varies according to local circumstances and hospital type, considerable variation between individual consultants is expected.

ACADEMIC MEDICINE

There are a significant number of academic physicians in nuclear medicine, with 40% holding at least a part-time academic contract.[12] They make an important contribution to the clinical work in their departments but have similar responsibilities to teaching and research as other academics, the exact balance being determined locally.

WORKFORCE REQUIREMENTS FOR CONSULTANTS IN NUCLEAR MEDICINE

Current workforce numbers

The 2003 Census reported that there were 62 consultants who gave nuclear medicine as their specialty (58 whole time equivalents (WTE)).[12] The picture is further complicated by the fact that some radionuclide work is delivered by specialists in other disciplines, as alluded to above. Very few of these appear in the nuclear medicine section of the Census data and most are only programmed to have a few sessions per week in the specialty. A survey carried out in 2000 for the Intercollegiate Standing Committee in Nuclear Medicine identified about 190 trusts providing nuclear medicine services, with an average of 2.2 consultants per trust.[2] This equates to at least 400 consultants involved in providing nuclear medicine services. However, the survey did not indicate how much of their time was devoted to nuclear medicine and, indeed, some trusts failed to identify any medical time at all for the service. A repeat survey is currently in progress, which should clarify the total number of WTE consultants devoted to nuclear medicine.[11] There are currently 229 individuals on the General Medical Council (GMC) specialist register for nuclear medicine.

Consultant programmed activities required to provide a specialist service to a population of 250,000

An allocation of 200 WTE consultants in the UK was proposed in the previous edition of this document.[13] This equates to 8.3 PAs per week for a population of 250,000 to maintain the current service. However, this does not take account of more recent developments.

Review of consultant job plans using the time estimates above will give a realistic indication of the workload that a consultant should be undertaking with their contracted PAs. Correlation with annual patient attendance data will also identify the increase in consultant establishment required to manage the local caseload reasonably and to maintain standards.

▪ Estimates of the potential increase in nuclear cardiology workload to meet guidance, combined with the time allocation detailed in Table 1, would suggest the need for an additional 2.3 clinical PAs per week to cover the expected increase in nuclear cardiology.[5]

▪ The currently recommended PET procedures would require 1.3 clinical PAs per week per 250,000 population – although indications for PET are still expanding.[14]

▪ A growth in the number of sentinel node localisation studies would require an extra 0.3 clinical PAs per week.

The total for these three workload areas alone is 3.9 additional clinical PAs per 250,000 population. Due to the nature of distribution of many nuclear medicine services it is likely that the 'true' population served by a nuclear medicine department is larger than that of the hospital in which the department is situated.

Assuming a ratio of 2.5 supporting activities for every 7.5 clinical activities, 1.3 supporting PAs should be added to the 3.9 additional clinical PAs.[15] Added to the previous figure of 8.3 PAs, this gives a total of 13.5 PAs per week per 250,000 population.

It could be argued that at least one more PA is needed to allow for the increased training and development work to implement this standard. However, some of the projected increase in workload will be offset by the extended role of other healthcare practitioners who, once fully trained, will be able to release some medical time and participate in the training themselves. There are, however, constraints on the implementation of this, at least in the short term (see below).

The time allocation calculated above relates to nuclear medicine activities carried out at consultant level, regardless of the specialty of the consultant. It does not distinguish whether the time is provided by nuclear medicine specialists or by other specialists with additional training, for example radionuclide radiologists or cardiologists.

National consultant workforce requirements

Retirement planning The Census indicated that 42% of current nuclear medicine consultants will reach 60 years within the next ten years.[12] It is likely that a similar percentage of other specialists contributing to the service will do likewise. The surveys in 2000 suggested that 100–120 consultants would need to be replaced by 2010.[2] Fifty percent would need to be fully trained in all aspects of nuclear medicine (imaging, non-imaging and therapy procedures). This implies that 10–12 new consultants need to be trained each year. This level of training is just sustainable within existing training numbers, taking into account the increased numbers of radionuclide radiologists in training.

European Working Time Directive The Census indicates that some specialists were exceeding the hours specified in the European Working Time Directive and suggested that a 27% increase in current consultant WTE numbers would be required to meet the directive targets.[12] This figure was scaled from the numbers responding (approximately two-thirds) to the question of 'actual hours worked', and a calculation of the excess hours required to be covered. It is accepted that there may have been some reporting bias in the survey, with those replying to the question being under greater pressure. However, the figure takes no account of the radiologists contributing to the service – a specialty with severe shortages – making it likely that this figure is an under- rather than overestimate of the workforce required to comply with the directive.

Discrepancies between hours worked and contracted time   The Census also identified discrepancies between contracted hours and hours worked.[12] It was clear that many were working in the specialty for periods well above their contracted sessions. With the potential reporting bias proviso as above, this Census indicated that a 38% increase in funded time was required just to meet current workload.

Workforce numbers required   It is assumed that the figure of 200 WTE consultants suggested in the previous edition of this document would cover the increase in consultant numbers required to meet the Directive and to avoid work above contracted hours. This was generally accepted as a realistic assumption for a consultant-led service for the workload envisaged in 2000. In addition:

■   Anticipated expansion of myocardial perfusion scintigraphy would require 89 WTE consultants.

■   Development of a PET service would require 50 WTE consultants.

■   Expansion of sentinel node imaging would require 11 WTE consultants.

■   There will be an additional requirement for the expansion of radioisotope therapy but the numbers are difficult to estimate because the degree of expansion will depend on the outcome of several clinical trials currently in progress.

The total requirement will, therefore, be about 350–360 WTE consultants for the whole of the UK.

As mentioned previously, not all consultants delivering nuclear medicine services work full-time in the specialty. The workforce required will be much larger and the exact size will depend on what fraction of time is contributed to the nuclear medicine service by radionuclide-trained consultants from other specialties. Consultants who do not work full-time in nuclear medicine can provide an important input into the workforce but it should be remembered that this entails a major increase in the total training requirement, as those doing the job will have to be trained to the same standard whether they do it for one day a week or five days a week.

The need for additional consultants will also depend on the extent of the work that can be undertaken by other healthcare professionals. The current drive to extend their roles will encourage MDT working and go some way towards alleviating medical workforce problems. However, there is currently a shortage of technologists and nurses in nuclear medicine in some parts of the country, which itself will need to be addressed before this initiative can be fully implemented. Cardiac, endocrine and breast nurse specialists are actively involved in some areas, but they too are in short supply with increasing demands on their time from their respective specialties. It is inevitable that in some areas the suggested intercollegiate 'hub-and-spoke' model of service delivery will have to be adopted, at least in the short term. It is also likely that the trained radionuclide radiologists will be required to spend a larger proportion of their PAs in delivering nuclear medicine services than presently, thus reducing the number required for replacement. This assumes that radiology pressures would permit this.

As indicated above, the current number of WTE consultants in the UK is 58, and an additional six consultants in other specialties give nuclear medicine as their second specialty. Interestingly, there are 229 individuals on the specialist register. Clearly there is a necessity for more consultants in this specialty but, in the short term, it is not possible to expand rapidly to the numbers outlined in this document. The College recommends a doubling of WTE physicians in the short to medium term. To provide 0.5 WTE per 250,000 population in the UK would mean 117 WTE, that is, an increase of 59 (101%).

CONSULTANT WORK PROGRAMME/SPECIMEN JOB PLAN

Activity	Workload	Programmed activities (PAs)
Direct clinical care		
General nuclear medicine studies and reporting*	See above, depends on casemix	**2–3**
Myocardial perfusion stressing*	8 patients	**0.8**
Myocardial perfusion scan reporting*	8 patients	**0.5**
PET imaging and reporting*	6 patients	**1**
X-ray conferences and cancer MDT meetings	2–5 per week	**0.5–1.5**
Inpatient therapy*	2 patients	**1**
Outpatient therapy clinic*	3 new patients plus 7 follow–up patients	**1**
Total number of direct clinical care PAs		**7.5 on average**
Supporting professional activities (SPA)		
Work to maintain and improve the quality of healthcare	Education and training, appraisal, departmental management and service development, audit and clinical governance, CPD and revalidation, research	**2.5 on average**
Other NHS responsibilities	eg medical director/clinical director/lead consultant in specialty/clinical tutor	**Local agreement with trust**
External duties	eg work for deaneries/Royal Colleges/specialist societies/Department of Health or other government bodies etc	**Local agreement with trust**

*These activities include justification of referrals, patient assessment, manipulation of drug therapy as appropriate, supervision of the test, telephone discussion with patients and colleagues and reporting.

The job plan will vary according to the casemix, an individual's areas of special expertise and the amount of specialist scientific, technical and nursing support available, for example whether the consultant or other staff administer radiopharmaceuticals. Where there is more than one consultant in a department, it would be expected that there would be flexibility in the job plan for rotation of sessions as required. This will facilitate maintenance of competence in less frequently performed procedures and allow cross-cover arrangements to be in place. In teaching departments some of the workload may be undertaken by trainees but appropriate supervision time must be allowed. See main body of text for more detailed guidance.

References

1. Royal College of Physicians. *Nuclear medicine: provision of clinical service*. Report of a working party. London: RCP, 1998.

2. Intercollegiate Standing Committee on Nuclear Medicine. *Nuclear medicine and radionuclide imaging: A strategy for provision in the UK*. London: RCP, 2003.

3. Hoefnagel CA, Clarke SEM, Fischer M *et al*. Survey: Radionuclide therapy practice and facilities in Europe. *Eur J Nucl Med* 1999;**26**:277–282.

4. British Nuclear Medicine Society. *Nuclear medicine generic quality guidelines for the provision of radionuclide imaging services*, April 2001. www.bnms.org.uk

5. Anagnostopoulos C, Harbison M, Kelion A, Kundley K *et al*. Procedure guidelines for radionuclide myocardial perfusion imaging. *Heart* 2004;**90** (Suppl 1):i1-10.

6. Royal College of Physicians. *The use of radioiodine in the management of hyperthyroidism*. London: RCP, 1995.

7. Royal College of Physicians. *Guidelines for the management of thyroid cancer in adults*. London: RCP, 2002.

8. Joint Committee on Higher Medical Training, Higher medical training curriculum for nuclear medicine. JCHMT, January 2003. www.jchmt.org.uk/nuclear/curr_nuclear.pdf

9. Royal College of Radiologists. *Structured training in clinical radiology, Appendix: curricula for subspecialty training*. RCR, 2000.

10. National Institute for Clinical Excellence. *Myocardial perfusion scintigraphy for the diagnosis and management of angina and myocardial infarction*. NICE Technology Appraisal 73, November 2003. www.nice.org.uk/TA073guidance

11. Nuclear medicine workload and resource survey currently being conducted by the National Radiological Protection Board, on behalf of the British Nuclear Medicine Society, The Institute of Physics and Engineering in Medicine, the Royal College of Physicians, the British Institute of Radiology, the Royal College of Radiologists and the National Radiological Protection Board.

12. Federation of the Royal Colleges of Physicians of the United Kingdom. *Census of consultant physicians in the UK 2003. Data and commentary*. 2003

13. Royal College of Physicians. *Consultant physicians working for patients: The duties, responsibilities and practice of physicians (2nd edition)*. London: RCP, 2001.

14. British Nuclear Medicine Society. *Clinical procedure guidelines*, October 2004. www.bnms.org.uk/guidelines.htm

15. Department of Health. *Consultant contract*, January 2004, paragraph 7.3. www.modern.nhs.uk/consultants/14680/Contract.pdf

Paediatric cardiology

i Description of the specialty and clinical needs of patients

Paediatric cardiology is a specialty concerned with all aspects of care of patients with congenital heart disease, from the fetus to adulthood. Paediatric cardiologists collaborate with adult cardiologists in the management of congenital heart disease in adolescents and adults. There is ongoing development of training and appointment of consultants with an interest in adults with congenital heart disease.

The incidence of congenital heart disease is eight in 1000 live-born babies and this has remained consistent over several decades. There have been great advances in the diagnosis and management of congenital heart disease in the last two decades. However, the provision of care has not kept up with these developments.

The paediatric cardiology specialist service attempts to meet the need for comprehensive assessment of patients, non-invasive investigations and invasive treatment in the form of intervention or surgery. There are a limited number of tertiary centres and care is usually delivered nearer to the patient's place of residence in the form of outreach hospitals. Outpatient clinics are arranged in conjunction with local consultant paediatricians.

The paediatric cardiology service has become increasingly subspecialised with developments in areas such as prenatal detection and treatment, interventional techniques, electrophysiological treatment of arrhythmias, treatment of pulmonary hypertension and cardiac transplantation, and non-invasive imaging such as three-dimensional echocardiography (ECHG) and magnetic resonance imaging (MRI).

ii Organisation of the service and patterns of referral

Primary, secondary and tertiary levels

The paediatric cardiology service is becoming integrated between primary, secondary and tertiary levels of care. It aims to provide a seamless transition for patients from primary to secondary care, then to tertiary care and back, based on agreed protocols.

Primary care   The main emphasis should be on the early detection and prevention of congenital heart disease but there are many limitations. In primary care, the symptoms of congenital heart disease must be recognised and appropriate referral made to secondary care for further assessment and treatment. An important area of management in primary care is the detection and differentiation of innocent from pathological murmurs.

Secondary care   Patients undergo evaluation of their symptoms and appropriate investigations are arranged. In many cases, the secondary care paediatrician is able to reassure patients, for example those with innocent murmurs. However, the vast majority of patients with suspected cardiac problems are referred to a tertiary care specialist either at the tertiary care centre or at an outreach clinic. It is important that such assessments in secondary and tertiary care are made quickly and efficiently.

Patients are evaluated by a secondary, or visiting tertiary, care specialist using two-dimensional ECHG. Much of the non-invasive assessment, diagnosis and treatment of patients with congenital heart defects can be carried out at the secondary care centres. Although this type of service has major advantages for patients, its delivery has stretched the services of the tertiary centres. This is because the expertise for managing congenital heart disease in outreach clinics is lacking at secondary care level and is largely dependent on tertiary care specialists.

Tertiary care This incorporates highly specialised investigation and treatment, including non-invasive diagnosis by specialised imaging techniques (eg two-dimensional and transoesophageal ECHG and MRI) and invasive procedures (eg diagnostic and interventional cardiac catheterisation, electrophysiology studies, pacemaker implantation and surgery). Invasive investigation and treatment and cardiac surgery are performed exclusively in tertiary centres. Some forms of treatment, such as cardiac transplantation, should be classified as even more specialised. Services for adolescents and adults with congenital heart disease are provided mainly in the tertiary centres.

Special patterns of referral

The pattern of referral of patients with congenital heart disease is variable. Some patients are referred by their GP to either the secondary or tertiary centre. The GP may see patients with a murmur or symptoms such as palpitations or chest pain and suspect these to have a cardiac origin.

Prenatal detection, not yet available comprehensively throughout the country, enables the diagnosis of congenital heart defect before the baby is born. This allows the parents to be much better prepared for the proposed management plan. The baby may be delivered at the tertiary centre and the treatment is then elective rather than on an emergency basis.

Some babies are referred from secondary care centres because of a suspicion of congenital heart disease. They are evaluated in the outreach clinic or at the tertiary centre clinic, either as outpatients or inpatients depending on their clinical condition. Children who need cardiac surgery are referred to the cardiac surgeon by the paediatric cardiologist, not by the GP or secondary care specialist.

A patient with suspected congenital heart disease should be referred to a secondary care specialist if considered non-urgent, for example for assessment of an asymptomatic murmur, or to a tertiary care specialist if urgent, for example if a baby is cyanosed or breathless.

Ways of working, clinical networks and community arrangements

Networks of care are being developed around the country. The aim is to produce a seamless pattern of care for the patient from the first point of contact with the healthcare system to whatever complex investigation or treatment is required. There is still a deficient network of care at the primary care level for congenital heart disease, but collaboration is better between secondary and tertiary care levels. These networks are based in a tertiary centre and its catchment population.

Paediatric cardiologists lead multidisciplinary teams (MDTs) in the tertiary care centres. In addition to various specialist medical staff, these involve nursing staff, outreach or cardiac liaison nurses, radiographers, technicians and play therapists. Paediatric cardiologists coordinate treatments with the cardiac surgeons and intensive care staff.

Outreach clinics are performed jointly by paediatric cardiologists and local paediatricians. Some centres have paediatricians with special expertise in paediatric cardiology and are able to offer non-invasive services for patients. This is very likely to develop into a more clearly defined service in most outreach hospitals in the future.

Patients with congenital heart disease usually require follow-up into adult life and facilities for this need to be better organised or, indeed, developed. In most cases these adult patients will need to be seen in tertiary care centres but as the service delivery is modified many will be seen in joint clinics in outreach hospitals.

The workload of paediatric cardiologists will continue to increase and secondary care specialists will have a hugely important role in the future. The demands of providing such a comprehensive service are enormous, particularly in an era of consultant appraisal and revalidation, while maintaining clinical competencies and keeping specialist knowledge up to date.

iii Working with patients/parents: patient-centred care

Because of the complex nature of many congenital heart defects, it is of great importance that paediatric cardiologists work closely with the parents of children with congenital heart disease and with adolescent or adult patients directly. The options of conservative management, medical treatment, interventional treatment or surgical treatment will need to be discussed with the parents or the patients or both. These discussions will involve cardiac liaison nurses who can offer further support and information to the patients or parents.

Information leaflets developed by hospitals or the British Heart Foundation (BHF) will help patients to understand their heart defect and its management. Local parent support groups also offer help. A considerable amount of information is available to patients and parents on the Internet and paediatric cardiologists and cardiac liaison nurses should be able to provide information about these websites.

iv Interspecialty and interdisciplinary liaison

Paediatric cardiologists work with many disciplines, including:

- paediatric cardiac intensivists
- anaesthetists
- other paediatricians or paediatric subspecialists
- paediatric intensive care nurses
- cardiac liaison nurses
- cardiac surgeons
- cardiac technicians
- radiographers
- pharmacists
- physiotherapists
- dietitians
- play specialists.

Paediatric cardiologists must work effectively with these specialists as they may need to be involved closely in the management of babies and children with congenital cardiac defects and other non-cardiac diseases.

v   Delivering a high quality service

Characteristics of a high quality service

■   responds to the demands of the patients

■   has sound quality assurance

■   maintains audit and clinical governance

■   keeps communication with patients' families at the forefront

■   has adequate backup from the IT department and good secretarial support.

Such care can only be delivered by an integrated MDT consisting of the specialists listed above and supported by service managers.

Information technology support is particularly important for maintaining databases of paediatric cardiac surgical activities, as emphasised in the Kennedy report.[1] Development of electronic patient records will be of great help.

Resources required for a high quality service

A high quality paediatric cardiology service cannot be provided if the service and resources remain stretched beyond their limits. The fifth joint report on cardiothoracic services made recommendations about service requirements, in particular highlighting the need for the number of paediatric cardiology consultants to increase from one per million to one per half million population.[2] This target has not been reached. The British Paediatric Cardiac Association (BPCA) and the specialist advisory committee (SAC) for paediatric cardiology have fully endorsed the standards and recommendations made in the Department of Health paediatric and congenital cardiac services review document and these recommendations need to be kept at the forefront when considering improvements of service.[3]

■   Patients need easy access to diagnostic services in secondary care units and coordinated access to tertiary care units.

■   Comprehensive investigation of patients in outreach clinics, up to the time of referral to the tertiary centre, forms an important bridge between primary and tertiary care.

■   Facilities for high quality non-invasive imaging are essential in the secondary care units.

■   Appointment of paediatricians with special expertise in paediatric cardiology will need to be an essential component of the service in the near future. Such paediatricians will need to have educational links with tertiary units for their professional development.

■   Rapid access clinics at both secondary and tertiary centres will need to be developed.

■   Access to specialised facilities such as transoesophageal and three-dimensional ECHG, MRI and spiral computed tomography (CT) scanning should be straightforward.

■   Care should be coordinated between the secondary care and tertiary care units and with the surgical unit for all patients, including adolescents and adults, with congenital heart disease.

■   Highly specialised nurses to coordinate management between secondary and tertiary centres, such as cardiac liaison nurses, will be needed.

vi   Quality standards and measures of the quality of specialist services

The SAC for paediatric cardiology has developed a competency-based curriculum for training in paediatric cardiology and is looking at methods of clinical assessment and competence. Curricula are being developed for subspecialty training in interventional techniques in fetal cardiology and in adult congenital heart disease, for example. A further curriculum is being developed for paediatricians who wish to expand their expertise in paediatric cardiology for the purpose of providing a paediatric cardiology service in a secondary care unit. The BPCA is working towards developing standards and measures of quality.

The SAC and BPCA have worked with the National Institute for Clinical Excellence (NICE) to develop guidelines for many interventional procedures, and other guidelines are being prepared (**www.NICE.org.uk**).

Paediatric cardiology has worked closely with United Kingdom Central Cardiac Audit Database (CCAD) to collect data on paediatric cardiac catheterisation, interventions and surgery. The CCAD is able to provide data for activity and the surgical results of all the units as a means of providing accurate patient information.

CLINICAL WORK AND/OR LABORATORY WORK OF CONSULTANTS IN PAEDIATRIC CARDIOLOGY

Direct clinical care

The exact pattern of working will vary from area to area. Paediatric cardiologists provide direct patient care in two ways:

▪ In the tertiary centre they provide comprehensive and coordinated care with other disciplines.

▪ In the outreach hospital, in collaboration with local consultant paediatricians, they provide an outpatient diagnostic imaging service for new patients and manage follow-up patients after a diagnosis of congenital heart disease has been made or treatment has been carried out at the tertiary centre.

Tertiary centre

Paediatric cardiologists are responsible for the assessment of patients presenting as acute emergencies or routine outpatient referrals; for performing procedures such as cardiac catheterisation and intervention; and for coordinating referral to cardiac surgeons. The exact pattern of working varies between regions.

Inpatient work   This will usually be at the tertiary centre. Regular ward rounds are essential in a consultant-led service; the frequency will vary depending on the number of inpatients. Generally, at least one ward round is carried out daily by a junior doctor but a consultant may also have a daily ward round, depending on how sick the patients are. Newly admitted babies with congenital heart disease are seen within a few hours of admission by the consultant paediatric cardiologist. If the baby is sick the consultant may review more than once during the day. In addition, the consultant will see patients both before and after diagnostic or interventional cardiac catheterisation procedures, and will perform these procedures.

In cardiac or paediatric intensive care unit (PICU) areas, paediatric cardiology consultants will review patients on a daily basis. They will have a major role in the management of these patients together with the intensivists. Patients undergoing cardiac surgery are usually admitted under the care of the cardiologists, although cardiac surgical consultants will see the patients both before and after the surgery. Paediatric cardiologists usually review surgery patients in the outpatient clinic after discharge from the ward. Increasingly, cardiac liaison nurses provide parents with additional support after discharge.

Prenatal detection   In some units, consultant fetal cardiologists provide this important service, whilst in others it is consultant paediatric cardiologists. This aspect of service is consultant-led or consultant-based, but there is no clearly defined pattern of working around the country. Pregnant mothers are scanned either because of suspicion of congenital heart defect in the fetus raised at an obstetric unit or because of a family history. All of this work is outpatient based and is highly complex.

Outpatient work   Outpatient work patterns and the workload vary between different hospitals. Each consultant may have one to two outpatient clinics per week in the tertiary unit. In addition, there may be rapid access clinics, for which the consultant on service for the week has responsibility. The clinics in the tertiary centre vary from a general mix of patients to disease-specific clinics such as new murmurs, cardiomyopathy and arrhythmia.

Counselling support/technician support/database   Fetal cardiology and paediatric cardiology require additional support from cardiac technicians to help with the inpatient and outpatient service. In fetal cardiology in particular, counselling support is essential. Following detection of heart defects in the fetus, counsellors/cardiac liaison nurses offer support to the parents to prepare them for the subsequent treatment of their child. Database and IT support are crucial in all aspects of congenital heart disease service.

Referral work   Consultants conduct referral work on a day-to-day basis as required. Referral letters for patients may be from GPs, secondary care specialists and other specialists within the tertiary centre.

Interspecialty and interdisciplinary liaison   Effective liaison with other subspecialists is essential to comprehensive patient care. These subspecialists are usually based in the tertiary centre and may include general paediatric surgeons, paediatricians, subspecialty paediatricians, neonatologists, paediatric intensivists, microbiologists, dentists and, most importantly, paediatric cardiac surgeons. Multidisciplinary teams are crucial to the delivery of care for patients with congenital heart disease. Team members consist of doctors, nurses, outreach nurses, play specialists, technicians and clinical managers. Nurses play a role in the wards, the outpatient clinic and in outreach services. Technicians perform investigations such as electrocardiograms, echocardiograms, stress testing, arrhythmia monitoring and invasive investigations such as haemodynamic monitoring. Paediatric cardiologists oversee these teams and investigations and are involved in their interpretation.

Case conferences   Joint case conferences are important in the management of patients. A consensus approach is adopted and discussion usually involves a team of paediatric cardiologists, cardiac surgeons, neonatologists and intensivists. These conferences are held weekly to decide on management of patients and act as educational meetings.

Number of patients   The number of patients under each consultant and the method of practice varies between hospitals. In some units, a paediatric cardiologist may be on service for a whole week, in which all the inpatients will be under his/her care. Other units admit patients under each consultant.

Specialised investigation and therapeutic procedure clinics   There are few such clinics in paediatric cardiology but the current trend is to develop pre-admission clinics for cardiac catheterisation, interventional procedures and surgery. Such clinics allow adequate time for the patient to receive full explanations of the proposed procedure in order to obtain informed consent. In the future, some of the clinics may be nurse-led to help the patients/parents prepare for the future plan of treatment.

Outreach centres

Outreach clinic services are offered by paediatric cardiologists within the catchment areas of most outreach hospitals. There are no outreach services in GPs' surgeries for paediatric cardiology.

Outpatient work   Each paediatric cardiologist undertakes a monthly commitment to an outreach clinic in several outreach hospitals. In collaboration with consultant paediatricians in the outreach hospitals, paediatric cardiologists provide outpatient facilities for either new patients referred for a cardiac opinion or for those who have been investigated and treated in the tertiary centre and have been discharged back to the outreach hospital for follow up. These patients do not then need to travel regularly to the tertiary centre and care is provided near to the patients' residences.

The outreach clinic workload is usually extremely heavy and the casemix varies. There can be a high proportion of patients for evaluation of murmurs and sometimes a high proportion of patients already diagnosed by a tertiary centre or paediatrician with special expertise in paediatric cardiology in the outreach hospital.

In the future, outreach work will need to be undertaken by consultant paediatricians with special expertise in paediatric cardiology with educational links to tertiary centres. Such service development will make the patient journey from the GP referral to a specialist opinion and completion of cardiac care of prime importance.

On call for specialist advice and emergencies

Paediatric cardiologists are available on call to advise trainees and to see patients immediately. These patients are usually newborn babies, or children with suspected congenital heart disease or previously diagnosed congenital heart disease. In these cases, the consultant will have to come into their base hospital out of hours to carry out emergency investigations and treatments. These range from ECHG, balloon atrial septostomies and, occasionally, diagnostic or interventional cardiac catheterisation.

Specialised facilities and services within the specialty

Paediatric cardiology relies heavily on specialised investigations carried out within their own service. Increased subspecialisation has resulted in paediatric cardiologists referring patients to other paediatric cardiologists for specific problems, such as electrophysiology studies.

In tertiary care centres, the facilities provided include:

- electrocardiography (ECG) services
- exercise stress testing
- ECHG and transoesophageal ECHG
- myocardial perfusion scanning

- MRI studies
- 24-hour arrhythmia and blood pressure monitoring
- tilt testing
- diagnostic and interventional cardiac catheterisation
- electrophysiology studies
- pacemaker implantation
- radiofrequency ablation
- implantation of intracardiac defibrillators
- cardiac surgery.

In secondary care outreach hospitals, the facilities provided include:

- ECG services
- exercise stress-testing
- two-dimensional ECHG
- 24-hour arrhythmia and blood pressure monitoring.

These specialised facilities require adequate space and highly qualified technical staff with the appropriate equipment.

Work to maintain and improve the quality of care

Leadership role and the introduction of service developments

Improving the quality of care requires integrated care pathways to be effective within the tertiary unit as well as within secondary care units. Service development requires working with NICE guidelines for some of the procedures and a MDT approach. Paediatric cardiologists must take a lead role in service development and exercise their team working and leadership skills.

Other work will involve duties in clinical governance, professional self-regulation, continuing professional development (CPD), education and training of other doctors and other staff in the department. Many consultants may undertake research work or management duties. All of these require the participation of consultants.

Education and training

Consultants paediatric cardiologists will be involved in training undergraduate students, senior house officers (SHOs) and specialist registrars (SpRs). The training programme for SpRs in paediatric cardiology is defined by a curriculum and requires competency assessments. It is organised by the specialty training committees of the deaneries. Paediatric cardiologists have an increasingly important role in the appraisal, assessment and mentoring of SpRs and other professionals to develop a highly competent team of healthcare workers.

Continuing professional development

Continuing professional development for paediatric cardiologists is regulated by the College.

Management duties

Paediatric cardiologists will be involved in local management as lead clinician or by undertaking other managerial work within each trust.

Regional and national duties

Paediatric cardiologists will have a role in the specialist training committees of the local deaneries. The National Society and the BPCA encourage involvement in educational, managerial and manpower negotiation.

There are regional specialty advisers in paediatric cardiology who represent the College and deal with issues related to reviewing job descriptions of new consultant posts. The Joint Committee of Higher Medical Training (JCHMT), through the SAC, deals with issues related to the curriculum and training of SpRs in paediatric cardiology. Paediatric cardiologists are represented on the SAC.

ACADEMIC PAEDIATRIC CARDIOLOGY

The role of the paediatric cardiologist in academic paediatric cardiology varies according to the setting. There are very few pure academic paediatric cardiologists as most are clinically based. Paediatric cardiologists are committed to teaching undergraduate students, and are involved in teaching the whole of the tertiary and secondary care centre teams. In the tertiary centre, the consultant may lead MDTs in clinical research.

WORKFORCE REQUIREMENTS FOR PAEDIATRIC CARDIOLOGY

The previous estimate indicated that there should be one paediatric cardiologist per million population.[4] The joint report of the British Cardiac Society and the Royal College of Physicians has recommended that there should be one paediatric cardiologist per 500,000 population.[2] The most recent Census showed that there were only 68 paediatric cardiologists in the UK.[5] Thus, the target of almost doubling the current consultant manpower will take a long time to achieve. It is possible that a shortened training curriculum combined with an increase in the numbers of SpRs and consultant posts would go some way towards achieving this target in a shorter period of time.

CONSULTANT WORK PROGRAMME/SPECIMEN JOB PLAN

Consultant paediatric cardiologists work in a variety of different clinical settings and possess a wide range of clinical skills. The job plan which follows can be regarded as general guidance.

Activity	Workload	Programmed activities (PAs)
Direct clinical care		
PICU ward rounds		1
Inpatient care plus referrals		1
Oupatient clinics		2–3
Specialised investigative or therapeutic procedures		2–3
Outreach clinics		2–3
Total number of direct clinical care PAs		7.5–8 on average
Supporting professional activities (SPA)		
Work to maintain and improve the quality of healthcare*	Education and training, appraisal, departmental management and service development, audit and clinical governance, CPD and revalidation, research	**2–3 on average**
Other NHS responsibilities	eg medical director/clinical director/lead consultant in specialty/clinical tutor	**Local agreement with trust**
External duties	eg work for deaneries/Royal Colleges/specialist societies/Department of Health or other government bodies etc	**Local agreement with trust**

*Within the team of paediatric cardiologists, any individual would expect to devote 2–4 PAs to a selection from the following activities:

■ lead clinician
■ audit
■ structured specialist training
■ general management
■ clinical governance and risk management
■ roles in the deanery, the BPCA and the College
■ membership of national subspecialty groups promoting quality issues in clinical care
■ IT – collecting reliable data in relation to clinical activities
■ cardiac networks.

References

1. Department of Health. *The report of the public inquiry into children's heart surgery at the Bristol Royal Infirmary 1984-1995: learning from Bristol (Cm 5207(I))*. London: DH, 2001.

2. Fifth report on the provision of services for patients with heart disease. *Heart* 2002;**88**(Suppl 3):iii1–56.

3. Department of Health. *Report of the paediatric and congenital cardiac services review group*, December 2003. www.dh.gov.uk/assetRoot/04/07/08/18/04070818.pdf

4. Provision of services for the diagnosis and treatment of heart disease. Fourth report of a Joint Cardiology Committee of the Royal College of Physicians of London and the Royal College of Surgeons of London. *Br Heart J* 1992;**67**(1):106–16.

5. Federation of the Royal College of Physicians. *Census of Consultant Physicians in the UK, 2003. Data and Commentary*. London: Federation of the Royal College of Physicians, 2003.

Palliative medicine

i   Description of the specialty and clinical needs of patients

Palliative medicine was recognised as a specialty in 1987 when specialist medical training programmes were established. This coincided with the rapid development of specialist palliative care services, which included new links between community, hospice and hospital care and between the NHS and the voluntary sector. Since 1995, the development of cancer services in line with the Calman-Hine report has given further impetus for specialist palliative care to be integrated with cancer services.[1] In particular, this has led to a rapid and continuing expansion in consultant posts – 350% since 1993.

As a consequence, many consultants in previously established posts are playing a key role in the strategic development of local services, and those taking up new appointments may be doing so without a fully developed or resourced service infrastructure. While this expansion has been primarily focused on cancer patients there is awareness that patients with non-malignant illness must have equitable access to specialist palliative care services.

Palliative care is the active total care of patients and their families by a multidisciplinary team (MDT) when the patient's disease is no longer responsive to curative treatment.[2] The majority of palliative care in the UK is provided within the clinical setting in which the patient is routinely managed, often in primary care rather than by specialist services. Ongoing specialist palliative care services are needed by a minority (15–30%) of people whose deaths are anticipated. Care may be provided directly by specialist services or indirectly through professional advice to the patient's carer. Referral is usually prompted by the presence of severe uncontrolled symptoms, major difficulties in adjusting to a terminal illness, or the need for inpatient terminal care.

Consultants in palliative medicine work within multidisciplinary specialist care teams and services. Traditionally, the vast majority of patients referred for specialist care have had advanced cancer but, while this remains the case for many services, the need for palliative medicine is not diagnosis-specific and is defined by the patient's and family's needs. An increasing proportion of patients with end-stage organ failure are now referred to specialist palliative care services, particularly in acute hospitals. Across the UK there is wide variation in the proportion of people dying from cancer who are seen by specialist palliative care services. In 2003 the range was 30–75%.[3] Around 20% of all cancer deaths occur in hospices or specialist palliative care inpatient units. The proportion of patients seen is determined partly by the availability of services, and rises as services expand. Referrals come predominantly from primary care (60%).

ii   Organisation of the service and patterns of referral

Primary, secondary and tertiary care

Primary and community care Palliative care for patients at home is provided by GPs and community nurses, with advice, where appropriate, from a community specialist palliative care team (of which there were 332 in the UK in 2003).[3] As cancer networks develop, the role of GPs in the care of cancer patients is becoming better developed and defined. It is expected that improved sharing of clinical information and clearer patient pathways will further develop the role of GPs in palliative care. The majority of patients would prefer to die at home if there were sufficient support.

Specialist palliative care teams in the community normally consist of clinical nurse specialists and at least part-time input from a consultant in palliative medicine. Where possible, other non-medical members such as a specialist social worker, occupational therapist and physiotherapist make a contribution. Each team typically covers a geographical area and liaises closely with the GPs and community nurses in that area.

Secondary care Every acute hospital should have a specialist palliative care team comprised of clinical nurse specialists (of which there are 249 in UK) and at least a part-time consultant in palliative medicine. In addition to advising on the care of individual patients, the consultant's role includes education, particularly for junior hospital doctors; the development of patient pathways and protocols; and participation in the strategic development of palliative care. The consultant will usually hold at least one outpatient clinic a week, possibly in addition to joint clinics with oncologists, and attend tumour site-specific team meetings.

Many consultants work in a hospital-based team and a community team, and may have responsibility for specialist inpatient beds which are often not on the site of the acute hospital.

No consultant should practise single-handed but 30% do at present, particularly in the hospital setting.[4] It is vital that the consultant has good links with colleagues in the surrounding network, including robust cover arrangements for absences and time spent on call. The consultant also needs adequate time for off-site continuing professional development (CPD) and for participation in clinical audit in collaboration with colleagues from surrounding units.

Tertiary care Many cancer services are organised on a 'hub-and-spoke' basis across a cancer network. Patient pathways lead patients to be referred to a cancer centre for radiotherapy and specialist medical oncology, while follow-up and chemotherapy are carried out at a more local cancer unit. In general, specialist palliative care services do not follow this model because they are organised geographically around patients' homes. The tertiary unit palliative care team will be fully involved with local residents and will have an advisory service for patients beyond the locality.

Every cancer centre needs at least one consultant in palliative medicine leading the delivery of specialist palliative care for inpatients. These consultants will spend a large proportion of time liaising with the local consultants in palliative medicine who know the patients already, to facilitate a transition back to local services.

Clinical networks and community arrangements

Specialist inpatient units Most specialist inpatient palliative care units are not on acute hospital sites, although a few are integrated into an acute hospital. Inpatient units admit patients with complex needs for symptom control and/or major emotional distress and/or family problems. Fifty percent of admissions are discharged and the average duration of stay is 13 days.[3] Patients are also admitted for inpatient terminal care if adequate support for a death at home cannot be provided.

The consultant in charge of a specialist inpatient unit will be supported by other medical staff, which may include non-consultant career grades (NCCG), clinical assistants and possibly a senior house officer (SHO), a specialist registrar (SpR) or both. Medical staff are non-resident on call. Patients who need acute management of reversible complications, such as neutropenic sepsis following chemotherapy, should not generally be admitted as there are usually only limited investigative facilities.

Supportive and palliative care networks   Services for cancer patients are now organised in 34 clinical networks. Palliative care services form part of supportive and palliative care networks which are subunits of cancer networks, although arrangements differ across the country to reflect local structures and meet local needs. The degree of integration within local cancer services is variable but increasing.

Patterns of referral   The majority of referrals to palliative medicine are made following the diagnosis of advanced, progressive and incurable disease. Referrals may come after a long period of disease-management in secondary care but 20% may follow an acute admission with no previous diagnosis. Referrals may be:

■   directly from the GP (60%) (when the terminal nature of the disease becomes apparent, where symptoms are difficult to control or there is high psychosocial need)

■   directly from a consultant in secondary care

■   from another specialist palliative care team in another setting or location

■   as a result of an enquiry by the patient or family (the family doctor or district nurse may be asked to make the referral).

Most inpatient services (216 in UK) have 24-hour specialist medical cover but admit patients within working hours only. Urgent referrals are normally seen within one working day. Admissions to specialist palliative care units can be arranged out of working hours, especially when patients are already known to the service or have been recognised as at risk of requiring emergency admission. Most services offer a 24-hour telephone advisory service to colleagues in the community and in hospital. They may provide specialist equipment (eg syringe drivers) for patients at home.

Most referrals need advice and support. Consultants in palliative medicine typically offer shared care with the GP in the community and with the referring specialist in a hospital setting.

Additional services available in specialist palliative care units:

■   bereavement services (339 in UK)

■   lymphoedema clinics (153 in UK)

■   complementary therapies in most units (eg massage and relaxation)[5]

■   art therapy in 50% of inpatient units

■   music therapy in 25% of inpatient units.

iii   Working with patients: patient-centred care

Patient choice and involving patients in discussions about their treatment

Palliative care has a patient-centred philosophy at its core and will aim to support the patient's views concerning end-of-life care. Patient choice in a multicultural society has been addressed in two documents produced by the National Council for Hospice and Specialist Palliative Care Services (NCHSPCS), known as the National Council for Palliative Care (NCPC) from November 2004.[6,7]

Opportunity for education, access to information and patient support groups

▪ Patient education is available from the Hospice Information service (**www.hospiceinformation.info**) and the NCHSPCS (**www.hospice-spc-council.org.uk** or **www.ncpc.org.uk**). They run projects interviewing patients and families about their hospice experience.[8]

▪ The Database of Individual Patient Experience (DIPEX) is a patient education website and has an end of life care section (**www.dipex.com**).

▪ Information is produced by, and available from, cancer support groups.

▪ User involvement at network and primary care trust (PCT) level is underway.[8]

▪ Patient-held records have been evaluated.[9]

▪ Patient support is provided via community nurse specialists in palliative care, sometimes called Macmillan nurses, and patients should also be supported by a dedicated social worker.[10]

▪ Local patient surveys, focus groups and the national patient survey provide valuable information for the development of services.

A number of charities offer information and support:

▪ Macmillan Cancer Line (**www.macmillan.org.uk**)

▪ CancerBACUP (**www.cancerbacup.org.uk**)

▪ National Cancer Alliance (**www.nationalcanceralliance.co.uk**)

iv Interspecialty and interdisciplinary liaison

Multidisciplinary team working

Clinical nurse specialists (CNSs) in palliative care Nurses with advanced qualifications and experience in palliative care are key members of the teams supporting patients in non-specialist settings.

Community CNSs are the largest professional group in community support teams. They assess the physical, psychological and social needs of patients at home, advise GPs and community nurses on the management of symptoms, and help to plan future management at home.

Hospital CNSs are the largest group in hospital support teams. Their key roles are to assess the needs of patients, advise on the management of symptoms and assist in planning for hospital discharge, whether to the patient's home, to a nursing home or to specialist inpatient palliative care. Some hospital-based CNSs work in a site-specific team for one type of primary cancer and provide supportive care for patients at all stages of the disease from diagnosis. They may offer advice and support during primary management and the advanced stages of the disease but some will handover patients to specialist palliative care if they have complex needs and advanced disease. Nurses with specific training, for example in the management of lymphoedema, run clinics for patients.

Specialist nurses based in a hospital or a specialist inpatient unit have an important liaison role in making the transition from the inpatient setting to the community as seamless as possible. Although they are rarely trained as counsellors, many CNSs provide considerable emotional and psychological support to patients and families. Community CNSs continue to support families in bereavement and refer individuals for whom bereavement is causing severe problems on to specialist services. Nurse specialists are part of the 24-hour on-call or crisis response teams provided by some community services.

Specialist social worker   Most inpatient services and an increasing proportion of other services include at least one specialist social worker. Their roles may include:

■   counselling and psychological support to patients and families, including children

■   advice on financial problems, including charitable grants and benefits

■   liaising with local authority social services in planning care after discharge

■   bereavement support, including complex and difficult bereavement problems

■   support for other staff within the specialist palliative care service.

Chaplain   Many patients and families seek spiritual help and support as death approaches, including those whose religion is non-Christian or who have no formal religious faith. The chaplain's role is increasingly to offer support tailored to the needs of the individual, to encourage religious leaders from other faiths to visit patients and to give comfort to patients facing death who do not have any religious affiliation.

Pharmacists   Specialist pharmacists provide an extremely useful resource for the specialty. Patients are frail, often with organ failure and in need of polypharmacy. In addition, many of the drugs prescribed in palliative care are used beyond their licence and some are specially formulated for individual patient needs.

Therapists and others   An increasing number of services involve physiotherapists, occupational therapists, clinical psychologists and a variety of complementary therapists in their teams. They may work with individual patients or provide group therapy, often in a day care setting. Physiotherapists and occupational therapists are important in the rehabilitation of patients with disability from advanced disease.

Conjoined services   Specialist palliative care may be conjoined potentially with all medical and surgical specialties in the hospital. It has an intimate relationship with primary care and works very closely with GPs and district nurses. Other closely linked bodies include:

■   major charities offering patient care (eg Marie Curie Cancer Care)

■   social services

■   nursing homes

■   voluntary bereavement services.

v   **Delivering a high quality service**

Since their inception, specialist palliative care services have aimed to provide a high quality of care, often using charitable funds to provide higher staffing levels and a better care environment than is usual within the NHS. More recently, services have been commissioned to a specification that usually includes quality standards. Such standards may be agreed regionally or nationally and are often verified by a peer review process or external accreditation.

Characteristics of a high quality service

■   24-hour access to the service, and clear referral and discharge criteria, based on need not diagnosis

■   a MDT including at least core specialists in palliative medicine, specialist nursing and social work

- patient access to the core specialties, and to other disciplines as appropriate, for physical, psychological, social and spiritual support
- evidence-based clinical management wherever possible
- clinical audit and research programmes to evaluate treatments and outcomes
- external and in-service education provision for professionals wishing to incorporate the palliative care approach into their practice and for those training in palliative care
- patient and family involvement in management plans and freedom for them to express their preference about where they wish to be cared for and where they wish to die
- support for carers and families through illness into bereavement and recognition of the needs of the bereaved.

Resources required for a high quality service

Referral

- means of receiving referrals rapidly (eg by fax and/or electronic transmission)
- dedicated administrative staff
- explicit standards specifying the interval from referral to first assessment for urgent and routine referrals.

Medical assessment

- early medical review, although not all new patients will be seen by the consultant in palliative medicine
- sufficient time for thorough medical assessment of a new patient, either in the outpatient clinic or on a domiciliary visit (at least an hour is normally required)
- access to medical notes and results of investigations carried out at other hospitals
- 24-hour medical advice available to colleagues in community and hospital settings
- support from suitably trained nurses
- dedicated administrative support
- rapid links to other medical disciplines, particularly clinical oncology and pain anaesthesia.

Day care

- dedicated day care space
- trained and experienced nursing support
- a separate clinical room in which medical assessment can be carried out
- facilities for minor procedures such as blood transfusion or interventional analgesia.

Inpatient care

- dedicated inpatient beds
- high ratio of nurses to patients (UK average 1.5:1)
- trained nurses with specialist skills and experience in palliative care
- dedicated social work support
- spiritual support
- access to other relevant professionals (eg pharmacist, lymphoedema specialist, physiotherapist, occupational therapist, clinical psychologist)

■ dedicated administrative support

■ other forms of support for staff, patients and families, such as complementary therapies, volunteers

■ overnight accommodation for families.

Education facilities and patient information

■ dedicated teaching space

■ audio-visual equipment

■ educational resources such as journals, books and videos in appropriate languages, access to computerised databases

■ staff with educational experience and relevant qualifications

■ information regarding medication regimens.

Links with colleagues

■ arrangements for communicating rapidly with the patient's GP and community nurse when the patient is discharged or dies

■ means for collaboration with colleagues in the community and in acute hospitals to support patients as their care moves between care environments.

Resources required in an acute hospital

Outpatient clinic

■ Facilities should allow the patient and any relevant family members to be seen together, if appropriate.

■ The consultant should be accompanied by at least one other member of the MDT.

■ The consultation should be unhurried and confidential.

■ There should be space for the patient and/or family members to talk separately with a clinical nurse specialist, social worker or other team member.

■ Specialist drugs should be dispensed promptly to avoid long waits for very sick patients.

■ There should be comfortable seating for patients to wait for transport or drugs.

Inpatient wards

■ There should be provision for private conversations with patients and with families, together or separately.

■ Each hospital should make policy decisions on whether the role of the consultant in palliative medicine is purely advisory, whether care is shared or whether the consultant in palliative medicine has admitting rights to hospital beds.

Resources required in specialist palliative care units

Facilities should be integrated wherever possible. The physical proximity of inpatient, outpatient and day care facilities promotes good communication and the efficient use of consultant expertise and time. If the community team base can be co-located, this further improves communication and allows the community clinical nurse specialists to keep links with their patients during admissions more easily. It is important that patients and families can access specialist units easily. Where a service covers a wide geographical area it may be more appropriate to have outlying day care units, or even to distribute the inpatient beds across one or more community hospitals, in addition to a hospice or NHS specialist palliative care unit.

Specialist inpatient unit

- an adequate number of single rooms, with en suite facilities where possible
- a comfortable, homely rather than clinical environment
- appropriate equipment for the care of weak, cachexic, debilitated patients (eg pressure-relieving mattresses, electrically operated beds and chairs, easily operated nurse call systems, individual telephones, TVs, assisted baths and showers etc)
- comfortable sitting rooms for patients and visitors
- self-catering facilities for hot drinks and simple snacks
- private rooms for interviews, counselling sessions
- dedicated space for viewing the deceased relative
- a chapel or spiritual room in which patients and families can pray, meditate or follow the rituals of their religion
- facilities for families to stay overnight.

Specialist day care centre

- a comfortable environment for people to meet socially
- facilities for a shared meal
- opportunities for creative therapy, such as art or music therapy
- at least one outpatient room in which patients can be medically assessed and nursing procedures performed
- an assisted bath and facilities for personal care
- appropriate space for complementary therapies such as massage.

In addition, because education is a major function for specialist palliative care, the specialist unit should provide space for teaching sessions and educational resources for use by the unit staff and students attending courses.

In every setting, consultants in palliative medicine and their supporting medical and non-medical teams must be provided with adequate office space, and computer and administrative support.

vi   Quality standards and measures of the quality of specialist services

These are defined by:

- *The NHS Cancer Plan* and the specific actions identified at regional and network level in both *The NHS Cancer Plan* and the subsequent *NHS plan – implementation programme*[11,12]
- *The manual of cancer standards* and the specific sections on standards in palliative care[13]
- guidance on supportive and palliative care by the National Institute for Clinical Excellence (NICE)[10]
- the College joint specialty committee on professional standards, London 2003 (**www.rcplondon.ac.uk**)
- the professional development committee of the Association of Palliative Medicine Physicians of UK and Eire (APM) (**www.palliative-medicine.org**).

CLINICAL WORK OF CONSULTANTS IN PALLIATIVE MEDICINE

Contribution to acute medicine

Consultants and SpRs in palliative medicine do not usually participate in the on-call rota for acute general medicine. Hospital support teams offer a consultation service for acute problems in palliative and terminal care during their normal working hours. Out-of-hours telephone consultation from a specialist inpatient service should be available.

Direct clinical care

The majority of inpatient specialist palliative care beds are funded by the voluntary sector and are located in free-standing hospices. In the UK there are 2,433 beds in the voluntary sector compared to 663 (25%) in NHS units. Nationally, there are 51 beds per million population. However, consultant posts are often shared with local district general hospitals (DGHs) or with trusts providing cancer services. NHS specialist palliative care units may be co-located with acute services. Consultant posts are often structured so that their input is spread between cancer services in cancer centres, cancer units within DGHs and within the community, in addition to responsibility for inpatient beds. Consultants in palliative medicine often carry out joint clinics with oncologists and attend tumour site-specific meetings.

Palliative care has a particularly close working arrangement with cancer services but since it is not diagnosis dependent the care networks also liaise with specialties other than oncology.

Community arrangements

Within the community, patients receive palliative care from their GPs. The role of the community palliative care team is advisory. Local arrangements vary but in some areas GPs with particular interest and expertise in palliative care have taken up posts as facilitators to promote training in palliative care among local GPs, or as local leads. Many specialist palliative care units employ GPs as clinical assistants, or have SHOs drawn from the vocational training scheme. This helps to develop considerable expertise in GPs and raises the local standard of palliative care at primary level.

Many consultants in palliative medicine are the sole consultant (30%) in their service. Although the number of trainees has increased (160 SpRs), the ratio of consultants to trainees and other medical staff remains high. Palliative medicine is often a consultant-delivered, as well as a consultant-led, specialty. A substantial proportion of specialist inpatient services are funded by the voluntary sector and more than half of consultants in palliative medicine have some or all of their sessions funded outside the NHS.

Consultants support inpatient units, day care, and community and hospital teams. A detailed workload study in 1997 indicated that one whole-time consultant would, on average, be responsible for 11 inpatient beds with 220 admissions per year; a home care service seeing 235 new referrals annually; a day hospice seeing 70 new referrals annually; and a hospital support team.[15]

Support teams both in the community and in hospital are often nurse-led. Some consultants will see all new referrals, others will see only a proportion. There is a wide variation in the proportion of time spent directly seeing patients, the time spent supporting and advising other members of the team and the time devoted to teaching, management and the strategic development of services in the area. On average, a consultant is likely to conduct at least two ward rounds per week, and devote two to three sessions to seeing outpatients, ward referrals or patients at home.

Multidisciplinary team meetings are key to team management of patients in palliative care, and consultants are likely to attend one to two per week. Increasingly, site-specific cancer services hold meetings of all the consultants concerned, therefore consultants in palliative medicine are being called upon to attend weekly or fortnightly meetings to discuss patients with lung, breast and other common cancers. Assessment of a new patient is time-consuming, often involving multiple physical symptoms, considerable emotional distress and complex family dynamics. Outpatient sessions allow up to an hour per new referral. Most consultants see one to two new patients and up to six follow-up patients in an outpatient clinic.

Many consultants work on more than one site. In addition, most provide both outpatient clinics and a domiciliary visit service. Considerable time is spent travelling, and liaising with GPs, hospital colleagues and other palliative care services. There is no participation in acute medical on-take work. Nevertheless, because many consultants work single-handed, those with responsibility for inpatients or for 24-hour care in the community may have an onerous on-call responsibility, sometimes seven days a week (see Table 1).[15] Some also carry out non-resident first on-call duties.

Table 1. Analysis of workload

Activity	Whole-time and maximum part-time consultants (99) Median hours and range
All activities*	49.5 (32–83)
Direct clinical	22.5 (2.5–51.5)
Indirect clinical	4.5 (0–16.5)
Teaching	3 (0–27.5)
Continuing medical education	1 (0–8.5)
Research	0 (0–19.5)
Administration and management	9 (0–23)
Other	4 (0–20)

*Mean hours for all activities = 51.3. On-call duties were not included.

Work to maintain and improve the quality of patient care

Leadership role and development of the service

- Joint clinics between oncologists or physicians and consultants in palliative medicine ensure that patients receive truly integrated management.

- Consultants in palliative medicine attend appropriate cancer site-specific multidisciplinary team (MDT) meetings.

- Palliative care services offer extended hours, in some cases a 24-hour service, to deal with crises.

- Hospice-at-home services provide an enhanced level of medical and nursing care for patients at home.

- Link nurse schemes offer additional training to one member of each ward or community nursing team so that they in turn can be resources for their colleagues

- Lymphoedema clinics improve the management of chronic lymphoedema, particularly following anti-cancer treatment.

Professional standards, education and training

- The APM has worked with the College to develop curricula for doctors at different levels of training. Specifically, it organises national meetings four times a year for all deanery regional specialty advisers involved in SpR training.

- The APM organises regular educational events four times a year, some with the Royal Society of Medicine.

- A mentoring scheme for new consultants is established.

- The professional development committee of the APM has produced guidance on CPD and clinical governance.

- The scientific committee of APM heads a research programme and liaises with the National Cancer Research Institute (NCRI).

- The professional standards joint specialty committee of the College has produced standards for good medical practice.

- NCCG committee highlights professional issues.

- The APM has contributed to all published NICE guidance to date for cancer sites, and to specialty guidelines (**www.nice.org**).

- Consultants contribute to several committees for the NCHSPCS.

- Consultants have leadership roles in regional work: writing and implementing strategies for service delivery and education in the supportive and palliative care networks.

- The Department of Health (DH) workforce team is involved in future planning of SpR and consultant numbers.

ACADEMIC MEDICINE

There are six academic departments of palliative medicine but increasing numbers of SpRs are doing higher degrees either during or after their clinical training.

The patient population is characterised by a short prognosis, an unstable clinical state, the need for polypharmacy and increasing cognitive impairment as death approaches. Therefore, conventional randomised controlled trials are difficult. Nevertheless, active research into methods of symptom control and into the cost-effectiveness of models of service delivery is being carried out. Academic departments make a major contribution to the delivery of clinical services and the clinical undergraduate and postgraduate teaching programmes. There is a clear need to support and develop the academic basis of palliative care.

WORKFORCE REQUIREMENTS FOR PALLIATIVE MEDICINE

The Census in 2003 identified 270 consultants (237 WTE) working in palliative medicine.[14] The median ratio of whole-time consultants to non-consultant medical staff (training and non-training) was 2:1. Although trainee numbers are increasing (160 SpRs in 2002), palliative medicine is predominantly a consultant-delivered service.

The majority of consultants have clinical responsibilities in more than one care setting. In 1997, 88% of consultants had responsibility for specialist inpatient beds, with a median of 11 beds per consultant.[15] The proportion of time spent in clinical work, both direct patient care and supporting other professionals in the team, was highest for part-time consultants but was more than 50% of the working week even for whole-time consultants. Non-clinical work, particularly teaching and strategic development of palliative care services, took an average of 39% of consultants' time. Few consultants had adequate time for CPD, audit or research.

In determining the consultant requirements in palliative medicine, a number of factors have to be taken into account:

  ▪ *An ageing population*   Cancer is the major diagnosis leading to referral for palliative care and is predominantly a disease of the elderly. World Health Organization (WHO) estimates suggest that the prevalence of cancer will increase markedly by 2010.

  ▪ *Trends in referral of patients with cancer*   Referral rates tend to rise as services become available, and reach 70% of the cancer population in some areas. A 70% referral rate has been used in calculating consultant requirements.

  ▪ *Increasing referral of patients with non-cancer diagnoses*   Research indicates that patients with non-malignant terminal illnesses have at least as many problems in terms of symptoms and social and psychological needs as those with cancer. In some services, referral of patients with non-malignant disease now accounts for 50% of referrals. A conservative estimate of 20% has been used.

  ▪ *A high proportion of female doctors in the specialty*   59% of consultants and 80% of SpRs are female. Many train part-time and a proportion wish to continue in part-time work as consultants.

  ▪ *The workloads measured in the 1997 survey*   These were too high to allow adequate time for CPD, audit, research and clinical governance and therefore did not facilitate the delivery of a high quality service.[15]

Based on calculations including all these factors, there should be a minimum of one WTE consultant in palliative medicine for every 160,000 residents (1.56 WTE consultants per 250,000 population). The current number of SpRs in training is intended to enable the specialty to reach this target by 2013.

Table 2. Minimum consultant requirements (England and Wales)

Cancer deaths/annum for 250,000 population	660
If 70% access specialist palliative care	462 referrals per year
Plus 20% non-cancer referrals	554 referrals per year
Requirement if one WTE sees 360 new patients year (APM calculation)	1.54 WTE
Minimum consultant requirement per 52 million population	320 WTE
Minimum consultant requirement	1 per 160,000 residents
Minimum consultant numbers, assuming 30% work part-time	1 per 120,000 residents

This calculation is in line with the Workforce Review Team for the DH who currently plan for 325 WTE consultants, or 455 including part-time consultants, by 2013. However, this does not take account of the new consultant contract (10 PAs per week) and the need to work within the European Working Time Directive. A pragmatic final estimate is two WTE per 250,000 population. This means that for England and Wales there will need to be 418 WTE consultants and 466 across the UK by 2013.

Table 3. The work of palliative medicine consultants generated by a population of 250,000 as programmed activities (PAs) (four hours)

Activity	Workload	PAs/week for 250,000 patients
Direct Patient Care		
Ward rounds	339 admissions/year	4–5
Outpatients	2 new patients/week plus 1–6 follow-ups	2
Hospital referrals	2–6 patients/week	
Community referrals	1 domiciliary visit/week	
Day care		3–5
MDT meetings with ward and community team	Ward: 1/week Community team: 1/week	2
On-call and weekend ward rounds		2
	Total direct patient care	13–16
Work to maintain and improve quality of care		6–8
	Total	19–24

CONSULTANT WORK PROGRAMME/SPECIMEN JOB PLAN

Recognised job patterns are:

- hospice with inpatients only
- hospice and community work
- hospice, community and acute hospital (the most common pattern)
- acute hospital and community
- acute hospital alone
- community service alone.

Inpatient work

- Consultants must conduct at least two ward rounds in a specialist inpatient unit per week, of which one is a MDT meeting.
- Teaching SpRs and other staff forms an important component of ward rounds.
- One WTE consultant is responsible for a median of 11 inpatient beds, admitting a median of 220 patients a year, of whom 188 will be newly referred.
- A consultant will see an average of 200–300 new and varied referrals each year.
- Full-time consultants spend a median of 4.5 hours per week in direct clinical care, which includes supervising specialist nurses, liaison with colleagues and case conferences.

Outpatient clinics

- Most consultants carry out one outpatient clinic per week.
- They see one to two new patients and up to six follow-up patients at each clinic.
- If a trainee takes part in the clinic they rarely see more than one to two new patients.

▪ Clinics may be held at an acute hospital, a palliative day care unit or attached to a specialist inpatient unit.

▪ Most consultants work flexibly and will see urgent referrals on any day of the week either as an outpatient or at home.

▪ Consultants working in cancer centres or cancer units will usually carry out one or more joint clinics with oncologists per week.

Specialised clinics

▪ Some consultants hold clinics for patients with pain problems, including non-malignant pain.

▪ Interventional procedures for pain control may be performed.

Home care

▪ Consultants make a wide range of domiciliary visits, on average one to two times a week.

▪ The median number referrals for patients at home is 235 per year.

▪ Service models vary: some consultants see all new referrals, in other services the majority are initially assessed by clinical nurse specialists.

▪ Typically, one session a week is spent supervising clinical nurse specialists in the community team.

On-call commitment

▪ Generally, the on-call commitment is onerous.

▪ Many consultants are first on call for specialist inpatient beds at least one in four.

▪ Many consultants work single-handed, and have second on-call rotas of 1:1.

▪ Sleep is rarely disturbed but the workload for the first on-call consultant during a weekend is significant. Time off in lieu is rarely included in job plans.

Table 4. Annual service activity undertaken or supported by one whole-time equivalent consultant[15]

Service	Median figures and ranges
Inpatient service	11 beds 220 admissions per year First on-call 1:3 (1:1 to 1:9)
Home care	235 new referrals (0–900)
Day hospice	70 new referrals (0–300)
Outpatient clinics	1 session per week (0–5) 44 new patients per year (0–300)
Domiciliary and hospital visits to patients	2 sessions per week (0–5) 45 domiciliary visits (0–700) 50 hospital visits (0–700)

CONSULTANT WORK PROGRAMME/SPECIMEN JOB PLAN

Activity	Workload	Programmed activities (PAs)
Direct clinical care		
Inpatients	11 beds 220 admissions per year	**2.5**
Outpatients	2 new patients per week	**1**
Home/domiciliary visits	1 per week	**0.5**
Day care	2–6 patients per week	**0.5**
Acute hospital support team		**1**
Multidisciplinary team meeting with ward and community teams		**1**
On call for specialist advice and emergencies and on call weekend ward rounds		**1**
Total number of direct clinical care PAs		**7.5 on average**
Supporting professional activities (SPA)		
Work to maintain and improve the quality of healthcare	Education and training, appraisal, departmental management and service development, audit and clinical governance, CPD and revalidation, research	**2.5 on average**
Other NHS responsibilities	eg medical director/clinical director/lead consultant in specialty/clinical tutor	**Local agreement with trust**
External duties	eg work for deaneries/Royal Colleges/specialist societies/Department of Health or other government bodies etc	**Local agreement with trust**

Note: most consultants in palliative medicine play a greater role in the strategic development of palliative care services locally than is common in other specialties and a high percentage (30%) are single-handed. This job plan does not represent the workload carried by the majority of consultants currently in post, and emphasises that the most common current pattern, whereby a single consultant carries responsibility for work in inpatient, community and hospital settings, is not sustainable other than in adequately staffed multi-consultant services.[4]

References

1. The Expert Advisory Group on Cancer to the Chief Medical Officers of England and Wales. *A policy framework for commissioning cancer services: Guidance for providers and purchasers of cancer services. (The Calman-Hine report chapter 4.5)*. London: Department of Health, and Cardiff: Welsh Office, 1995.

2. World Health Organization. *WHO definition of palliative care*, 2002. www.who.int/cancer/palliative/definition/en/

3. Hospice information. *Minimum data set 2003* and *Hospice* and *Palliative care facts and figures 2003*. www.hospiceinformation.info/factsandfigures.asp

4. The Federation of the Royal Colleges of Physicians of the United Kingdom.*Census of consultant physicians in the UK, 2002. Data and commentary*. London: The Federation of the Royal Colleges of Physicians of the United Kingdom, 2002.

5. Marianne Tavares. *National guidelines for the use of complementary therapies in supportive and palliative care.* London: The Prince of Wales's Foundation for Integrated Health and The National Council for Hospice and Specialist Palliative Care Services, 2003.
    www.fihealth.org.uk also at www.hospice-spc-council.org.uk/public/complementary-guidelines.pdf

6. Firth S. *Wider horizons: care of the dying in a multi-cultural* society. London: National Council for Hospice and Specialist Palliative Care Services, 2001.

7. Mount J et al. *Palliative care services for different ethnic groups.* London: National Council for Hospice and Specialist Palliative Care Services, 2001.

8. National Council for Hospice and Specialist Palliative Care Services. *Our Lives not our illness: User involvement in palliative care (Briefing bulletin 6).* London: National Council, 2002. www.ncpc.org.uk/Publications/B_B.htm

9. Cornbleet MA, Campbell P, Murray S, Stevenson M et al. Patient-held records in cancer and palliative care: a randomised, prospective trial. *Palliat Med* 2002;**16**(3):205–12.

10. National Institute for Clinical Excellence. *Improving supportive and palliative care for adults with cancer.* National Institute for Clinical Excellence, March 2004. www.nice.org.uk/page.aspx?o=1100017

11. Department of Health. *The NHS cancer plan: a plan for investment, a plan for reform.* London: DH, 2000.

12. Department of Health. *NHS plan implementation programme.* London: DH, 2000.

13. Department of Health. *Manual of cancer services assessment standards: consultation document.* London: DH, 2000. (Specific section on palliative care in 2001 update.)

14. The Federation of the Royal Colleges of Physicians of the United Kingdom.*Census of consultant physicians in the UK, 2003. Data and commentary.* London: The Federation of the Royal Colleges of Physicians of the United Kingdom, 2003.

15. Makin, W et al. What do Palliative Medicine Consultants do? *Palliat Med* 2000;**14**(5);405–409.

Rehabilitation medicine

i   Description of the specialty and clinical needs of patients

Rehabilitation medicine helps people with disabilities achieve and maintain their optimal physical, psychological and social function. The primary aims of the specialty are to empower the disabled person, to assist them in reducing the impact of their disability and to promote their full inclusion into society. This process can only be delivered through an integrated multidisciplinary team (MDT) with the central involvement of the disabled person and their family. Rehabilitation medicine focuses on education and training of the disabled person, in which the consultant in rehabilitation medicine has a key role to play.

Disability in childhood and the elderly are largely under the aegis of the specialties of paediatrics and geriatrics respectively. Rehabilitation medicine has developed as a specialty primarily to meet the needs of disabled people through the intervening period of adult life. Although the basic principles are not age specific there is good evidence that adults with disabilities require different rehabilitation programmes from those required by children and elderly people. However, many aspects of the specialty, particularly relating to technical aids, provision of wheelchairs, orthotics or prosthetics, are relevant to people of all ages.

Rehabilitation medicine covers a considerable number of disabling conditions. In adulthood, most arise from injury or disease within the central and peripheral nervous system, such as traumatic brain injury, spinal cord injury, stroke, multiple sclerosis, Parkinson's disease and motor neurone disease. Although there are greater numbers of people with musculoskeletal disabilities, only a relatively small number require the specialist skills of rehabilitation medicine, and many are looked after by specialists in rheumatology and general practice. Other conditions arising in childhood, such as cerebral palsy, spina bifida, myopathies and dystrophies, will continue into adulthood and young people will need support, advice and assistance. Rehabilitation medicine also deals with the needs of people requiring lifelong technical assistance following amputation or with congenital limb deformity. Technological provision such as environmental control equipment and the prescription of wheelchairs, prosthetics and orthotics are not disease specific and cover a considerable range of disabilities.

The type of disability has a bearing on the type of service required. At the onset of an acute illness, such as multiple sclerosis or traumatic brain injury, people generally require a more medical model of care. However, for those with static conditions, or once maximum functional improvement has been gained, services move towards a long-term, supportive and community-focused role based on a social model of disability. The rehabilitation team should continue to support and empower the disabled person and their family, help them manage their own disability and prevent secondary complications, and provide the necessary support and treatment when clinical intervention is required.

ii   Organisation of the service and patterns of referral

Rehabilitation medicine is a relatively new specialty and is still quite under-developed in many parts of the UK.[1] However, there has been some growth at tertiary, secondary and community levels. There are now a number of specialist rehabilitation centres, which generally serve an area with a population of around two to four million. These specialist regional centres tend to take tertiary referrals for more complex or severe disabilities. Services have developed mainly because of the rarity of some complex conditions but also because of the scarcity of appropriately trained and specialist physicians, therapists and nurses. Regrettably, not all parts of the UK have access to such a tertiary centre.

At the secondary level many hospitals now have a dedicated stroke unit. There is good quality evidence of the efficacy of such units.[2] Some have now extended their role and become broader based rehabilitation units. These need support from community teams and the ability to refer to a specialist tertiary centre.

Disabled people themselves have been increasingly vocal in promoting more accessible and local services. Some parts of the UK have seen the development of community-based rehabilitation teams. In some areas there are outreach teams from the tertiary centre or teams focused around a local stroke unit at the district general hospital (DGH). Teams may have a diagnosis-specific orientation such as multiple sclerosis or head injury, or will have a more generic orientation, perhaps concentrating on specific age groups. Some have been developed for a specific purpose such as early stroke discharge. Unfortunately, there is no coordinated provision of community rehabilitation services across the UK. Services are often patchy and fragmented.

Historically, services in primary care have consisted of individual therapists working in relative isolation. This is still largely the case although a number of specialist nurses and therapists have emerged in recent years. There are now a number of specialist nurses working with people with multiple sclerosis, Parkinson's disease, epilepsy and dystonia. However, the evidence for the effectiveness of stroke units has highlighted the importance of coordinated MDT working and it is hoped that in the future there will be more community teams rather than individuals working alone.[2]

Rehabilitation medicine has emerged largely from other hospital specialties, and physicians are normally hospital based. There is little tradition of rehabilitation physicians working within the community but this is slowly changing and there are now a small number of community-orientated rehabilitation medicine posts.

In common with many other medical specialties, referral to specialist services may come from primary care physicians or consultant colleagues. However, because of the multifaceted nature of rehabilitation many professions allied to medicine, such as physiotherapy, occupational therapy, speech therapy and clinical psychology, will also refer into specialist services, either directly to specialist colleagues or to the service as a whole. Ideally, disabled people should be able to self-refer to such services but current government policy makes this difficult.

iii   Working with patients: patient-centred care

Patient choice, opportunities for education and promoting self-care

Patient-centred care is central to the ethos of rehabilitation medicine. Individual disabled people must be integral to the decision-making process of their own rehabilitation programme. Rehabilitation depends on setting achievable goals in a realistic timescale. Such goals must be relevant to the needs and wishes of the disabled person. If the disabled person, and often their family, is not involved in the goal-setting process then proper rehabilitation is not taking place. Thus, in this specialty more than most, patient choice is central to the delivery of the service.

The rehabilitation programme should educate the disabled person about their condition and treatment possibilities so that they are able to make their own choices. In the longer term, the aim of the programme is to enable the person to be in charge of the management of their own condition through education and training. In some cases, such as those with severe cognitive damage, such self-empowerment is not possible and an advocate must be involved.

Patient support groups and the role of the carer

Disability is usually not about one individual but about the whole family network. Many disabled people need additional assistance from their family and many require a complex care package with a variety of professionals visiting the home. It is the duty of the MDT to involve not only the disabled person in their rehabilitation programme but also the carer. Many teams have found it useful to develop an individual within the team whose main role is to support and listen to the needs of the carers. In this context, patient support groups can be a major help to the disabled person, their family and, indeed, the rehabilitation team. Many support groups around the UK are an integral part of the rehabilitation support network. They have a particular role in providing good quality accessible information and can often provide peer support and counselling services.

Patients with chronic conditions

Many disabled people have lifelong requirements for rehabilitation and disability support services. If the ultimate aim of these services is to enable the disabled person to be in charge of their own management then it is appropriate for them to have full access to their own clinical records and preferably to hold these records themselves. This would promote communication between the disabled person and the variety of professionals with whom they have contact. Rehabilitation medicine should lead the way in developing the role of the expert patient.

iv Interspecialty and interdisciplinary liaison

Rehabilitation medicine cannot work without a full MDT. There is now clear evidence of the effectiveness of such a team over and above individual therapists working in isolation. This is the case in the context of stroke and such evidence is emerging in the context of traumatic brain injury, and multiple sclerosis.[3,4,5] The key to MDT working is that professional roles are somewhat blurred, particularly as the rehabilitation goals are set to the wishes of the disabled person rather than the wishes of an individual department. The key members of a MDT are likely to be:

- *Nurses* Rehabilitation nurses have a crucial role as they are with the person 24 hours a day, at least in the post-acute inpatient setting. They carry over the skills learned in therapy into daily tasks. There are an increasing number of specialist nurses who are either disease specific (eg multiple sclerosis) or symptom specific (eg incontinence), and who work in hospital and community settings.
- *Occupational therapists* Occupational therapists work on strategies to promote independent daily living, and advise on appropriate aids and adaptation to facilitate such independence. Occupational therapists work closely with colleagues in the community to facilitate reintegration of the individual at home and to help them maintain a state of maximum independence.
- *Physiotherapists* Physiotherapists concentrate on restoring and maintaining joint range, muscle power and balance in order to facilitate walking. They often have a key role in the provision of wheelchairs and suitable seating and play an important part in pain relief or promoting strength and cardiovascular fitness.

■ *Speech and language therapists*   Speech and language therapists work on all aspects of communication including language, phonation, articulation and the use of communication aids. They have developed particular expertise in aspects of swallowing and often take the lead in the management of dysphagia.

■ *Dietitians*   Dietitians work closely with speech and language therapists to ensure correct diet. Many disabled people have changing metabolic requirements, particularly when recovering from an acute injury, and the role of the dietitian can be vital at both early and later stages.

■ *Clinical psychologists*   Clinical psychologists are responsible mainly for assessing the psychological impact of disability and work to ameliorate psychological or behavioural problems through a variety of retraining programmes. Clinical neuropsychologists are a central part of any team dealing with traumatic brain injury and it is doubtful that a neurobehavioural unit could function without neuropsychological input.

A number of other therapists and professionals assist the rehabilitation team, including social workers, counsellors, art and music therapists, prosthetists, orthotists and bioengineers. There is an increasing emphasis on technological advances to support people with disabilities, particularly in wheelchairs, environmental control, and communication aids. Appropriately trained bioengineers are vital in a modern rehabilitation team.

Rehabilitation medicine has key links with a number of other medical and surgical specialties, for example:

■ paediatrics and geriatrics

■ orthopaedic surgeons for joint surgery, tenotomies and amputations

■ general surgeons and gastroenterologists to initiate and supervise PEG feeding

■ ear, nose and throat (ENT) surgeons for tracheotomy management

■ anaesthetists for pain management and sedation for minor procedures

■ neurologists for epilepsy management and diagnostic advice

■ neurosurgeons for immediate management after traumatic brain injury and ongoing advice with regards to shunts and intrathecal pumps

■ psychiatrists for the assessment and management of mood and behaviour in conjunction with clinical psychologists

■ urologists for the management of continence.

This is not an exhaustive list but illustrates the wide range of skills required by the rehabilitation physician and team in order to use the expertise of other specialists in a timely and appropriate fashion.

Rehabilitation medicine services also need links with primary care and other community services. This is particularly important in times of re-integration into the community after an acute event such as stroke or traumatic brain injury. The GP and the primary care team will need to be involved in discharge arrangements and ongoing care packages. Other community-orientated services, such as consumer groups, voluntary sector, education, employment, housing and social services, are vital. Finally, there is a growing need for rehabilitation services to work with legal colleagues to assist those in the process of seeking compensation.

v Delivering a high quality service

Characteristics of a high quality service

A high quality rehabilitation medicine service will have a robust MDT which works as a cooperative automaton, with each individual respecting and understanding the skills of the others. Such team working needs to be developed and fostered. Good listening, communicating and negotiating skills, both within the team and between different professionals, are essential to full coordination of the process of care. Many teams have recognised that a named case manager or key worker within the team can provide a useful coordinating and continuity function. In addition, systems for information storing and resolution of conflict between team members are crucial in a high quality service.

Resources required for a high quality service

Specialised facilities

Inpatient unit

- For a population of 250,000, the needs of adults in the age range of 16–65 are likely to require 15–20 beds. (Fifteen beds constitute the minimum that is likely to be viable for a MDT.) The beds must be located together in order to provide an appropriate environment for rehabilitation and to make best use of the rehabilitation nursing complement.
- Some single room accommodation will be needed but sufficient space must be available for therapy, recreation and social activities, team meetings, case conferences and individual therapy.
- The inpatient unit must have immediate access to acute medical services, psychiatry, neurology, rheumatology, orthopaedics, urology, dietetics and enteral feeding services. The usual range of radiology and pathology services should be available on the same site.
- The unit must have a supply of wheelchairs, including electric chairs, immediately available for patients on the unit and have access to specialist orthotics, special seating and wheelchair clinics.

Outpatient facilities   Specialist rehabilitation has traditionally been provided on a tertiary basis. Whilst conventional outpatient facilities may meet the needs of some patients undergoing rehabilitation, the majority need access to the MDT. Therefore, day assessments, case conferences or outreach visits are often more appropriate.

Whatever the pattern of outpatient services, the consultant will need access to:

- gymnasium and hydrotherapy resources
- light and heavy workshops
- orthotics and prosthetics (amputee rehabilitation)
- specialist wheelchairs and seating
- counselling services
- psychology services
- driving assessment and training services
- sexual and genetic counselling services
- local education and employment training services
- vocational rehabilitation services
- social services.

Assistive technology services These services currently include communication aids, environmental control units, electric wheelchairs, smart controllers and switch access facilities. All services are developing rapidly and need to store demonstration equipment for assessors to access easily. Efficient repair, replacement and emergency back-up services are required and can be supplied via commercial contact or via in-house provision. For the latter option, workshops and storage facilities are required.

Workforce requirements: clinical and support staff

Consultant workforce See *Workforce requirements for rehabilitation medicine* below.

Non-medical workforce Section iv highlighted the key members of the MDT. The exact number of these team members will clearly depend on the size and scope of the individual unit. A post-acute unit will, for example, need a higher ratio of 24-hour nursing staff than a later-stage step-down unit that works towards integrating people back into the community. Obviously some key members such as occupational therapists and social workers will become more involved at the time of hospital discharge and when the individual is back at home. Here, it is simply important to state that a rehabilitation team must have access to an appropriate range and appropriate numbers of specialist nurses, therapists and clinical psychologists.

vi   Quality standards and measures of the quality of specialist services

The developments in quality standards and measures of the quality of services in rehabilitation medicine are summarised comprehensively in the supplement on clinical governance published in *Clinical rehabilitation*.[5] The College proposed the following two standards for the specialty:

- All patients entering a rehabilitation programme should have a set of goals established and agreed between the team and the patient/family within a defined time from entry.
- All patients enrolled in a rehabilitation programme should have at least one agreed outcome measure assessed on admission and discharge from the programme.

These specifically represent the multidisciplinary nature of the specialty. There have been several publications on standards and guidelines in recent years. The *National clinical guidelines on rehabilitation following acquired brain injury*, published jointly by the College and the British Society of Rehabilitation Medicine (BSRM), provides a comprehensive framework for the management of an important patient group and complements the guidelines for the management of head injuries published by the National Institute for Clinical Excellence (NICE) in June 2003.[6,7] It is envisaged that these evidence-based guidelines will underpin the development of rehabilitation services for this client group over the next decade.

The BSRM published *Clinical Standards for specialist inpatient rehabilitation services in the UK*, *Clinical standards for specialist community rehabilitation services in the UK* and, more recently, *Amputee and prosthetic rehabilitation – standards and guidelines*.[8,9,10] Guidelines for prescription and provision of special seating systems are expected. Guidelines on management of adults with spasticity using botulinum toxin were published in April 2001.[11]

The diversity of the patient population undergoing rehabilitation means that no single outcome measure can be applied. Hard outcomes, such as the percentage discharged to their own home or returned to work, are frequently reported but provide no graded assessment for those not quite achieving them. Global disability measures such as the Barthel Index or Functional Independence

Measure (FIM) are used increasingly but they have well-recognised floor and ceiling effects and are sometimes of little relevance to the intervention. Goal attainment scores are being explored as a means of assessing success in meeting individual goals but provide little comparative information. At present, best practice entails identification of a range of suitable validated measures, relevant to the rehabilitation provided, which are then applied as uniformly as possible.

All services, and this is no less true of rehabilitation medicine, need clear service specifications so that providers, purchasers and consumers understand what is being provided. Among the main factors that influence quality of service are critically and regularly audited documented standards and a robust consumer voice. A strong, committed and informed management structure is critical to safeguard the quality of the service.

CLINICAL WORK OF CONSULTANTS IN REHABILITATION MEDICINE

Contributions made to acute medicine

Increasingly, consultants in rehabilitation medicine have found it more effective to practise solely in the specialty rather than combining rehabilitation with acute medicine. The practices are totally different and the demands of acute medicine often override the timescale for rehabilitation medicine and make it more difficult to practise the latter effectively.

However, rehabilitation medicine specialists can assist acute medicine services by providing timely advice and ensuring that people who have become disabled progress through the various facets of their care without undue delay. They need to ensure that providers of emergency or acute services can access post-acute services rapidly when required, ensuring that the disabled person is in the most appropriate environment for treatment at each stage of recovery.

Direct clinical care

Inpatient work

Inpatient work will vary depending on the type of specialist rehabilitation being provided. The following list is amalgamated from a spectrum of sources:

- *Ward rounds*   A multidisciplinary weekly ward round for 20 beds takes four to five hours. One programmed activity (PA) should be allowed for each ward round.
- *Referral work*   10–12 referrals may be seen per week, requiring one to two PAs.
- *Interdisciplinary liaison*   This is the hallmark of rehabilitation medicine and requires considerable communication and listening skills in an inpatient rehabilitation unit (one PA per week). Rehabilitation medicine overlaps with almost every other surgical and medical specialty, demanding a great deal of time for interspecialty liaison. Probably two PAs per week is spent negotiating, discussing and planning with other colleagues, both medical and non-medical.
- *Case conferences*   There are two to three per week, lasting one to two hours (one PA).

Outpatient work

Conventional clinics   As mentioned previously, these are not particularly appropriate to the specialty as it is largely tertiary based. Where they are still in use, two to six new patients or four to eight follow-up patients may be seen in a session of one PA.

Special clinics   These are conducted either on the specialised unit or by outreach. Examples include:

▪ school leavers clinic (in conjunction with paediatrics)

▪ prosthetic amputee rehabilitation (specialised unit)

▪ specialised wheelchair seating (specialised unit or outreach)

▪ electric indoor/outdoor powered chairs (specialised unit or outreach)

▪ environmental control assessment (outreach)

▪ spasticity clinic

▪ incontinence clinic

▪ disease specific clinics, eg multiple sclerosis.

Acute general medical clinic   Very few rehabilitation medicine consultants are involved in acute take. Those that do acute on-call work tend to refer patients on to their specialist colleagues and only follow up those with chronic disabling conditions.

Non-acute general medical clinic   For the above reason there are few rehabilitation medicine consultants who do non-acute general medical clinics.

Specialist investigative and therapeutic procedure clinics

At present, these are mainly concerned with spasticity, for example botulinum toxin clinics and phenol blockade services (local and intrathecal). Splinting, tracheostomy and percutaneous endoscopic gastrostomy (PEG) insertion are done in conjunction with other specialties or as multidisciplinary clinics.

Specialist on call

All consultants running specialist inpatient facilities need to be part of an on-call rota. The exact rota depends on the number of consultants involved and the experience of junior staff. With a unit of 20 beds, a consultant may be on call one in two or one in three, but it is unlikely that they will need to come into the hospital more than once a month.

Other specialist activity including activities beyond the local services

There are a number of other specialist activities that can be undertaken by a consultant in rehabilitation medicine. Many examples have been referred to in previous sections. Assessments for disabled drivers, for example, are linked to rehabilitation medicine services. Patients with neurological disabilities who require specialised urodynamic and fertility advice will be seen in conjunction with appropriate specialties.

Services outwith the base hospital

Domiciliary work entails two to three visits per week. Hospice work is not a particular feature of rehabilitation medicine at present but there is an overlap with palliative care in certain rapidly progressive conditions such as motor neurone disease. Some other services have been outlined in the description of outpatient work.

Clinically related administration

At least one PA per week should be allocated for administration. Necessary resources include IT systems with full Internet access and appropriate secretarial services. It is also worthy of note that many rehabilitation medicine physicians in tertiary units have a proactive management role and are, in effect, clinical directors of their unit.

Work to maintain and improve the quality of care

This work encompasses duties in clinical governance, professional self-regulation, continuing professional development (CPD) and education and training of others. For many consultants at various times in their careers it may include research, serving in management and providing specialist advice at local, regional and national levels.

ACADEMIC MEDICINE

There is an increasing evidence base for the efficacy of rehabilitation. Excellent evidence from randomised, placebo-controlled studies shows the efficacy of multidisciplinary rehabilitation in the context of stroke.[2] There is also emerging evidence of the efficacy of rehabilitation techniques in the context of traumatic brain injury, multiple sclerosis and community-orientated rehabilitation.[3,4,12] However, there remains a clear need for further evidence with regard to the efficacy of individual techniques and different therapeutic approaches. Regrettably, the academic base of rehabilitation medicine remains fragile and threatened. There are only a handful of designated academic units in the UK and very few full-time academic positions. Increased cooperation and collaboration between the nursing, therapy, and medical undergraduate and postgraduate programmes is necessary, and will require improved liaison between universities within the major teaching centres. There should be greater realisation that other research methodologies may be as appropriate as the randomised placebo-controlled study. Single-case designs and greater reliance on qualitative methodologies are highly relevant to the development of a broader academic base in rehabilitation medicine.

It is good to see that many medical undergraduate curricula now contain compulsory teaching on rehabilitation medicine but more emphasis on education and training in this specialty is still needed at undergraduate and postgraduate level.

WORKFORCE REQUIREMENTS FOR REHABILITATION MEDICINE

As a general statement, the specialty would wish to see one whole time equivalent (WTE) consultant physician per 250,000 of the population.[13] However, a survey of the medical staffing in rehabilitation medicine in 2000 showed that not one health region in the UK currently meets this minimum standard. There are a total of 133 consultants whose main specialty is rehabilitation medicine, and a further 25 consultants with a different main specialty who also practise in rehabilitation medicine.

It remains difficult to confirm the accuracy of these figures because of the heterogeneity of the specialty and the significant number of part-time staff and rehabilitation physicians who also hold appointments in other specialties (eg neurology, rheumatology or geriatric medicine).

To fulfil the target of one consultant per 250,000 demands 195 WTE by 2010 for England and 233 for the UK. The current figure is 125 WTE (head count 133). This would require a significant increase in the number of consultant appointments. Although the calculations are not evidence based, this would seem to be a reasonable target. When viewed over a 10-year period, rehabilitation medicine has shown the second highest expansion rate at about 150% (Census 1993–Census 2003).[14] Despite this, there remains a great urgency in the appointment of new consultant posts, which is proving to be difficult at a time when there is significant expansion in several other acute specialties, with pressure to meet government targets.

The National Service Framework (NSF) on Long-Term Conditions is expected to be published in 2005. It is important that adequate resources are available to provide the service as recommended in the NSF. A sub-group will make workforce recommendations and it is envisaged that innovative ways of delivering the service may be presented.

The number of specialist registrars (SpRs) in the UK is around 65. In the last two years there has not been any increase in the number of national training numbers (NTNs). At the moment the specialty is broadly in balance with regard to the SpR to consultant ratio. However, if, as is hoped, there is an increase in the number of consultants in the field then there will need to be an associated increase in the number of SpR training posts.

CONSULTANT WORK PROGRAMME/SPECIMEN JOB PLAN

The work programme/job plan for consultants in rehabilitation medicine will vary widely. The job plan for a consultant working in a post-acute rehabilitation facility, for example, will obviously have a different emphasis than a consultant working mainly in a primary care or community setting. The BSRM has recently produced draft model job specifications and job plans for different settings (available from the BSRM). Thus, the following table can be viewed as a broad indication of some of the activities appropriate in a work programme/job plan and the relevant number of PAs that should be allocated to each activity.

Activity	Workload	Programmed activities (PAs)
Direct clinical care		
Inpatient: ward rounds	20 beds	**1 per ward round**
Referrals	10–12 per week	**1–2**
Multidisciplinary meeting/case conferences etc	Variable	**2–4**
Outpatient clinics, including specialised clinics	2–4 new patient 4–8 follow-up patients	**1 per clinic**
Outreach work from base hospital	Various	**1–2**
Work in another specialty	Not often required	**–**
Work in general medicine/acute take	Not often required	**–**
Work in academic medicine	Few academic appointments	**0–4 (more for full-time academic appointments)**
Clinical administration	Variable	**1–2**
Total number of direct clinical care PAs		**7.5 on average**
Supporting professional activities (SPA)		
Work to maintain and improve the quality of healthcare	Education and training, appraisal, departmental management and service development, audit and clinical governance, CPD and revalidation, research	**2.5 on average**
Other NHS responsibilities	eg medical director/clinical director/lead consultant in specialty/clinical tutor	**Local agreement with trust**
External duties	eg work for deaneries/Royal Colleges/specialist societies/Department of Health or other government bodies etc	**Local agreement with trust**

References

1. British Society of Rehabilitation Medicine. Manpower survey, April 2000.

2. Langhorn P, Williams BO, Gilchrist W, Howie K. Do stroke units save lives? *Lancet* 1993;**342**:395–398.

3. Semylen JK, Summers SJ, Barnes MP. Traumatic brain injury: Efficacy of multi-disciplinary rehabilitation. *Arch Phys Med Rehabil* 1998;**79**:678–683.

4. Freeman JA, Langdon DW, Hobart JC, Thompson AJ. The impact of rehabilitation on disability and handicap in progressive multiple sclerosis: Randomised controlled trial. *Ann Neurol* 1997;**42**:236–244.

5. Turner-Stokes L. Clinical governance in rehabilitation medicine. The state of the art in 2002. *Clin Rehabil* 2002; **16**(Suppl 1):13–20.

6. Royal College of Physicians and British Society of Rehabilitation Medicine. *Rehabilitation following acquired brain injury: national clinical guidelines* (Turner-Stokes L, ed). London: RCP, BSRM, 2003.

7. National Institute for Clinical Excellence. *Head injury – triage, assessment, investigation and early management of head injury in infants, children and adults*, June 2003. www.nice.org.uk/page.aspx?o=56817

8. Turner-Stokes L, Williams H, Abraham R, Ducket S. Clinical standards for specialist inpatient rehabilitation services in the UK. *Clin Rehabil* 2000;**14**(5):468–480.

9. Turner-Stokes L, Williams H, Abraham R. Clinical standards for specialist community rehabilitation standards in the UK. *Clin Rehabil* 2001;**15**(6):611–623.

10. British Society of Rehabilitation Medicine. *Amputee and prosthetic rehabilitation – standards and guidelines*, 2nd edition. Report of a working party. London: British Society of Rehabilitation Medicine, 2003.

11. Barnes M, Bhakta B, Moore P *et al. The management of adults with spasticity using botulinum toxin: a guide to clinical practice.* London: British Society of Rehabilitation Medicine, 2001.

12. Barnes MP, Radermacher H. *Community rehabilitation in neurology: a summary of the evidence of the efficacy of community rehabilitation.* Cambridge: Cambridge University Press, 2003.

13. Royal College of Physicians. Physical disability in 1986 and beyond. *J R Coll Physicians Lond* 1986;**20**(3):160–94.

14. The Federation of the Royal Colleges of Physicians of the United Kingdom. *Census of consultant physicians in the UK, 2003. Data and commentary.* London: The Federation of the Royal Colleges of Physicians of the United Kingdom, 2003.

Renal medicine

i Description of the specialty and clinical needs of patients

Renal medicine, or nephrology, involves the care of patients with all forms of renal tract disease. A major component of the service is the management of patients with acute or chronic kidney failure, and this element of the service is often used in assessing workforce requirements. In addition, nephrologists provide care for patients with kidney diseases without impairment of excretory kidney function, including proteinuria and nephrotic syndrome. Nephrologists work closely with urologists in providing care for patients with haematuria, recurrent urinary tract infection, kidney stone disease, urinary tract obstruction and neurogenic bladder, and with obstetricians in managing kidney disorders in pregnancy. The care of children with kidney disease is coordinated by paediatric nephrologists, and particular support is required for the transition to adult renal services.

Kidney disease is a long-term condition for many patients, and can impact on all apsects of life. The care, support and treatment of patients with end-stage kidney failure is an important aspect of adult renal service provision. A significant part of this service involves the early detection of kidney problems, and the prevention and management of progressive kidney disease. A coordinated approach involving access to, and support from, the whole range of health professionals is required to ensure that nutritional, lifestyle, social and psychological needs are met alongside the management of biochemical and metabolic disorders. The complexity of renal healthcare requires integrated multiprofessional working to provide a high quality service.

There has been a sustained increase in the number of patients receiving renal replacement therapy (RRT) in the UK. The National Kidney Research Fund (NKRF) reported that 19,307 patients were receiving dialysis in the UK in 2002, representing a 20% increase since the 1998 National Renal Survey.[1] The National Service Framework (NSF) for Renal Services highlights the fact that treatment rates for established kidney failure are slower in England than in other comparable countries, indicating ongoing unmet need.[2] The main growth in recent years has been in hospital-based haemodialysis, with little change in the number of patients receiving peritoneal dialysis. In parallel, there have been significant changes in the co-morbidity of patients accepted onto RRT programmes.

Transplantation rates have been sustained by increasing living donor kidney transplantation. Nephrologists work closely with transplant surgeons in the provision of renal transplant services, and are involved in the assessment of potential recipients, evaluation of potential living donors, pre- and post-operative care, and long-term follow up of patients following kidney transplantation.

ii Organisation of the service and patterns of referral

Primary, secondary and tertiary levels

Access to renal services is required at primary, secondary and tertiary levels at different stages of a patient's journey with kidney disease.

Primary care The early detection and prevention of kidney disease requires close collaboration between primary care practitioners, nephrologists and other specialists in secondary care. There is increasing emphasis on the management of risk factors for kidney disease, including early detection and treatment of diabetes and hypertension, and provision of clear guidance on the indications for referral to hospital. Late referral of patients with progressive renal impairment remains a problem. The College joint specialty committee for renal disease is currently preparing guidelines on referrral of patients with kidney disease to secondary care.

Secondary care The provision of care for patients with renal failure is largely hospital based, but the importance of involving primary care trusts in the commissioning and delivery of the service is recognised. Referrals to secondary care arise from GPs and from other specialists in secondary care including diabetologists and urologists.

Tertiary care During the 1960s and 1970s, RRT programmes in the UK were provided by a small number of renal units based in tertiary referral centres covering large catchment populations. In the 1980s and 1990s, there was a significant increase in renal services, provided to some extent by an increase in satellite units. There are currently 53 main adult renal units (not including satellite units) in England, five in Wales, 10 in Scotland and three in Northern Ireland. Referral to a tertiary centre may be required for creation of vascular access for haemodialysis, management of chronic renal failure where there is co-morbidity, management of acute renal failure, and renal transplantation. In 2002 there were 21 transplant centres in England, 26 in the UK.

Clinical networks

The level of renal service provision in different hospitals varies considerably, and networks have often evolved according to local geography. Some district general hospitals (DGHs) do not have a consultant nephrologist. Others have a nephrologist on a sessional basis, perhaps providing support for a satellite dialysis unit but unable to provide 24-hour cover for renal problems. Some hospitals may have consultant nephrologists who provide on-call cover for renal medicine, and often provide cover for general internal medicine (GIM), but who require access to a tertiary centre for renal transplantation. Haemofiltration for the urgent management of acute renal failure can be performed in many intensive care units, but subsequent transfer to a hospital with specialist nephrology input may be required.

Relationship with other services/agencies

The multidisciplinary team (MDT), which delivers healthcare to kidney patients, is represented by a number of professional bodies. The British Renal Society (BRS) (**www.britishrenal.org**) is a multiprofessional group created to improve standards of care for kidney patients and their families. The BRS established a multiprofessional national renal workforce planning group in 2001 with representation from a number of agencies. These include:

- The Renal Association (**www.renal.org**)
- British Association for Paediatric Nephrology (**www.bapn.uwcm.ac.uk**)
- British Transplant Society (**www.bts.org.uk**)
- British Society for Histocompatibility and Immunogenetics,
- Royal College of Nursing Nephrology Nurses Forum (**www.rcn.org.uk**)
- European Dialysis and Transplant Nurses Association/European Renal Care Association (**www.edtna-erca.org**)

■ British Dietetic Association/Renal Nutrition Group (**www.bda.uk.com**)

■ British Association of Social Workers (**www.basw.co.uk**)

■ British Psychological Society (**www.bps.org.uk**)

■ Association of Renal Technologists (**www.artery.org.uk**)

■ Renal Pharmacy Group (**www.renalpharmacy.org.uk**)

■ Neonatal and Paediatric Pharmacists Group (**www.nppg.demon.co.uk**)

■ Association of Renal Managers (**www.armmanagers.org**)

■ Society for District General Hospital Nephrologists

■ Vascular Surgical Society of Great Britain and Ireland.

iii Working with patients: patient-centred care

Patient choice and involving patients in decisions about their treatment

The onset of kidney disease is often a major life-changing event. Patients, families and carers should have their needs assessed on a regular basis to ensure that appropriate support is provided to enable them to be involved in decisions about their treatment. The consultant nephrologist is central to ensuring that optimum support is provided by the MDT, and that patients have access to the knowledge and expertise that they require.

A key requirement for involving patients in decisions about their treatment is the ability to offer a choice of treatment options. This is particularly important when considering the modality of RRT for treatment of established renal failure. The need to provide information in a range of languages appropriate to the local population, and to take account of religious needs, for example when considering dietary advice, is widely recognised.

Opportunities for education and promoting self-care

Renal units provide information to patients and their carers through direct consultation with members of the MDT, information in the form of leaflets, books and videos, and dedicated education sessions.

Patients should be offered opportunities for self-care whenever possible, for example, when choosing the modality for RRT. Peritoneal dialysis and home haemodialysis offer greater opportunities for independence but decisions about treatment must take account of the impact on carers and home and family life. Whilst conferring independence and allowing flexibility, home haemodialysis does require considerable motivation and can put enormous emotional strain on the patient's family or partner.

Access to information, patient support groups and the role of the expert patient

Many renal units have active kidney patients' associations which provide information and support at a local level. At a national level, 63 kidney patients' associations come together as the controlling council of the National Kidney Federation (NKF). The NKF campaigns for improvements to renal provision and treatment, and provides support services for patients. It provides information through its website (**www.kidney.org.uk**), the magazine *Kidney Life*, leaflets on kidney disease, and the National Kidney Patients' Helpline.

The NKRF (**www.nkrf.org.uk**) supplies information booklets and factsheets on a range of kidney conditions and launched the National Kidney Helpline in October 1999 to offer advice from healthcare professionals on all aspects of kidney disease. It provides support for kidney patients through patient grants and dissemination of information on kidney disease. The NKRF has highlighted the opportunities offered by the expert patient task force (**www.doh.gov.uk/cmo/progress/expertpatient**), set up by the Department of Health (DH) in 1999 to design a programme that would bring together the work of patient and clinical organisations in developing self-management intiatives.

Patients are encouraged to keep informed about the results of investigations. Record sheets are available from the NKF so that patients receiving treatment for kidney failure can monitor their own results.

iv Interspecialty and interdisciplinary liaision

Multidisciplinary team working

During the course of their illness, patients with kidney disease encounter numerous professional staff who each contribute to their management and care. Patients' varied needs may form a focus at different times for renal physicians, renal nurses and healthcare support assistants, renal dietitians, renal social workers, renal clinical psychologists, renal counsellors, renal clinical technologists, renal pharmacists, occupational therapists and physiotherapists, renal transplant and vascular surgeons, transplant coordinators and the histocompatibility and immunogenetics service. Renal unit managers and administrators have a key role in ensuring that patients have access to members of the MDT.

Access to the circulation or peritoneum in haemodialysis and peritoneal dialysis respectively are essential for dialysis provision. Dialysis access is best provided by a MDT including surgeons responsible for the creation of access, renal physicians and renal nurses, and radiologists with vascular imaging and interventional skills for the provision of vascular access.

Working with other specialists

Nephrologists often provide support for patients who develop kidney problems in other units and hospitals, particularly in intensive treatment units (ITU), cardiothoracic units, and liver and vascular units, where acute renal failure is common. Diabetes and immune-mediated kidney disease are the commonest causes of chronic renal failure, and nephrologists need to work closely with diabetologists and immunologists. The multisystem consequences of kidney failure, for example the increased risk of cardiovascular disease and metabolic bone disease, mean that patients with kidney failure require the support of many other specialists. The increasing number of elderly patients on RRT programmes often require the skills of physicians specialising in geriatric medicine. Close working with renal transplant surgeons is essential for delivery of a renal transplant service. Renal pathologists provide essential support to nephrology and transplant services.

Consultants whose primary specialty is renal medicine may work in additional specialties. Additional specialties declared by nephrologists in the 2002 Census included acute medicine, general medicine, diabetes, endocrinology, metabolic medicine, hepatology, obstetric medicine and transplantation medicine.[3]

Working with non-consultant medical practitioners

Currently, non-consultant career grade (NCCG) practitioners provide valuable support to many renal programmes. A survey conducted to inform the BRS workforce planning exercise indentified 37 NCCG practitioners in renal medicine in the UK. Each practitioner provided, on average, 9.4 sessions per week, the majority of which were devoted to the management of dialysis patients.

v Delivering a high quality service

Characteristics of a high quality service

A high quality service is one in which patients, their families and carers have timely access to the full range of renal healthcare professionals (see the workforce requirements section below), and the services they offer. The service should meet the standards set out by the Renal Association in *Treatment of adults and children with renal failure: standards and audit measures.*[4]

Resources required for a high quality service

Specialised facilities

The Renal Association document *Treatment of adults and children with renal failure: standards and audit measures* identified five major components to renal medicine, with different essential requirements:[4]

1. *Renal replacement therapy*   The most significant element of work concerns preparing patients with established renal failure for RRT and medical supervision of these patients for the remainder of their lives.

   The facilities should provide for an annual acceptance rate of 120–130 per million population, and offer patients a choice of modality according to their needs. These should include hospital-based haemodialysis, haemofiltration or haemodiafiltration, home haemodialysis, continuous ambulatory peritoneal dialysis, automated peritoneal dialysis and renal transplantation. Active non-dialytic management of the patient with established renal failure, including nutritional, medical and psychological support, should be available. Decisions not to institute or to discontinue dialysis should be made jointly by the patient and consultant nephrologist after consultation with relatives, the family practitioner and members of the caring team. Physicians have identified a requirement of 37 specialist beds per million population.[5]

   All equipment used in the delivery and monitoring of RRT should comply with the relevant standards for medical equipment. Designated space is required for the support and training of patients opting for home-based treatment.

   Haemodialysis patients should be able to dialyse three times per week at a convenient time at a local unit, with at least 80% of patients using an arteriovenous fistula. Haemodialysis machines should be replaced after seven years' service or after completing 50,000 hours operation, whichever is first. Water used in preparation of dialysis fluid must meet requirements for bacterial and chemical contaminants. It has been estimated that at least 50 haemodialysis stations are required per million population.[5] Facilities for isolation and segregation of patients must meet the DH guidelines for renal dialysis and transplantation units.[6]

   Transplant units should have four beds per million population for new transplants, one-third of which should be single-bed cubicles. The beds should be within a single ward, with beds to provide dialysis. There should be 24-hour access to operating theatres, laboratory support including histocompatibility and human leukocyte antigen (HLA) antibody testing, haematology, biochemistry, virology, bacteriology and pathology. Imaging services required include routine X-ray, angiography, ultrasound, computed tomography (CT), magnetic resonance imaging (MRI) and radioisotope scanning.

2. *Emergency work*   Emergency work predominantly concerns the treatment of acute renal failure and medical emergencies arising from an established renal failure programme. Renal wards admitting patients with acute renal failure require either a designated high dependency unit (HDU) where, in addition to RRT, the following are available: close nursing supervision, oxygen, continuous electrocardiogram and oxygen saturation monitoring, automated blood pressure monitoring, and central venous pressure monitoring facilities and expertise. Patients with multiple organ failure and those who are haemodynamically very unstable require access to an intensive care unit.

3. *Routine nephrology*   This relates to work associated with the immunological and metabolic nature of kidney disease, which involves investigative procedures in an inpatient setting. It is estimated that 10 inpatient beds per million population are required with access to the full range of immunology, haematology, biochemistry, virology, bacteriology and pathology support.

4. *Investigation and management of fluid and electrolyte disorders*   This makes up a variable proportion of the nephrologist's work, depending on the other expertise in the hospital.

5. *Outpatient work*   This consists of the majority of general nephrology together with clinics attended by pre-dialysis, dialysis and renal transplant patients. Patients with progressive renal failure should be managed in a clinic with multidisciplinary support from dietitians and specialist nurses. Education and preparation for dialysis, including referral for timely formation of vascular access, should be available. In addition to monitoring and optimising kidney function, renal transplant clinics should provide management of cardiovascular risk, osteoporosis, post-transplantation pregnancy, and prevention and detection of skin malignancy.

In addition, renal units should have the IT support necessary to perform internal audit and to submit required data to the UK Renal Registry.

Workforce requirements: clinical and support staff

Patients with kidney disease must have certain dependencies on doctors, nurses and other health professionals.

- *Renal physicians* provide a wide range of clinical services for patients with kidney disease. A key element of their role is leadership, ensuring close collaboration between colleagues in the MDT and in other services.

- *Renal nurses and healthcare support assistants* provide patient and carer education, support and advocacy. Renal nurses often develop specialist practice roles, acquiring the skills and competencies to manage kidney patients at different stages of their illness and on particular RRT modalities. Healthcare assistants work within the nursing team in skilled roles, usually within a discreet area of practice.

■ *Renal dietitians* provide advice on the changing dietary requirements of patients with kidney disease, optimising nutrition and assisting in the management of hyperphosphataemia and cardiovascular risk factors.

■ *Renal social workers* care for the needs of patients at the interface of health and social services, addressing the practical, economical, social and psychological problems of patients with kidney disease and their families and carers.

■ *Renal clinical psychologists* offer psychological assessment and intervention for patients with kidney disease and their families and carers, as well as clinical supervision and training of direct care staff.

■ *Renal counsellors* provide services and interventions, often related to emotional distress, bereavement and loss, and enhancing patients' ability to make informed decisions about their treatment.

■ *Renal clinical technologists* manage and assure high specification dialysis and water treatment equipment. Their role often extends to educating patients and staff, advising on the design, installation and commissioning of new dialysis facilities and necessary administrative and/or IT support.

■ *Renal pharmacists* have a key role in the management of medicines for patients with kidney disease, who often require a large number of medications. Pharmacists are involved in education of patients and healthcare professionals, discharge planning, medicines review schemes, development of protocols and financial risk assessment.

■ *Renal unit administrators and managers* have responsibilities for coordinating the complex logistics of a renal programme involving a diverse range of staff, equipment and consumables. The professional background and job description of renal unit administrators and managers varies considerably.

■ *Renal transplant surgeons* are responsible for leading a renal transplantation service, providing the best quality of life for suitable RRT patients. Renal transplantation is complex, and patients and carers often need the skills of all the other members of the transplant team.

The UK Transplant Coordinators Association advises on the job specification, training and accreditation, accountability and workforce requirements of transplant coordinators (**www.uktca.co.uk**).

The histocompatibility and immunogenetics service should be headed by a Grade C clinical scientist or medical consultant with relevant histocompatibility and immunogenetics qualifications and experience, and supported by healthcare scientists who have completed a recognised training scheme.

vi   Quality standards and measures of the quality of specialist services

Specialist society guidelines

■ *Treatment of adults and children with renal failure: standards and audit measures.*[4]

■ *Good practice guidelines for renal dialysis/transplantation units: prevention and control of blood-borne virus infection.*[6]

■ *Standards for solid organ transplantation in the United Kingdom.*[7]

National Institute for Clinical Excellence (NICE) guidelines

▮ *Renal failure – home versus hospital haemodialysis (No. 48).*[8]

▮ *Central venous catheters – ultrasound locating devices (No. 49).*[9]

▮ *Renal transplantation – immuno-suppressive regimens (adults) (No. 85).*[10]

▮ *Management of Type 2 Diabetes – Renal Disease, prevention and early management (Guideline F).*[11]

CLINICAL WORK IN RENAL MEDICINE

Contributions made to acute medicine

The Census in 2002 reported that 52% of consultant nephrologists have a regular on-call commitment for unselected emergency medical admissions, with 57.1% providing continuing care for most or all patients admitted on an emergency take, and 84.5% dealing with GIM outpatient clinics or outpatient follow up.[3] Consultant nephrologists with GIM commitment report an average of 38 patients per week, of which 11.5 are followed up by the admitting nephrologist.

Direct clinical care

Inpatient work

Different models of providing inpatient care have developed according to local need and numbers of consulant nephrologists. In small units with two or fewer consultant nephrologists (3.5% of consultant nephrologists are single-handed), consultants may provide continuing cover for all inpatient apects of renal medicine. In larger units, individual consultants may either provide continuing cover for subspecialty interests (for example general nephrology, transplantation, vasculitis), or they may rotate cover for all inpatients, devoting time to other activities (research, management, teaching, audit) when not directly involved in inpatient care.

The College Joint Specialty Committee for Renal Disease has set standards recommending that a consultant should see every patient admitted under him/her within 24 hours of admission, and a diagnosis and treatment plan should be reviewed and agreed.[12] Consultant nephrologists should, therefore, visit the wards daily to see new admissions and new referrals from other specialties. The Census in 2002 reported that consultant nephrologists spend, on average, eight hours per week on ward duties.[3]

Outpatient work

The Census reported that consultant nephrologists spend, on average, 10.8 hours per week in outpatient clinics related to renal medicine.[3] This equates to two to three clinics per week, and is likely to reflect a mixture of general nephrology, pre-dialysis, haemodialysis, chronic ambulatory peritoneal dialysis (CAPD), renal transplant and specialty clinics (eg diabetic nephropathy). The number of patients seen will vary considerably depending on the clinic and the support staff available. For example, a new patient with established renal failure may require one hour of consultant time if they are seen in a clinic without support staff, but might spend half an hour with the consultant and half an hour with other staff, including specialist nurses, a dietitian and a phelobotomist if they are available, in a dedicated pre-dialysis clinic. Similarly, a follow-up patient with established renal failure may need to spend 10–30 minutes with a consultant, depending on the availability of specialist support staff who might advise on management of anaemia, dialysis access and diet.

Specialist investigative procedures

The Census reported that consultant nephrologists spend, on average, 1.1 hours per week on special procedures.[3] These include renal biopsy, temporary and permanent central venous line insertion, and peritoneal dialysis (PD) catheter insertion. The procedures are often shared with radiologists and surgeons.

Specialist on call

On-call work for renal medicine is often high intensity, particularly because of the need to support patients with acute renal failure. A frequency of one in five or less is recommended. Consultants need 24-hour support from a full emergency haemodialysis service.

Specialist activity beyond the local services

Many consultant nephrologists provide cover for satellite dialysis units and give telephone advice or accept referrals from neighbouring hospitals that are unable to provide 24-hour nephrology cover.

Clinically related administration

Clinical activity in renal medicine often generates administrative duties which demand 50–100% of the time spent on direct clinical care. For example, following a renal transplant clinic the consultant nephrologist will need to check laboratory results on all patients, arrange admission or rearrange follow-up if unexpected results are identified, contact patients and/or GPs concerning any alterations to treatment, and dictate and sign relevant correspondence.

Work to maintain and improve the quality of care

This work encompasses duties in clinical governance, professional self-regulation, continuing professional development (CPD) and education and training of others. For many consultants at various times in their careers it may include research, serving in management and providing specialist advice at local, regional and national levels.

Leadership role and development of the service

The increasing numbers of patients needing treatment for kidney disease underlines the importance of planning for expansion and development of serivces. Such development must be led by renal physicians to ensure the MDT meets NICE guidance and the recommended standards of the Renal Association and the NSF, and to evaluate innovative approaches to service delivery. Leadership is usually provided by the clinical director. Depending on the size of the unit, clinical leads may take on local management duties in specific areas such as dialysis or transplantation, or may take a lead in audit.

Education and training

Training renal physicians to meet the requirements for consultant expansion is essential, and consultants need sufficient time to supervise and appraise trainees. All renal physicians are involved in education and training, and many will act as educational supervisors within their hospital or take on specific roles within their deanery or for the College. Renal physicians must also participate in appraisal and continuing medical education (CME). Systems for menoring new consultants are encouraged.

Regional and national work

Participation of renal physicians in regional and national work is important to ensure that patients have equitable access to a high quality service across the UK, and that opportunities for teaching and research are widely available. These roles, which are usually for a fixed term, can be onerous and it is essential that arrangements for covering local duties are agreed with colleagues and managers.

Collectively, these roles in service development and provision, audit, education and training, mentoring, appraisal and professional development ensure that requirements for clincial governance are met. Overall responsibility for clinical governance usually rests with the clinical director.

ACADEMIC MEDICINE

Clinical contribution to the NHS

The BRS reported that in 2001, 21% of renal physicians held academic appointments, each contributing an average of 0.5 WTE each.[13] Of the 312 consultants in renal medicine identified in the College Census in 2002, 217 held NHS contracts, 68 held NHS/academic contracts and 27 held academic/research contracts. The Census reported that consultants in renal medicine spend, on average, 4.5 hours per week on academic or research duties, 1.6 hours per week on teaching undergraduates, and 1.4 hours per week teaching postgraduates.[3]

Teaching and research

Renal medicine has a strong track record in teaching and research. Many specialist registrars (SpRs) undertake a period of formal research training, and many NHS consultants supervise research alongside academic colleagues. Academic renal physicians often train in laboratory science and work closely with basic scientists. The introduction of recombinant human erythropoietin as a treatment for renal anaemia is an example of how advances in cell and molecular biology translate into improved treatment for patients.

WORKFORCE REQUIREMENTS FOR RENAL MEDICINE

The Census of consultant physicians in the UK, 2003 identified 334 consultants in renal medicine in the UK (307 WTE).[14]

The BRS established a multiprofessional national renal workforce planning group in January 2001 to prepare recommendations for establishments and staffing levels across each professional group involved in renal healthcare. The report was published under the auspices of the Royal College of Nursing, the Royal College of Physicians and the Royal College of Paediatrics and Child Health.

The report provides a detailed review of the curent workforce and provides a specialist workforce plan for adult renal services to 2010.[13] A summary of the findings is presented in the appendix. The Renal Association has calculated that by 2010, 570 WTE will be required in the UK, this equates to 2.45 WTE per 250,000 population, which will require an increase of 86%.

However, requirements will vary across the UK, being influenced by factors such as ethnicity and age which impact on the prevalence of kidney disease.

CONSULTANT WORK PROGRAMME/SPECIMEN JOB PLAN

The majority of consultant nephrologists work in excess of 40 hours. The Census in 2003 identified 192 (59%) consultant nephrologists exceeding 40 working hours per week, who worked, on average, 67.3 hours per week.[14] It has been calculated that a 22% increase in WTEs would be needed simply to enable existing consultants to meet the European Working Time Directive. To formulate a job plan for a 48-hour week requires acknowledgement that alterations to current working practices, in parallel with an urgent expansion in consultant numbers, are needed. Consultants may need to vary their working week by sharing responsibilities in certain areas with colleagues, but with individual consultants providing a lead for some activities. For example, responsibility for ongoing care at a satellite dialysis unit often rests with one consultant, whereas another consultant may provide a lead for specialist procedures, thereby maintaining expertise in this area.

The work programme is based on working patterns reported in the Census 2003 and the guidance from the central consultants and specialists committee of the British Medical Association.

Activity	Workload	Programmed activities (PAs)
Direct clinical care		
Outpatient work	Patients per clinic 3–6 new, or 2–16 follow up	**2–4**
Inpatient work	Daily review of new referrals 2–3 ward rounds per week	**3–4**
Specialist investigative procedures		**0.25**
Specialist on-call	1:5	**1–2**
Specialist activity beyond the local services		**0–2**
Clinically related administration		**1–2**
Medical on call	1:10	**0.5–1**
Total number of direct clinical care PAs		**7.5 on average**
Supporting professional activities (SPA)		
Work to maintain and improve the quality of healthcare	Education and training, appraisal, departmental management and service development, audit and clinical governance, CPD and revalidation, research	**2.5 on average**
Other NHS responsibilities	eg medical director/clinical director/lead consultant in specialty/clinical tutor	**Local agreement with trust**
External duties	eg work for deaneries/Royal Colleges/specialist societies/Department of Health or other government bodies etc	**Local agreement with trust**

Appendix: A summary of the findings of the British Renal Society workforce planning group

Table 1. Estimated consultant requirements

| | | 2001 Actual | | 2001 Required*** | |
	Population	Consultant posts 2001*	WTE in nephrology	Consultant posts	WTE in nephrology
England	50.19	227**	161	429	305
Wales	2.95	13	9	25	18
England and Wales	53.14	240	170	454	323
Northern Ireland	1.68	10	7	14	10
Scotland	5.11	40	28	44	31
Total	59.93	290	206	512	364

* College Census 2001[15]
** Includes one consultant in Her Majesty's Forces
*** *Consultant physicians working for patients*, second edition, p240.[5] Consultant requirements for 2001 are based on an estimate of the nephrology needs of a population of one million and take into account the service contribution of trainees and NCCGs and the demands of general medicine, academic commitments and part-time working for personal reasons.

Table 2. Total number of specialist renal healthcare practitioners and WTE in 2001 in England and the United Kingdom

| | England | | United Kingdom | |
	Total	Renal WTE	Total	Renal WTE
Renal physicians	226	161	290	206
Renal transplant surgeons	68	42	81	51
Renal transplant donor coordinators	67	50	87	59
Renal histocompatibility scientists				
Consultant scientists	12	8	14	9
Healthcare scientists	180	111	252	151
Renal dietitians	142	118	180	147
Renal social workers	56	43	73	55
Renal clinical psychologists	6	2	7	3
Renal clinical technologists	173	173	225	225
Renal pharmacists	66	28	97	34
Renal administrators and managers	55	43	65	50
Nurses				
Haemodialysis	1,895	1,541	2,330	1,894
Peritoneal dialysis	215	175	250	203
Ward based (renal and transplant)	1,529	1,243	1,834	1,491
Healthcare assistants				
Haemodialysis	712	570	876	701
Peritoneal dialysis	44	35	51	41
Ward based (renal and transplant)	621	497	746	597

Table 3. Current and recommended specialist renal staff to patients on renal replacement therapy (RRT) ratios

Professional group	Current workforce ratios	Recommended workforce ratios
Renal physicians	1 physician per 131 RRT patients (1 WTE in nephrology per 185 RRT patients)	1 physician per 75 RRT patients (1 WTE in nephrology per 100 RRT patients)
Transplant surgeons	1.35 surgeons pmp (0.85 WTE pmp)	2 surgeons pmp (1.2–1.5 WTE pmp)
Dialysis access surgery	1 consultant vascular access session per 120 haemodialysis patients	1 dialysis access session per 120 patients on dialysis. Equates to 1 WTE surgeon per 350 cases per year
Donor transplant coordinators	1 WTE pmp	1 WTE pmp and 1 WTE per 20 live donor transplants
Histocompatibility and immunogenetics scientists	1 WTE consultant clinical scientist per 4,231 RRT patients and 1 WTE healthcare scientist per 260 patients on RRT	1 WTE consultant clinical scientist/medical consultant per 1,200 RRT patients and 1 WTE healthcare scientist per 135 RRT
Renal nurses and healthcare assistants (HCAs)		
Haemodialysis	1 WTE per 5.1 haemodialysis patients	1 WTE per 4.5 haemodialysis patients
Skillmix	2.7 nurses: 1 HCA	1.5 nurses: 1 HCA
Peritoneal Dialysis	1 WTE per 24 community dialysis patients	1 WTE per 20 community dialysis patients
Skillmix	2.5 nurses: 1 HCA	5 nurses: 1 HCA
Renal wards (includes transplant wards)	1.2 WTE per bed	1.4 WTE per bed
Skillmix	2.5 nurses: 1 HCA	2.5 nurses: 1 HCA
Dietitians	1 WTE per 260 RRT patients	1 WTE per 135 Haemodialysis patients*
Social workers	1 WTE per 693 RRT patients	1 WTE per 140 RRT patients
Clinical psychologists	1 WTE per 15,233 RRT patients	1 WTE per 1,000 RRT patients
Clinical technologists	1 WTE per 59 haemodialysis patients	1 WTE per 50 maintenance haemodialysis plus 1 WTE per 20 home haemodialysis
Pharmacists	1 WTE per 1120 RRT patients	1 WTE per 250 RRT patients plus 1 WTE per 60 transplants per annum
Managers/administrators	1 WTE per 382 dialysis patients	1 WTE per 150 dialysis patients

*Inpatient dietetic care requires additional support as quantified in table 3.9.5
PMP = per million population

Table 4. Workforce requirements for England

	England							
	2001 Establishment		2001 Required		2006 Projected		2010 Projected	
	Total	Renal WTE	Total	Renal WTE	Total	Renal WTE	Total	Renal WTE
Renal physicians	226	161	429	305	600	426	696	494
Renal transplant surgeons	68	42	105	75	105	75	105	75
Renal transplant donor coordinator	67	50	68	50	112	83	112	83
Histocompatibility scientists								
Consultant scientist	12	8	39	26	54	36	63	42
Healthcare scientist	180	111	370	231	517	323	598	374
Renal dietitians	142	118	382	318	530	442	618	515
Renal social workers	56	43	297	229	406	312	470	362
Renal clinical psychologists	6	2	93	31	132	44	153	51
Renal clinical technologists	173	173	221	221	395	395	493	493
Renal pharmacists	66	28	294	125	411	175	475	202
Renal administrators and managers	55	43	134	105	211	165	260	203
Renal nurses								
Haemodialysis	1,895	1,541	1,731	1,407	2,862	2,327	3,578	2,909
Peritoneal dialysis	215	175	267	217	371	302	444	361
Ward based (renal and transplant)	1,529	1,243	2,507	2,038	3,485	2,833	4,034	3,280
Renal healthcare workers								
Haemodialysis	712	570	1,173	938	1,943	1,554	2,425	1,940
Peritoneal dialysis	44	35	56	45	78	62	93	74
Ward based (renal and transplant)	621	497	1,040	832	1,446	1,157	1,675	1,340

Table 5. Workforce requirements for the United Kingdom

| | United Kingdom | | | | | | | |
	2001 Establishment		2001 Required		2006 Projected		2010 Projected	
	Total	Renal WTE	Total	Renal WTE	Total	Renal WTE	Total	Renal WTE
Renal physicians	290	206	512	364	688	488	803	570
Renal transplant surgeons	81	51	130	89	130	89	130	89
Renal transplant donor coordinator	87	59	87	59	144	98	144	98
Histocompatibility scientists								
Consultant scientist	14	9	48	32	64	43	75	50
Healthcare scientist	252	151	468	282	629	379	734	442
Renal dietitians	180	147	464	380	636	521	738	605
Renal social workers	73	55	356	272	475	365	555	427
Renal clinical psychologists	7	3	106	38	143	51	168	60
Renal clinical technologists	225	225	272	272	463	463	583	583
Renal pharmacists	97	34	425	152	574	205	669	239
Renal administrators and managers	65	50	165	127	51	193	312	240
Renal nurses								
Haemodialysis	2,330	1,894	2,127	1,729	3,357	2,729	4,223	3,443
Peritoneal dialysis	250	203	312	254	435	354	524	426
Ward based (renal and transplant)	1,834	1,491	2,958	2,405	4,112	3,343	4,760	3,870
Renal healthcare workers								
Haemodialysis	876	701	1,441	1,153	2,275	1,820	2,860	2,288
Peritoneal dialysis	51	41	65	52	91	73	109	87
Ward based (renal and transplant)	746	597	1,228	982	1,706	1,365	1,978	1,528

References

1. National Kidney Research Fund. *Renal services for dialysis: commissioner and provider perspectives.* A position paper by the National Kidney Research Fund, 2002.

2. Department of Health. *The National service framework for renal services. Part one: dialysis and transplantation.* London: DH, 2004.

3. The Federation of the Royal Colleges of Physicians of the United Kingdom. *Census of consultant physicians in the UK, 2002. Data and commentary.* London: The Federation of the Royal Colleges of Physicians of the United Kingdom, 2002.

4. The Standards and Audit Subcommittee of the Renal Asscociation on behalf of the Renal Association and the Royal College of Physicians of London in collaboration with the British Transplant Society, Intensive Care Society and the British Association of Paediatric Nephrologists. *Treatment of adult patients with renal failure. Recommended standards and audit measures.* Third edition. London: Renal Association and Royal College of Physicians, 2002.

5. Royal College of Physicians. *Consultant physicians working for patients.* Second edition. London: RCP, 2001.

6. Department of Health. *Good practice guidelines for renal dialysis/transplantation units: prevention and control of blood-borne virus infection.* Recommendations of a working group convened by the Public Health Laboratory Service (PHLS) on behalf of the DH. London: DH, 2002.

7. British Transplantation Society. *Standards for solid organ transplantation in the United Kingdom.* Second edition. London: British Transplantation Society. 2003.

8. National Institute for Clinical Excellence. *Renal failure - home versus hospital haemodialysis (No. 48),* September 2002. www.nice.org.uk/page.aspx?o=36747

9. National Institute for Clinical Excellence. *Central venous catheters – ultrasound locating devices (No. 49),* September 2002. www.nice.org.uk/page.aspx?o=36752

10. National Institute for Clinical Excellence. *Renal transplantation – immuno-suppressive regimens (adults) (No. 85),* September 2004. www.nice.org.uk/page.aspx?o=221103

11. National Institute for Clinical Excellence. *Management of Type 2 Diabetes - Renal Disease, prevention and early management* (Guideline F), March 2002. www.nice.org.uk/page.aspx?o=39385.

12. Royal College of Physicians. *Good medical practice for physicians.* London: RCP, 2004. www.rcplondon.ac.uk/college/pa/prof_gmpfp.htm

13. British Renal Society. *A multi-professional renal workforce plan for adults and children with renal disease. Recommendations of the National Renal Workforce Planning Group,* 2002. www.britishrenal.org/workfpg/WFP_Renal_Book.pdf

14. The Federation of the Royal Colleges of Physicians of the United Kingdom. *Census of consultant physicians in the UK, 2003. Data and commentary.* London: The Federation of the Royal Colleges of Physicians of the United Kingdom, 2003.

15. The Federation of the Royal Colleges of Physicians of the United Kingdom. *Census of consultant physicians in the UK, 2001. Data and commentary.* London: The Federation of the Royal Colleges of Physicians of the United Kingdom, 2001.

Respiratory medicine

i   Description of the specialty and clinical needs of patients

Respiratory medicine is concerned with diagnosis, treatment and continuing care of patients with a considerable and challenging range of pathologies. They include:

- asthma
- chronic obstructive pulmonary disease (COPD)
- diffuse interstitial lung disease
- sarcoidosis
- asbestos related conditions including mesothelioma
- cystic fibrosis
- tuberculosis
- management of chronic and acute respiratory failure
- sleep disordered breathing
- pneumonia
- pulmonary disorders in the immunocompromised host
- bronchiectasis
- pulmonary hypertension
- pulmonary haemorrhage
- pulmonary embolism
- allergic lung disorders
- disorders of the pleura (including malignancy, pleural effusion and pneumothorax)
- pulmonary manifestations of systemic disease
- genetic and developmental lung disorders
- a major commitment towards lung cancer, being the most common cancer in both males and females in the uk

Subspecialty interests also include:

- lung transplantation
- cystic fibrosis
- HIV/AIDS
- occupational lung disease
- palliative care and intensive care.

In addition, most respiratory physicians have a major commitment to the care of patients admitted as medical emergencies and conduct inpatient and post-take ward rounds. The expectation that all patients with respiratory disease have the option of being reviewed during their inpatient stay by a respiratory specialist represents a considerable increase in workload.

ii   Organisation of the service and patterns of referral

Primary, secondary and tertiary levels

Primary care and community respiratory medicine   Some GPs with an expertise in respiratory medicine provide asthma and chronic obstructive pulmonary disease (COPD) clinics within their surgeries, often serviced by nurse specialists. Such services should be developed further in collaboration with the local respiratory physicians and integrated with local services in secondary care. One area in particular where this is possible is respiratory rehabilitation.

Secondary care/inpatient service   Respiratory medicine provides a hospital-based service and respiratory physicians have a major commitment to the care of patients admitted as medical emergencies on unselected medical take. All district general hospitals (DGHs) have at least one consultant with a special interest in respiratory medicine and most have two or three. The prevalence of respiratory diseases and inpatients under the care of other disciplines, both medical and surgical, with problems requiring respiratory specialist input have a significant impact upon workload.

Tertiary care   Patients with certain conditions such as cystic fibrosis are usually managed in regional centres. Surgical and radiotherapy services are usually based in regional or subregional centres. Supraregional centres exist for the investigation of occupational lung disease, the management of patients with pulmonary hypertension and patients requiring assisted ventilation, and the assessment and management of patients requiring lung transplantation.

Most patients requiring admission are referred by their GP or via the A&E department. Most outpatient referrals are from GPs, specialist colleagues in the hospital and the A&E department. Suspected cases of lung cancer need to be seen within two weeks.[1] Facilities and resources need to be in place to enable all urgent referrals to be seen promptly. Patients with other life-threatening conditions such as severe asthma may need to be seen even more urgently.

Special patterns of referral   The British Thoracic Society (BTS) is working to achieve a countrywide network of regional centres to coordinate and, where appropriate, to provide specialist care. Each centre should provide access to specialist services for thoracic surgery, sleep-related respiratory disorders, ventilatory support, cystic fibrosis, pulmonary hypertension and lung transplantation. These centres would be ideally placed to provide specialist advice on other rare respiratory disease and coordinate national programmes of research.

The BTS is also working closely with the Royal College of General Practitioners (RCGP) in the development of GPs with a special interest (GPSI) in respiratory disease.

iii   Working with patients: patient-centred care

Patient choice and involving patients in decisions about their treatment

It is enshrined in *Good medical practice* that patients should be involved in decision-making about their treatment.[2] This is particularly important where potentially harmful drugs may be used such as in the treatment of lung cancer but also in the use of oral steroids and other immunosuppressants in respiratory disease. Respiratory physicians are totally committed to this and have led the way in regular discussions and educational sessions on ethical matters at BTS summer meetings for the last few years. Discussions have often included problems presented by ethnic and religious differences.

Access to information, opportunities for education and promoting self-care

Asthma care has led the way for the development of self-management plans, the proper administration of which includes significant education for patient groups. This has been developed by respiratory physicians jointly with the National Asthma Campaign and the British Lung Foundation.

In every respiratory clinic in the country there are locally produced and national information leaflets available, often produced by the British Lung Foundation and/or the National Asthma Campaign.

All patients have access to their own notes on request, but where clinically delicate information is involved respiratory physicians have developed training programmes for breaking bad news, both in the context of lung cancer and other potentially fatal conditions such as interstitial lung disease.

Patients with chronic conditions and the role of the expert patient

Asthma, COPD, cystic fibrosis and interstitial lung disease are followed up in respiratory outpatient clinics and in primary care. The BTS has long supported the British Lung Foundation in developing *Breathe Easy* patient-run patient support groups for these chronic conditions. The Cystic Fibrosis Trust helps patients and families with cystic fibrosis. Respiratory physicians are heavily involved in this group.

The concept of the expert patient is likely to be extremely helpful in the development of self-care and support for patients and families where chronic respiratory conditions are a problem.

iv Interspecialty and interdisciplinary liaison

Multidisciplinary team working

Respiratory nurse specialists make an invaluable contribution to the services that respiratory units are able to offer and the quality of those services. Respiratory nurse specialists undertake many roles, including running asthma clinics, providing education for patients with asthma, and liaising with GPs and nurses in the community. In many districts the respiratory nurse specialists supervise the domiciliary nebuliser service, and assist in the assessment and monitoring of patients requiring long-term domiciliary oxygen. In some units respiratory nurse specialists have the primary role in supervising patients with COPD who are selected for hospital-at-home care, and in running the pulmonary rehabilitation service (this is likely to increase sharply within the next few years). Respiratory nurse specialists may be employed full-time to supervise patients requiring domiciliary non-invasive ventilation (NIV) and continuous positive airway pressure (CPAP) for sleep-related breathing disorders. In small units respiratory nurse specialists may undertake many of these tasks together, whereas in large units often one or more respiratory nurse specialists may be required for each service.

Tuberculosis (TB) liaison health visitors (nurses) organise and conduct the contact tracing service when patients with TB are identified and, in many cases, supervise treatment to check it is being taken correctly and chase up patients who default from treatment.

Lung cancer nurse specialists provide an invaluable counselling service to patients and their relatives when a diagnosis of lung cancer is made, and advise patients and other healthcare workers on the general management of symptoms caused by lung cancer. In some cases they will visit patients at home or may liaise with other nurses who provide the domiciliary service.

Respiratory function technicians undertake lung-function testing of various levels of complexity. In some units they are involved in the sleep service and in exercise testing.

Physiotherapists play an important role in the management of both inpatients and outpatients with respiratory diseases. They teach patients with cystic fibrosis and bronchiectasis how to undertake postural drainage and help patients with hyperventilation to control their breathing.

Respiratory physiotherapists help in cystic fibrosis and bronchiectasis clinics. They may run rehabilitation courses or treatment for hyperventilation. They often help run NIV services and have a major input to the care of ward patients with respiratory failure.

Working with other specialists

Respiratory medicine specialists work as members of a multidisciplinary team (MDT). The team includes career grade and doctors in training, ward-based and outpatient nurses, respiratory nurse specialists, physiotherapists, secretaries and respiratory lab technicians. Members of the team liaise with many other specialties, particularly with imaging, histopathology and radiology in hospital, and with the local thoracic surgery and oncology units, local palliative medicine services and social services.

Clinical networks have been established for lung cancer management and others may follow. There are already strong links between secondary care and primary care with respect to lung cancer care, TB care and asthma care. Other links are likely to develop, to enable early discharge of patients with COPD and pulmonary rehabilitation, and through smoking cessation clinics. Respiratory medicine welcomes the development of GPSIs in respiratory disease.

Respiratory medicine specialists also work as members of a MDT in palliative care and some are responsible for HIV work. Close clinical liaisons have been developed between respiratory physicians and disciplines where multisystem disease often affects the lung. These include rheumatology, haematology, genitourinary medicine (GUM), renal medicine and oncology.

v   Delivering a high quality service

Characteristics of a high quality service

A high quality service implies that inpatients and outpatients receive prompt, expert, effective and compassionate care and, with few exceptions, the care they need should be available locally. This requires a well-motivated, well-staffed team that has access to suitable facilities. Respiratory specialists should not work in isolation and must have appropriate dedicated support staff. Respiratory nurse specialists have a crucial role.

For referrals, there should be a respiratory physician available 24-hours a day for advice. Referral letters should be reviewed by the respiratory physicians and explicit standards concerning reasonable time from referral to first appointment for urgent and non-urgent patients should be followed.

Resources required for a high quality service
Specialised facilities
Inpatient unit

▪ a fully staffed high dependency unit (HDU)/acute lung unit in every DGH.

Outpatient clinics

▪ sufficient consultation and examination rooms for clinicians and respiratory nurse specialists

▪ dedicated outpatient area with rooms large enough for patient, consultant, medical students or other trainees

▪ natural lighting and additional lighting

▪ quiet room for bereavement counselling

▪ efficient imaging department in close proximity to the respiratory services

▪ bronchoscopy suite

▪ seminar room for unit meetings and multidisciplinary lung cancer meetings

▪ flexible appointment system

▪ experienced respiratory nurse specialists to assist in clinic

▪ pharmacy service available to meet needs identified in clinic

▪ adequate secretarial staff

▪ fully supportive pulmonary function laboratory.

Therapeutic services Many consultants offer therapeutic services in addition to their routine respiratory work and job descriptions should recognise this. Nurse specialists may offer a valuable contribution in many areas and consultant sessional contributions will vary.

▪ long-term oxygen therapy and other domiciliary oxygen treatment

▪ treatment of sleep disorders (especially CPAP)

▪ pulmonary rehabilitation service, including the organisation of programmes, patient assessment and participation, utilising outpatient and day care facilities

▪ terminal care, incorporating terminal care beds with a specified commitment from the respiratory physician

▪ nebuliser services and asthma support services

▪ NIV/acute respiratory failure in the form of a respiratory HDU in larger centres (perhaps five programmed activities (PAs) per week for the consultant, and consultant supervision accounting for up to 2.5 PAs per week in winter, less in summer)

▪ treatment of neuromuscular disorders (assisted ventilation) using laboratory and inpatient services

▪ NIV outpatient service (increasingly needed for COPD patients and patients with neuromuscular disorders).

Diagnostic services Investigation of patients with respiratory disorders requires access to specialised facilities, including a bronchoscopy suite, for diagnostic (bronchoscopy, transbronchial biospy, medical thorascopy) and therapeutic (brachytherapy, endobronchial stenting, laser treatment or electrocauterising) procedures. Facilities for the investigation of sleep-related breathing disorders (overnight oximetry and sleep rooms) and their treatment (funded supply of CPAP machines) may be required. With the increasing provision of NIV, both in hospital and in the patient's home, specialised facilities and support are necessary.

vi Quality standards and measures of the quality of specialist services

The concept of a quality driven service with standards of care clearly defined in contracts is a framework in which the quality of respiratory medicine for a community can be improved. The standards should be set in relation to:

▪ referral system

▪ outpatient clinics

▪ thoracic surgery

▪ outpatient treatment

▪ inpatient care

▪ discharge from the respiratory service

▪ training of medical and nursing staff

▪ the availability of the appropriate facilities and equipment

▪ administration, information and education for patients

▪ storage and handling of medical records.

The contracting process should include the use of treatment guidelines when constructing local arrangements for referral, for shared care and for clinical audit criteria, which are necessary for quality control. Possible outcome measures include quality of life assessments and patient satisfaction questionnaires. Guidelines produced by the BTS, and in association with others where appropriate, cover all the major conditions. Recent guidelines from the National Institute for Clinical Excellence (NICE) for COPD care and obstructive sleep apnoea will soon be joined by NICE guidelines for TB treatment.

CLINICAL WORK OF CONSULTANTS IN RESPIRATORY MEDICINE

Contributions made to acute medicine

Most respiratory physicians working in DGHs and teaching hospitals have a commitment to general medicine in addition to caring for patients with respiratory disease. The commitment varies from hospital to hospital, dependent on local practices and staffing levels. Most spend at least 60% of their time on respiratory work, and some undertake respiratory work exclusively. Approximately one-third of all acute medical admissions have respiratory problems.

Direct clinical care

Inpatient work

Consultants usually undertake at least two ward rounds per week (two sessions) with the respiratory team. Teaching and training are an important component of the ward rounds. With the development of HDUs and specialist care, it is likely that daily ward rounds will become necessary. This could be shared between the consultants on the unit but it is likely to involve each consultant in an additional 0.5 PAs per week. In addition, consultants conduct post-take ward rounds in respect of unselected medical admissions, according to the on-take rota. Ward referrals are seen on the wards or in outpatient clinics as required.

In general, each consultant team should have no more than 20–25 inpatients under their care. However, with the current drive for patients to be admitted under the care of appropriate specialists, and with the wide seasonal variation in the admission of patients with respiratory disease, respiratory physicians often have more than this number. This has implications for the appointment of additional respiratory physicians. The inpatient work of the majority of respiratory physicians predominantly involves the investigation and management of patients admitted acutely but also includes the investigation and management of patients admitted electively. Many units are able to offer a self-admission policy to patients with conditions such as cystic fibrosis, lung cancer or asthma.

Referral work   Respiratory physicians undertake a considerable amount of referral work for patients under the care of other specialists in the hospital (0.5–1 PA needs to be set aside for this).

Interspecialty and interdisciplinary liaison   Respiratory physicians caring for patients with lung cancer attend weekly MDT meetings with oncologists, thoracic surgeons, pathologists and radiologists, requiring one to two hours. Some consultants have close links with the intensive therapy unit (ITU) and attend regular meetings. Consultants offering other specialist services such as transplantation assessment and follow up have close links with thoracic surgeons.

Outpatient work

Most consultants undertake three outpatient clinics a week though some undertake four or five.

New patients   Two new patients (general or specialist) can be seen per hour per consultant.

Follow-up clinic   Five patients per hour can be seen for general work, fewer if juniors are working alongside. Three to four patients per hour can be seen for specialist work.

Specialty clinics   It is difficult to be prescriptive about the number of patients that can be seen by a consultant and his/her team as this depends largely on the nature of the patients and on the size and experience of the team. A consultant working alone in a clinic is often expected to see six new patients or 15 follow-up patients, or a combination of the two. Such numbers are increasingly difficult to justify, and it is difficult to offer a high standard of care to those numbers of patients. Trained assistants such as Calman trainees in their final two years, associate specialists or experienced staff grades should see slightly fewer patients. Junior Calman trainees or senior house officers (SHOs) should see a fraction of these numbers. The number of new patients and follow-up patients seen with complex respiratory problems could be much less than suggested above.

General medical clinics   Respiratory physicians working in DGHs may see new general medical referrals and most see follow-up general medical patients following discharge from hospital. The numbers seen are as above.

Specialist investigative and therapeutic procedure services

Bronchoscopy   Most respiratory physicians undertake one bronchoscopy session each week. The number of sessions needed will depend on the demography of the local population. No more than six bronchoscopies can be undertaken in one session, fewer if complex procedures are added such as transbronchial biopsy or if junior doctors are being trained. Additional sessional requirements are needed where there is a regular commitment to therapeutic procedures such as brachytherapy, endobronchial stenting, laser treatment or electrocautery.

Medical thoracoscopy   This is a growing service offered by respiratory physicians and may require 0.5–1 session per week with two patients per session.

Sleep-related breathing disorders   This is a rapidly developing subspecialty. Many units are able to offer a basic overnight oximetry service though they do not hold dedicated clinics. Some units now offer a comprehensive sleep service and hold dedicated clinics for patients with sleep-related breathing disorders, both for diagnosis and monitoring of patients receiving CPAP treatment. The provision of a comprehensive sleep service requires the provision of one to two sleep rooms and a funded supply of CPAP machines. Consultants providing a comprehensive sleep service spend at least one session a week on this work.

Domiciliary assisted ventilation service   This is provided by specialist centres and, increasingly, in large DGHs. The sessional commitment varies enormously depending on the number of patients seen. With the introduction of domiciliary NIV for patients with COPD, in addition to the use of this therapy for patients with neuromuscular disorders, it is likely that the sessional commitment of consultants offering this service will increase significantly.

Occupational lung diseases   Relatively few units have consultants who offer a comprehensive occupational lung disease investigation service. Consultants working in such units probably spend at least two to three sessions per week on this work.

Specialist services within the specialty

Examples of specialist services provided at a local level:

Lung cancer   Most respiratory physicians investigate and provide supportive care for patients with lung cancer. This is included in their inpatient and outpatient sessional commitment, although the introduction of MDT meetings has added one to two hours per week to this. The lead lung cancer physician spends at least 0.5 PAs per week coordinating services. If clinicians provide a chemotherapy service, 0.5 PAs per week needs to be allowed for this.

Pulmonary rehabilitation service   This is a rapidly developing service in which patients are seen one to two times a week for six to eight weeks for education about their condition, support and a supervised exercise programme. The service is largely provided by respiratory nurse specialists and physiotherapists, though may include dietitians and occupational therapists. The lead clinician probably needs to allocate 0.5 PAs per week for this.

Sleep-related breathing disorders   See above.

NIV for acute respiratory failure   NIV is rapidly being established as a routine service in most hospitals. Although the service is largely provided by trained nursing staff and physiotherapists, consultant supervision of this service is essential and accounts for up to 2.5 PAs per week in the winter months, fewer during the summer. In most hospitals one consultant takes the lead role in supervision of the service and, depending on the number of patients requiring NIV, could spend two PAs a week on this. In large centres, where NIV is also used to assist with the weaning of patients on ventilators in the ITU, more sessions would be required and the service could be provided in a respiratory HDU with up to five PAs per week for the consultant in charge. The rapid and necessary growth in acute lung units and HDUs to maintain those needing respiratory support outside ITUs has significantly increased the involvement of respiratory physicians.

Pulmonary TB contact tracing   In most units, consultants see and manage patients with pulmonary TB, although one consultant needs to take the lead for supervision of the contact tracing service and management of difficult cases such as multidrug-resistance. The lead clinician is likely to need to spend 0.5–1 PA per week on this, depending upon the numbers of local cases.

Assessment of patients for nebulisers and oxygen therapy   This is largely undertaken by a respiratory nurse specialist and the time spent by consultants on this work is encompassed in their normal outpatient commitments.

Specialist clinics   Many consultants offer dedicated clinics for patients with asthma, bronchiectasis and interstitial lung diseases. This may be in addition to their usual three clinics per week.

GP X-ray reporting service   The commitment necessary for consultants providing this service is 0.5 sessions per week.

Examples of specialist services provided at a regional or supra-regional level:

Cystic fibrosis   Patients with cystic fibrosis are usually cared for in large regional centres, although some units provide care for small numbers of patients and others share the care with the regional centre. Most large centres require the services of at least one whole time equivalent (WTE) consultant physician and supporting staff. Consultants supervising the care of only a few patients probably need to allocate one PA per week.

Lung transplantation   There are four centres in England where lung transplantation is undertaken. Each centre requires a consultant physician specialising in the assessment and management of patients post-transplantation. At least five PAs per week are necessary.

Domiciliary assisted ventilation service   See above.

Occupational lung diseases   See above.

Services outwith the base hospital   Some consultants undertake outpatient clinics in hospitals other than their base hospital, either at a city's central chest clinic or specialised clinics at another hospital. Some consultants provide general medical/respiratory clinics in outlying towns in rural areas. In general terms, the time commitment for such clinics is included in their usual three clinics per week, though travel time must be included.

On call for specialist advice and emergencies

Very few DGHs are able to provide continuous specialist advice from on-call consultant physicians in respiratory medicine, though specialist advice is usually available. Larger centres are able to provide such advice from on-call physicians and the frequency of the on-call work depends on the number of consultants in the unit or city if a city-wide service is provided.

Work to maintain and improve the quality of care

This work encompasses duties in clinical governance, professional self-regulation, continuing professional development (CPD), education and training of others. For many consultants, at various times in their careers, it may include research, serving in management, and providing specialist advice at local, regional and national levels.

Leadership role and development of service

There are many service developments that deliver improved patient care, for example:

▪ *Multidisciplinary clinics and MDT meetings* – largely depend on organisational factors.

▪ *Hospital-at-home schemes for patients with COPD* – require the appointment of respiratory nurse specialists but this is offset by the savings in inpatient costs.

▪ *Development of pulmonary rehabilitation services* – requires the appointment of respiratory nurse specialists or respiratory physiotherapists.

▪ *Nurse-led outpatient clinics.*

▪ *Acute lung unit* – assisted ventilation for patients with COPD has been shown not only to reduce length of stay but also to improve survival and reduce ICU workload.

ACADEMIC MEDICINE

Each region should have an academic centre adequately staffed to coordinate regional teaching and research. Teaching should include undergraduate and postgraduate contribution to the specialist registrar (SpR) training programme. Research should range from basic laboratory work through human studies to clinical trials. The BTS research committee and the BTS/Medical Research Council (MRC) clinical trials group currently run nationwide multi-centre trials involving interested centres.

WORKFORCE REQUIREMENTS FOR RESPIRATORY MEDICINE

Clinical programmed activities required in respiratory medicine for a nominal DGH of 250,000

Emergency medical take   The specialty will be on call typically one in five with SpRs. In the average DGH, twice-daily post-take ward rounds are necessary in order to cope with increasing numbers and to keep to the College recommendation of <25 patients per round. Approximately one-third of the activity takes place outside the normal working day as defined in the 2003 consultant contract so, on average, 16 PAs per week are spent on post-take ward rounds. A further four PAs per week will accrue in administration time as a result of these ward rounds. The specialty's share of these 20 PAs will therefore be four PAs per hospital.

General medical follow-up clinics   A DGH of 250,000 admits 230–250 patients per week. The one in five share per specialty will therefore be 45–50 per week. The percentage of these patients requiring follow-up will vary across the country, but will typically be around 25–40%, that is 12–23 patients per week. Some of these will need more than one follow-up visit, and so the average DGH will need to provide two PAs of this activity per specialty (32 follow-up patients at four patients per hour). Allowing for administration time, this amounts to three PAs per hospital.

Ward referrals   A DGH of this size typically generates 10 ward referrals per week to respiratory medicine from other specialties. At 30 minutes per new patient, this is two PAs per hospital.

Ward rounds   Each consultant will need to perform two ward rounds per week in addition to the on-call ward rounds. Each ward round generates its own share of administrative duties including discharge-planning meetings, meetings with relatives and so on. One PA per consultant is needed for this activity.

Lung cancer   There are strict performance targets relating to lung cancer. Incidence varies across the population. In an average DGH of 250,000, 10 PAs are required to deliver the relevant quality standards for a DGH with an average standardised mortality ratio (SMR) for lung cancer. This includes time spent in MDT meetings, time spent as lead clinician for lung cancer, and the necessary bronchoscopy sessions. In DGHs with SMRs for lung cancer significantly above average, up to 12 PAs per week will be required, therefore 8–12 PAs per hospital (average 10) are required.

General clinics in respiratory medicine   A DGH of this size will generate typically 900 new non-cancer referrals per year in respiratory medicine. A consultant is able to provide clinics for 40 weeks per year. The consultant will see seven new patients per PA, requiring 3.2 PAs. Respiratory medicine is a specialty with a significant burden of chronic conditions and there are typically three to four follow-up patients for every new patient seen. Allowing each follow-up patient half the time of a new patient, a further 5.6 PAs are required. Finally, allowing 0.25 PAs per clinic for administration (screening referrals, following up results, dictating and signing letters) makes 11 per hospital.

Table 1. Specialised services within the specialty

Service	PAs per DGH per week
Acute NIV	1–2
Terminal care	0.5–1
Nebuliser assessment	0–0.5
Oxygen assessment	0.5
Sleep	1–2 in addition to any clinics
Pulmonary rehabilitation	0.5
Home ventilation support	0.5
Hospital-at-home services for COPD	0–1 depending on availability
Occupational respiratory medicine	0.5
Cystic fibrosis	0.5
TB treatment and contact tracing	0.5–2 depending on incidence
Total	**6–11 (assume 9 on average)**

Conclusion   An average of 39 consultant PAs are required to provide the services above, identified as being on a per-hospital basis (ie all activity listed above apart from respiratory ward rounds). Each consultant will provide one further PA in ward rounds and work related to running of the respiratory ward(s). Assuming a 7.5 PA contract, one PA of which is taken up by respiratory ward rounds, the 39 PAs of work for each DGH serving 250,000 population requires six consultants for its delivery.

Workforce requirements

The calculation above demonstrates the requirement for six respiratory physicians for an average DGH serving 250,000 population. The total requirement for the consultant respiratory workforce is 1,236 WTEs.

The flexible working party of the BTS surveyed all members in 2003, and published the results in *Thorax*.[3] This revealed that 39% of current SpRs are female and that, of these, over 50% plan to work part-time. Respiratory physicians are unusual in that a higher than average percentage perform sessional commitments in other specialties including emergency medicine, intensive care and palliative care. Because of these two factors it is anticipated that by 2012, 1.4 actual consultants will be required to equate to one WTE consultant. The actual number of respiratory physicians required to deliver a quality service in respiratory medicine for England and Wales is therefore 1,851 consultants.

In January 2004 there were 560 consultants working in respiratory medicine in England and Wales (data on file with BTS workforce committee). Based on the current stock of national training numbers in England and Wales it is anticipated that by 2012 there will be approximately 910 consultants in the specialty. Therefore, without significant further expansion or international recruitment, by 2012 there will still be fewer than half the number of consultants required to deliver a quality service in respiratory medicine.

CONSULTANT WORK PROGRAMME/SPECIMEN JOB PLAN

Activity	Workload	Programmed activities (PAs)
Direct clinical care		
Outpatient clinics		3
Ward rounds		2
Specialist investigative/ therapeutic procedures/ bronchoscopy		1
Clinically related administration		1–2
General medical on-call/ post-take ward rounds/MDT meetings		0.5–1.5
Total number of direct clinical care PAs		**7.5 on average**
Supporting professional activities (SPA)		
Work to maintain and improve the quality of healthcare	Education and training, appraisal, departmental management and service development, audit and clinical governance, CPD and revalidation, research	**2.5 on average**
Other NHS responsibilities	eg medical director/clinical director/lead consultant in specialty/clinical tutor	**Local agreement with trust**
External duties	eg work for deaneries/Royal Colleges/specialist societies/Department of Health or other government bodies etc	**Local agreement with trust**

References

1. Department of Health. *The NHS cancer plan: a plan for investment, a plan for reform.* London: DH, 2000.

2. General medical council. *Good medical practice: protecting patients, guiding doctors.* London: GMC, 2001.

3. Abstracts of the British Thoracic Society winter meeting. 3–5 December 2003, London, United Kingdom. *Thorax* 2003;**58**(Suppl 3):iii1–100.

Rheumatology

i **Description of the specialty and clinical needs of patients**

Rheumatology deals with the investigation, diagnosis, management and treatment of patients with arthritis and other musculoskeletal conditions. The term 'musculoskeletal conditions' incorporates over 200 disorders affecting joints, bones, muscles and soft tissues. These include inflammatory arthritis, soft tissue conditions, autoimmune rheumatic disorders, osteoarthritis, spinal pain and metabolic bone disease. While a large number of musculoskeletal conditions are confined to the musculoskeletal system, many also affect other organ systems, making their management complex.

Arthritis and musculoskeletal conditions affect one in five people in the UK.[1] Of these more than two million people visited their GP in the last year because of osteoarthritis.[2] Around 387,000 people in the UK have rheumatoid arthritis.[2] Musculoskeletal conditions affect people of all ages, gender and race. There is a common perception that all musculoskeletal conditions are long term and persistent and that nothing can be done to treat them, when in reality modern treatments can be highly effective. Conditions can vary dramatically in their severity and different joints can be affected. A range of effective management options are available and in all cases the person with arthritis needs to be at the centre of the decision-making process about the most appropriate treatment options.

Rheumatology is a multidisciplinary specialty and the rheumatology department works in close liaison with orthopaedic surgeons, physiotherapists, occupational therapists, podiatrists and specialist nurses amongst others. Rheumatology requires interdisciplinary knowledge and awareness of new research in internal medicine, immunology, orthopaedics, neurology and pain management, rehabilitation, psychiatry and professions allied to medicine. Training may also include specialist experience in paediatric and adolescent rheumatology and sports medicine.

In 2002, the National Institute for Clinical Excellence (NICE) approved the use of biologic therapies for people with severe rheumatoid arthritis. This development has had a significant impact on the work of rheumatologists and on resources and staffing, as patients on these drugs need careful monitoring and have to be registered on the British Society for Rheumatology's Biologics Register (BSRBR), which monitors the long-term safety of patients on biologic therapies.

ii **Organisation of the service and patterns of referral**

Primary, secondary and tertiary levels

Primary care   In the last year, 8.9 million adults in the UK (19% of the adult population) attended their GP for arthritis or a related condition.[1] Most of these are non-inflammatory problems such as back pain and osteoarthritis which can usually be managed effectively in primary care. Referral to secondary care is appropriate for the small minority with 'red flags', or where there is diagnostic uncertainty or the need for further specialist investigation with the view to intervention (eg surgery). Current evidence suggests that many patients referred to orthopaedic surgeons do not need an orthopaedic opinion and, even amongst those on a surgical waiting list, 10–15% do not need an operation.[3] Increasingly, some form of triage by practitioners with special interests (usually

GPs or physiotherapists) is being used as a way to improve the efficiency and appropriateness of the referral process (see **www.doh.gov.uk/pricare/gp-specialinterests**). This approach has been shown to have tangible benefits for patients, including reduced waiting times, convenient access, high levels of patient satisfaction, reduction in waiting times for orthopaedic referral and increased conversion rate for surgery.

Secondary care Secondary care rheumatology services are provided largely by consultant rheumatologists and the multidisciplinary team (MDT) which works alongside them. Clinics may take place within a general outpatient department or a dedicated rheumatology unit. The majority of rheumatologists practise whole-time in the specialty, however, some 16% of rheumatologists also practise general internal medicine (GIM) and approximately 9% have a commitment to rehabilitation medicine.[4] Although many patients' conditions and treatment can be managed within primary care, others benefit from the diagnostic expertise and skills of a specialist hospital unit, including education, medication, and investigative and therapeutic procedures. Some areas offer a 'hub-and-spoke' model of service provision, whereby members of the rheumatology MDT come out of the 'hub' to do regular clinics within primary care settings.

Tertiary care There is provision for specialised services that cover the needs of a small group of patients with rare conditions who may require specialised investigation or management not available in a local hospital setting. Examples of these are tertiary referral for complex connective tissue diseases, rare metabolic bone disease and other rare musculoskeletal conditions. These services allow access to a multiprofessional team, skilled and experienced in certain conditions which may include specialised surgery such as cardiac surgery, neurosurgery and hand surgery, and to a specialist rheumatology MDT including rehabilitation therapists, specialist nurses, podiatry and orthotics services. Tertiary care services also include specialist paediatric and adolescent rheumatology clinics in centres of excellence for complex paediatric conditions.

Clinical networks and community arrangements

The development and delivery of a rheumatology service needs to take account of the needs of the local population and the current local service provision, including the skills and interests of practitioners. Activities of those delivering the service are not prescriptive and will depend upon how the service is configured. Various models for incorporating practitioners with special interests into rheumatology services have been implemented, including hospital-based triage, GP initial assessment clinic, and physiotherapy-led back pain services. National guidelines (eg for back pain and chronic pain) are a useful starting point for developing integrated care packages but work best if guidelines are customised to the needs of the local health economy.

Relationship with other services/agencies

The nature of the rheumatology specialty means that close collaboration with other services and agencies as well as the MDT is vital in order to provide a patient-centred service. Therefore, all rheumatology departments work closely with other departments including social services, occupational therapy, physiotherapy, dietetics and chiropody. An effective working relationship between rheumatologists and providers of other services is vital to the model of patient-centred care embraced by the rheumatology community, as it ensures quick and appropriate access to the treatments and services that the patient requires.

The key voluntary sector organisations with an interest in rheumatology issues have developed excellent collaborative methods of working. Arthritis Care, the National Rheumatoid Arthritis Society (NRAS), the British Society for Rheumatology (BSR) and the Arthritis Research Campaign (**arc**) have worked together on a number of specific campaigns under the auspices of the Arthritis and Musculoskeletal Alliance (ARMA), including submissions to NICE appraisals and lobbying work on access to biologic agents including anti-TNFalpha. Rheumatology teams may also work closely with other patient support organisations such as the National Osteoporosis Society and Lupus UK.

Complementary services

Complementary therapies have become more popular and more widely available over the last few years. Although conventional treatment is safe and effective for most people, for some, drugs and surgery cannot fully control the symptoms of arthritis. People are increasingly concerned about the side effects of some of the more potent drugs. Complementary therapies cannot cure arthritis but they may ease pain, stiffness and some of the side effects of taking drugs. It should be noted that some herbal remedies may have side effects of their own and it may be wise to consult a rheumatologist before embarking on any such therapy, although they may have little or no knowledge of the remedy concerned.

There are a wide variety of complementary therapies available for people with arthritis and musculoskeletal conditions. They range from ancient systems of medicine such as acupuncture and homeopathy to treatments such as chiropractic, osteopathy and reflexology. Treatments are described as complementary when they have not been used traditionally in conventional medical settings. Rheumatologists would wish to be kept informed of patients undergoing complementary therapies as they may affect other medicines that have been prescribed.

iii   Working with patients: patient-centred care

Involving patients in decisions about their treatment

'The era of the patient as the passive recipient of care is changing. Health professionals and patients should be genuine partners seeking together the best solutions to each patient's problems.'[5]

The patient should, when at all possible, be an equal partner in decisions about appropriate treatments and therapies to help manage their condition. Not only will this contribute to the patient feeling that they have been treated as a 'person' rather than a 'patient', but also they are more likely to comply with any treatment offered if they understand and feel happy with the course of treatment agreed upon.

Availability of clinical records/results

With increased emphasis on access to personal information in society in general, there is a growing demand from patients to have access to their clinical records on demand. Furthermore, if patients are to be more actively involved in their treatment they need to be fully aware of records and results in order to make fully informed decisions.

In an increasing number of cases, particularly where disease-modifying anti-rheumatic drugs (DMARDs) including biologic therapies are being used, patients are being asked to keep a personal diary and to self-report any adverse events that they experience in the course of treatment. In this way patients are becoming an equal partner in producing their own records. There is certainly a trend towards greater patient access to records and results within rheumatology services. Patients are often encouraged to keep monitoring cards on which recent relevant blood tests and drug dosage changes are recorded.

Ethical and religious considerations

Rheumatology departments should consider the potential needs of the local population and may consider the following when planning local services:

- Literature should be provided in other languages and alternative formats. The Birmingham Arthritis Resource Centre has audio information available to borrow in Gujurati, Bengali, Punjabi, Urdu, Arabic and Chinese. They can be contacted by telephone on 0121 464 2708.

- Local support groups and services that may be able to provide additional advice and support for people from different ethnic groups should be explored.

- A translator may be needed when a diagnosis is given and decisions about treatment are being made. Different trusts will have different local arrangements for providing this support.

- Female patients may wish to be seen by a female doctor for ethical or religious reasons and to have access to chaperones when requested.

- Services should aim to allow patients to uphold their religious beliefs, keep religious festivals, holy days or follow rituals of prayer. Some examples of this might be a flexible appointments system or allowing patients to express a preference to see a female consultant where possible. The new system of electronic booking may well introduce this flexibility.

Access to information

Voluntary organisations working across the UK with and for people with arthritis produce a wide range of patient literature on arthritis and other musculoskeletal conditions, and related topics such as independent living, diet and exercise. The **arc** and Arthritis Care regularly produce information of a consistently high quality which is easily digestible.

The **arc** publishes over 80 booklets, leaflets and information sheets about arthritis. Medical practitioners, hospital departments or GP surgeries can order large quantities of educational material and, as part of **arc**'s commitment to raising awareness and educating the public and medical profession about rheumatic diseases, all their medical and patient literature is available free of charge. Orders can be placed via their website (**www.arc.org.uk**). Patients can also order their own literature via the site free of charge.

Arthritis Care, the UK's largest voluntary sector organisation working with and for people with arthritis, also produces a wide range of patient information booklets, many of which have won British Medical Association Patient Information Awards. Patients can order free of charge via their website (**www.arthritiscare.org.uk**).

Patients should be informed of the potential advantages and disadvantages of searching the Internet for general research and information on their condition, particularly at the early stages of diagnosis, as some of the unsolicited information may not be helpful. Members of the rheumatology team should guide patients to websites of trusted organisations such as those above.

Opportunities for education

Arthritis Care offers a range of courses to people with arthritis and musculoskeletal conditions. These include a popular course called 'Challenging arthritis' which promotes independence and taking control of arthritis, and was used by the Department of Health (DH) as a model for their expert patient programme. Personal development courses, courses specifically aimed at young people, and an arthritis awareness course for employers are also available. Details of their local arthritis care groups and courses in their area can be found via the website (**www.arthritiscare.org.uk**).

The DH's new expert patient programme brings together the valuable work of patients and clinical organisations in developing self-management initiatives. More than half of the primary care trusts (PCTs) in England are now either actively implementing the expert patient programme or have committed to joining in the near future. Initial pilot groups set up between 2001–2004 will be extensively evaluated and the programme will then be mainstreamed and rolled out across the NHS between 2004–2007.

Supporting patients to manage their condition

People who have a chronic condition of any kind may experience similar issues. Fatigue and depression are often strongly linked to chronic conditions and, unlike other symptoms, are often invisible. Patients may deal with the diagnosis and day-to-day experience of managing their conditions in different ways, and rheumatology departments may provide access to counselling services where appropriate and available.

Voluntary sector organisations such as Arthritis Care provide information and support for patients via their helpline or via email: **help@arthritiscare.org.uk**, and through local group activities and membership schemes. They also run specific information and support services for young people. Other disease-specific organisations such as the National Rheumatoid Arthritis Society, National Osteoporosis Society and Lupus UK provide useful resources, membership schemes, information helplines and informative websites.

The role of the carer

The care arrangements that are in place for a person with arthritis or other musculoskeletal conditions vary significantly between individuals. Care and support at home can range from the help of a friend, partner or child to professional care that is paid for by the individual or provided by local social services.

Members of the rheumatology MDT involved in making decisions about an individual's treatment will need to know about arrangements at home and will take great care to respect the individual's feelings. There are related issues of professional ethics and confidentiality and any involvement that a relative or friend has in a patient's treatment should be based firmly on the wishes of the patient.

Carers who provide day-to-day support for somebody with arthritis or another musculoskeletal condition may benefit greatly from knowing more about the condition and may need some support themselves. Again, voluntary sector organisations may be able to offer free information and support. Carers UK, a UK wide organisation offering support to carers, can be contacted via their website (**www.carersonline.org.uk**). The Arthritis Care booklet *Reaching independence* also offers useful advice.

iv   Interspecialty and interdisciplinary liaison

The rheumatology specialty has embraced the concept that in order to provide the best standards of care for patients' needs, access to a MDT must be made available. Also, as some musculoskeletal conditions require treatment and management outside the rheumatology department, effective interspecialty working relationships are essential, for example between rheumatologists and orthopaedic surgeons. In several areas acute back pain services have been established, often run by a physiotherapist working closely with medical and surgical backup, resulting in rapid access for patients and reduced surgical spinal outpatient waiting lists.

The provision of dedicated rheumatology practitioners is becoming ever more important. In many units specialist rheumatology nurse practitioners are an important link between the patient and primary and secondary care. They are key to ensuring that patients are made aware of the range of services available locally and helping them to make considered decisions about treatment options. They also manage their own patient caseload, run management and education clinics, and perform joint injections.

General practitioners with special interests (GPSIs) also usually work as part of a MDT which aims to provide an integrated service spanning primary and secondary care. Practitioners working in isolation, unsupported by a clinical team, pose a potential clinical governance risk. It is the responsibility of the local rheumatologists, hospital trusts and PCTs to ensure that practitioners with special interests working within the clinical service have appropriate training and experience, evidence of continuing professional development (CPD) in their specialist area, and adequate clinical facilities and support. As with all practitioners, robust and transparent procedures for clinical governance, audit, evaluation and accountability are essential.

v   Delivering a high quality service

Characteristics of a high quality service

In conjunction with several users of services, the ARMA has identified certain basic principles and characteristics that are necessary to provide a high quality patient-centred rheumatology service. These form the basis of the ARMA Standards of Care project.[6]

   ▪ Access to services is fundamental. Rheumatology services should offer access to consistently high quality and prompt services across the country without any postcode limitations. All patients should have access to services and receive treatment and care on the basis of need. All services should be fully physically accessible and should be located and designed appropriately for people with a range of mobility impairments. Patients with musculoskeletal conditions should receive early assessment and diagnosis from an appropriately trained specialist (usually a rheumatologist) as well as speedy access to appropriate treatments and services. Patients should have rapid access to appropriate healthcare professionals for further management.

   ▪ Access to high quality information for people with musculoskeletal conditions is a key priority. People should have access to information on health conditions, treatments and their potential side effects, support services and signposting, for example helplines for further information and support at all stages of care.

   ▪ Of crucial importance in the delivery of high quality services is the principle that services should be centred on the needs of users. All healthcare services should be designed to improve quality of life, preserve independence, limit the impact of the condition on a person's work and or/daily activities, and empower people with musculoskeletal conditions to manage their condition effectively. In order to enhance continuity of care, people with musculoskeletal conditions should be able to see the same healthcare professionals wherever possible.

■ People with musculoskeletal conditions should be regarded as equal partners in decision making regarding their own healthcare options. People should have access to local user-led self-management training courses and support networks or self-help groups.

Basic resources required for a high quality service

In order to provide a high quality patient-centred service there are several resources which rheumatology services should offer:

Outpatient facilities

■ All services should have appropriate access including disabled parking and 'drop-off' points, appropriate disabled seating and toilets, and a suitable waiting area for patients.

■ There should be sufficient consulting rooms and examination rooms and a clean area should be available for procedures such as epidurals and joint injections.

■ When necessary, nursing assistance should be available to help with procedures such as intra-articular injections.

■ Where local arrangements include drug-monitoring clinics they may be undertaken by an appropriately trained nurse or other healthcare professional with specialist rheumatology expertise.

■ There should be an adequate booking system for outpatient appointments, flexible enough to allow for fluctuations in doctor availability and adequate for both urgent and long-term appointments.

■ Some units provide day case facilities in rheumatology departments. These can provide facilities for many patients requiring lengthy treatments that may include intravenous infusions and joint injections. These units allow patients to have their treatment administered in a more relaxed and friendly environment away from the hospital ward or rheumatology outpatient department.

■ Changes in clinical practice, patient expectation and financial pressures have resulted in a trend for care to be provided in outpatients. This means that more patients with severe complicated disorders are being managed as outpatients, and procedures such as joint injections and epidurals are usually undertaken on an outpatient basis. Provision of patient information is very important to any rheumatology service and should be readily available. There is an increasing quantity of patient literature available from the **arc**, Arthritis Care and other specialist societies. Addresses and contact numbers of useful support groups and information on social security should also be provided. Patients should be given written instructions on how to manage their conditions.

■ Referral to departments of physiotherapy, occupational therapy, appliances and orthotics, chiropody and social work should be straightforward. Patients should be able to have blood tests and X-rays at the time of their outpatient visit. Haematology, biochemistry, immunology and microbiology services are needed. Facilities for electrophysical tests should be available. Polarising light microscopy must be available, either within the department or in one or other of the laboratory services. Convenient and speedy mechanisms for cross-referral to other specialties, in particular orthopaedics, should be available. Many rheumatologists also run combined clinics with orthopaedic surgeons, respiratory physicians, renal physicians and paediatricians.

▪ A rheumatology service should provide appropriate imaging facilities including access to a magnetic resonance imaging (MRI) scanner and a computed tomography (CT) scanner, facilities for isotope bone scans and bone densitometry.

▪ Departments should provide means whereby professional (but non-medical) advice can be given to patients or carers by telephone, usually by an experienced senior nurse trained in telephone helpline work. This may be provided on an answerphone basis or by direct telephone access at set times.

▪ The need for close liaison between primary care teams and secondary care teams has become more important as shared care of patients on second line or cytotoxic and biologic therapies is now accepted practice. A senior liaison nurse is most useful in supporting non-specialist groups with telephone helplines, visits to surgery and ensuring printed protocols and record cards are provided. BSR guidelines on the monitoring of people on DMARDs might be provided to GPs to ensure uniformity of monitoring standards and to help the primary care team in the management of these patients. The new General Medical Services GP contract determines that 'near patient testing' may impact on systems of drug monitoring in place locally.

Inpatient facilities

▪ Many patients with rheumatoid arthritis or connective tissue disorders will require inpatient care as a direct consequence of their disease or its treatment at some stage. Medical care during admission should involve, and usually be directed by, the rheumatologist.

▪ Inpatient facilities (including items such as cutlery and bedding) should be appropriate for patients with all levels of physical disability. Self-medication, which empowers patients to retain control of their treatment whilst allowing education regarding the action and side effects of their drugs should be encouraged.

Staffing support

▪ Consultant rheumatologists should not work in isolation and should have access to appropriate support staff including specialist practitioners. The availability of TNFα for rheumatoid arthritis has made this need for adequate support from nursing and administrative staff even more important, due to the time involved in administering the drugs and in the paperwork for registering patients and providing follow-up data for the BSRBR. Therefore, the BSR has published a set of business cases for the funding of TNFα in order that rheumatologists can put forward cases for adequate resources.

▪ A rheumatology department should have dedicated physiotherapy and occupational therapy sessional time and access to hydrotherapy.

▪ A rheumatology department must have access to adequate secretarial staff of sufficient experience and grade to be able to deal with patient enquiries and to arrange appointments. A rheumatology service follows a large number of patients over a long period of time, many of whom may require urgent specialist access between appointments. Secretarial and medical records staff have important roles in coordinating this care.

Innovative approaches in rheumatology practice

There are many examples of good practice in rheumatology services across the country. Many areas have developed priority and referral guidelines for common musculoskeletal conditions. These guidelines form the basis of electronic bookings, which are now available for some rheumatology, physiotherapy and bone densitometry referrals and will be introduced nationally for all referrals by 2005. These fully booked appointments, made at the time of GP consultation and decision to refer, may increase patient choice and satisfaction by giving patients the opportunity to choose when and at what time to attend appointments and also increase efficiency of hospital resources.

Many units now run a rheumatology advice service for GPs and patients about the management of musculoskeletal conditions. GPs can be empowered to manage rheumatological conditions in primary care. Therefore, the patient gets the treatment they need from their GP quickly and without having to be unnecessarily referred to secondary care, avoiding lengthy waiting lists.

vi   Quality standards and measures of the quality of specialist services

Specialist society guidelines

The BSR commissions and produces its own clinical guidelines which are published under the publications, guidelines and library section of the BSR website (**www.rheumatology.org.uk**). The BSR standards, guidelines and audit working group looks at existing guidelines and assesses whether they need to be updated. The working group also commissions new guidelines for treatments and therapies for arthritis and other musculoskeletal conditions. All new BSR guidelines have to be auditable. Examples of current BSR guidance are biologic therapies for rheumatoid arthritis, monitoring of second line drugs, and epidural steroids for spinal pain. BSR guidelines are all measured against the Appraisal of Guidelines research and Evaluation (AGREE) standard.

Following the issuing of NICE guidance on anti-TNFα for people with rheumatoid arthritis, many rheumatologists have experienced difficulty in obtaining appropriate funding for patients who fulfil the criteria for treatment.[7] Although there is an obligation for trusts and PCTs to fund compounds approved by NICE, in practice funding remains difficult, particularly for administrative and nursing support in administering therapy. The set of business cases produced by the BSR can help rheumatologists secure the necessary funding. These can be found on the BSR website.

Several patient organisations produce excellent literature intended for people with arthritis and musculoskeletal conditions. Please see section iii for further details.

National Institute for Clinical Excellence guidelines

The BSR has been actively involved in producing submissions for several NICE technology appraisals. On a number of occasions BSR has adopted a successful joint working approach with the ARMA and its members in order to give a balanced submission response from the whole arthritis community. BSR also works closely with the College on NICE appraisals. Previous NICE appraisal topics which the BSR has had involvement with include cox II inhibitors for osteoarthritis and rheumatoid arthritis; etanercept and inifliximab for rheumatoid arthritis; and anakinra for rheumatoid arthritis. The BSR is also currently contributing to the NICE guideline on osteoporosis. Some of BSR's previous submissions to NICE appraisals can be found on the BSR website under the policy and campaigns section (**www.rheumatology.org.uk**).

ARMA Standards of Care project

The BSR is contributing to the ARMA Standards of Care project which aims to identify reasonable expectations of care and services for all people with musculoskeletal conditions, including access to quality services for all people with musculoskeletal conditions, timely diagnosis and treatment, information, services which are centred on the needs of users, independence and self-determination.[6]

CLINICAL WORK AND/OR LABORATORY WORK OF CONSULTANTS IN RHEUMATOLOGY

Contributions made to acute medicine

As part of the hospital acute physician team, 16% of consultant rheumatologists practise GIM. The BSR, in reference to potential conflict between specialty care (largely outpatient) and general medicine (largely inpatient), maintains that no single-handed consultant rheumatologist should be expected to do GIM. This negotiation will become part of the new consultant contract arrangements.

2003 consultant contract

Consultants opting for the new consultant contract will have negotiated contractual work plans. In many cases, year one negotiations have not run smoothly and the BSR has produced guidance and examples of job templates to facilitate this process for year two arrangements (2005 negotiations). This advice and job plan guidance is not designed to be comprehensive and rheumatologists have also been referred to the DH job-planning guidelines available on the DH website (**www.dh.gov.uk/Home/fs/en uk**).

Job plan examples are available from the BSR for the work of a full-time consultant with GIM, without GIM, and for those in research.

Sessions of four hours previously considered to be a notional half day (NHD) are now known as programmed activities (PAs). Job plans are based on a template of 10 PAs together with allowances for predictable on-call work.

Where the physician also has a general medical commitment and participates in the on-take rota with post-take rounds, the number of clinics is usually reduced accordingly. Undergraduate and postgraduate teaching or supervision of specialist registrars (SpRs) will also reduce the number of patients seen by the consultant in a clinic.

Direct clinical care

Outpatient work

Workload figures are based on recommendations of best practice from the BSR.

A full-time consultant rheumatologist would be expected to undertake four to five clinics weekly and those performing GIM up to four. These would include routine and special clinics and activities such as combined clinics with orthopaedic surgeons or paediatricians. The exact number will depend on other duties, the geography of the service (eg split sites), responsibility for a rehabilitation unit and administrative duties.

Ideally, 30 minutes should be allocated for a new patient and 10–15 minutes for a follow-up appointment. If junior staff are shared with general medicine then they may be absent from clinics depending on their on-call rota and clinic structure. Numbers booked will need to take this into account.

Numbers of patients

New patients　It is suggested that six to seven new patients should be booked into a clinic for a single consultant. Five of these patients would be routine or soon bookings, with one always held for urgent cases. The optimum number depends on casemix.

Review clinics　10–15 review patients is considered a reasonable load for a single-handed consultant depending on casemix.

Mixed clinics　One new patient takes the time of two review patients, depending to an extent on casemix.

The impact of additional staff in a rheumatology clinic　Junior staff see fewer patients than a consultant, who must also oversee their work. It is recommended that for each GP clinical assistant, senior house officer (SHO) or SpR, the number of additional patients booked per clinic should be as follows:

	New patients	*or* Review patients
GP clinical assistant	3–4 extra	*or* 7–10 extra
SHO/SpR	2 extra	*or* 7 extra
Experienced SpR	4 extra	*or* 10 extra

This is to allow time for supervision by the consultant.

When a rheumatology specialist practitioner (nurse, physiotherapist or occupational therapist) is present and can undertake monitoring or some procedures, a consultant can see more patients.

The impact of teaching in outpatient clinics

To allow for teaching in a clinic there should be about 25% fewer patients.

Inpatient work

Time should be allowed for day case work and for the small number of patients who are admitted acutely ill with rheumatological conditions due to complications of such conditions or their treatment.

On-call work

Many large rheumatology departments have their own consultant on-call rota. This is essential if the trainees have on-call commitments. Even where consultant rheumatologists have no acute general medical responsibility there are rheumatology emergencies. Some may be dealt with by the acute on-call team but consultant rheumatologist advice should always be available. Providing an emergency opinion service to A&E departments may also be an appropriate on-call activity.

Work to maintain and improve the quality of care

This work encompasses duties in clinical governance, professional self-regulation, CPD, education, apprasial and training of others.

Service developments that deliver improved care

Rheumatology services have evolved in recent years to operate around a patient-centred model of providing treatment and care. Developments include specialist nurse-led clinics, back pain services, the introduction of dedicated rheumatology day units, physiotherapy triage systems and combined clinics with orthopaedics.

Leadership role and the introduction of service developments

Rheumatologists have a responsibility to develop and guide the MDT; to hold team meetings; plan service developments; and introduce new treatments and management plans as they are developed. Rheumatologists frequently have major roles in medical management within their trusts.

Education and training

Rheumatologists are often involved in the formal training of undergraduate medical students and postgraduate medical doctors. Specialist registrar rotations require a structured curriculum-based training programme and such programmes are in place for hospitals involved in this training process.

Opportunities for education and training are widespread in the rheumatology specialty. The BSR has an education and training committee and the **arc** an education subcommittee. The BSR holds an annual meeting usually attended by more than 1,400 people. The meeting features a large exhibition, keynote speakers, the latest education updates, and cutting-edge clinical case reports. Abstract presentations report breaking news and the latest scientific advances in the specialty. The most important aspect of the meeting is the opportunity for people working in the field to communicate and learn about the latest developments in rheumatology. The BSR also offers several education courses across the year for health professionals working in the rheumatology specialty. All of these courses and meetings are important in providing opportunities for CME.

Mentoring and appraisal of medical staff and other professional staff

Within the specialty, appraisal follows individual trust requirements and is often carried out within clinical disciplines, for example doctors appraised by doctors and nurses by nurses, or within departments. Given the multidisciplinary nature of the rheumatology team, there may be an interest in introducing 360-degree multidisciplinary appraisal but, as yet, there are no national models for this approach. The BSR has also developed a peer review scheme which operates at a local and regional level between hospital and community trusts.

Clinical governance

Specialists in rheumatology aim to offer patients high quality patient-centred care for their individual clinical needs. Systems for clinical governance vary between trusts and are increasingly likely to become based on best practice as defined by ARMA standards of care and BSR guidelines.

Research – clinical studies and basic science

Research within the specialty occurs both within academic institutions and in rheumatology departments within district hospitals. Rheumatology research may be funded by grants for national bodies, for example **arc**/Medical Research Council, or through the NHS research and development programme. The specialty is developing a range of nationally recognised programmes to attract DH research and development funding. Developments in research include the BSRBR which was set up to monitor the long-term safety of people taking biologic agents for musculoskeletal conditions.

Regional and national work

The BSR has set up several regional groups across the UK, with the aim of meeting to consider local issues and sharing good practice. The BSR has developed an effective working relationship with the College, including representation on its joint specialty committee for rheumatology. The rheumatology community is developing effective links with parliament and the DH, and regularly responds to NICE appraisal consultations and other consultations from the DH and associated bodies such as the Commission for Healthcare Audit and Inspection (CHAI). The BSR has a very active external relations department.

ACADEMIC MEDICINE

Rheumatology has an active research base with many flourishing academic departments throughout the UK. These departments are often associated with departments of immunology and/or pathology. International recognition of the UK's contribution in this area has come in the form of the Albert Lasker prize to Professors Feldmann and Maini based at the Kennedy Institute, Imperial College London.

It is vital to maintain a flow of clinicians who can bridge the gap between the laboratory bench and the clinic, and one must be mindful of the need to establish conditions which facilitate both good clinical training and the acquisition of laboratory skills.

Clinical contribution to the NHS

Nearly all academic rheumatologists in the UK provide support for their clinical colleagues in the NHS, undertaking both outpatient clinics and providing some ward cover. This contribution is important and likely to continue but it is also essential that an academic rheumatologist is not overwhelmed by NHS commitments.

Teaching

Academic rheumatologists often play the lead in organising undergraduate and or postgraduate teaching of rheumatology within individual medical schools. This effort is clearly vital in terms of providing undergraduate students with a good grounding in diseases of the musculoskeletal system and in encouraging an academic approach to this important subject. Likewise, postgraduate students need to be inspired by their academic teachers and encouraged to continue their career in musculoskeletal research.

Research

It is only through a more profound understanding of the aetiopathogenesis of musculoskeletal disease that we will ultimately develop more specific forms of therapy with fewer side effects. Thus, a key role for the academic rheumatologist is to develop programmes of research into the causes, methods of assessment and therapies of musculoskeletal disease. The UK has a number of outstanding academic units with international research reputations.

Other academic duties

Most academic rheumatologists serve on a variety of committees, both NHS and more overtly academic. These range from clinical and/or research governance committees at a local level to national research committees such as those run by the **arc** or the Wellcome Trust.

WORKFORCE REQUIREMENTS FOR RHEUMATOLOGY

Consultant programmed activities required to provide a service in rheumatology for a population of 250,000

The consultant requirement, measured as the number of PAs, needed to provide a service depends on the volume of inpatient and outpatient work. The figures below are based on an epidemiological needs-based assessment of the number of incident and prevalent cases of musculoskeletal conditions likely to present to primary care, and the proportion of these cases who would benefit from assessment, treatment and follow-up in secondary care.[8] The assessment is based on providing services to adults (aged 16 and over) in a total population of 250,000.

Cases seen by rheumatologists can be broadly divided into four main categories: inflammatory disorders of joints and connective tissues; osteoarthritis; back pain; and other regional and widespread pain syndromes (soft tissue rheumatism).

The following assumptions were made:
- 90% of incident cases of inflammatory disorders should be referred to a rheumatologist.
- 60% of prevalent cases should be under hospital review 2.5 times per year on average.
- Of the 40% of prevalent cases not under regular review, 10% would be referred as new cases each year.
- 5% of incident cases of osteoarthritis would be referred for rheumatology assessment.
- 2.5% of prevalent cases of osteoarthritis would be referred for assessment each year.
- 70% of new patient referrals would be seen on one further occasion.
- 5% of those aged under 45 and 10% of those aged over 45 with incident back pain would be referred to secondary care.
- Of those referred to secondary care, 75% would see a rheumatologist.
- Of those seen by a rheumatologist, 50% would have one further appointment.
- 7% of those with incident regional or widespread pain would be referred to a rheumatologist.
- 50% of those referred would be seen on one further occasion.

Based on these assumptions a population of 250,000 would generate the following workload per annum:

	New cases	Follow-up cases
Inflammatory disorders	84	2,190
Osteoarthritis	502	351
Back pain (including osteoporosis)	500	250
Regional and widespread pain	657	328
Total	1,743	3,119

If we assume that a consultant can see six new or 12 follow-up patients per clinic (as described above) then this volume of outpatient work equates to 551 clinics per year. If we assume that a consultant provides four and a half clinics a week for 44 weeks per year then one consultant can provide 198 clinics per year. Thus, a population of 250,000 requires 2.8 whole time equivalent (WTE) consultants. This equates to one consultant per 90,000 population.

According to the database held by the **arc** Epidemiology Research Unit at the University of Manchester, there were 469 consultants with a commitment to rheumatology in England and Wales as at 1 September 2003. Based on the latest population estimate for England and Wales of 52,455,000 this is equivalent to one rheumatologist per 111,844 of the population.[9] The majority of consultants with a commitment to rheumatology practise whole-time. However, approximately 16% of consultant rheumatologists also have a commitment to general medicine and 9% have a commitment to rehabilitation. There are 50 academic posts. Assuming that maximum part-time consultants work full-time, and allowing for part-time consultants and for sessional commitments to academic work, general medicine or rehabilitation, there are 365 WTEs in rheumatology in England and Wales, equivalent to one per 143,712 of the population. This represents a 10% increase in WTEs since 2001.[10]

To achieve one WTE consultant rheumatologist per 90,000 population would require a total of 583 consultants. On the basis of the current figure of 365 WTEs in England and Wales, there is currently a shortfall of 217 as at 1 September 2003.

CONSULTANT WORK PROGRAMME/SPECIMEN JOB PLANS

Rheumatologist with GIM

Activity	Workload	Programmed activities (PAs)
Direct clinical care	3–4 outpatient clinics and associated administration (1.25 PAs per clinic)	3.75–5
	2 GIM and specialty ward rounds	2
	Patient-related administration, relatives and contact	0.5–1
On call	Peri and post take ward rounds weekdays and weekends – predictable and unpredictable – (1:8)	1–2
Total number of direct clinical care PAs		7.5 on average
Supporting professional activities (SPA) Work to maintain and improve the quality of healthcare	Education and training, appraisal, departmental management and service development, audit and clinical governance, CPD and revalidation, research	2.5 on average
Other NHS responsibilities	eg medical director/clinical director/lead consultant in specialty/clinical tutor	Local agreement with trust
External duties	eg work for deaneries/Royal Colleges/specialist societies/Department of Health or other government bodies etc	Local agreement with trust

Rheumatologist without GIM; on-call rheumatology rota

Activity	Workload	Programmed activities (PAs)
Direct clinical care	3–5 outpatient clinics and associated administration (1.25 PAs per clinic)	3.75–6.25
	Ward round, inpatient referrals and MDT	1
	Monthly combined clinic with orthopaedics	0.25
	Patient-related administration	0.5–1
On call	Annualised on call – predictable and unpredictable	0.5
Total number of direct clinical care PAs		7.5 on average
Supporting professional activities (SPA) Work to maintain and improve the quality of healthcare	Education and training, appraisal, departmental management and service development, audit and clinical governance, CPD and revalidation, research	2.5 on average
Other NHS responsibilities	eg medical director/clinical director/lead consultant in specialty/clinical tutor	Local agreement with trust
External duties	eg work for deaneries/Royal Colleges/specialist societies/Department of Health or other government bodies etc	Local agreement with trust

Full-time academic clinical rheumatologist; on-call rheumatology rota

Activity	Workload	Programmed activities (PAs)
Direct clinical care – acute trust	Specialist patient clinics plus associated administration	1.25–2.5
	1 ward round and inpatient referrals	1.0–1.5
On call	Annualised on call predictable and unpredictable on rheumatology rota	0.5
Total number of direct clinical care PAs		3.5 on average
Research academic sessions – university	6 full academic sessions	5–6
Supporting professional activities (SPA) Work to maintain and improve the quality of healthcare	Education and training, appraisal, departmental management and service development, audit and clinical governance, CPD and revalidation, research	1.5 on average
Other NHS responsibilities	eg medical director/clinical director/lead consultant in specialty/clinical tutor	Local agreement with trust
External duties	eg work for deaneries/Royal Colleges/specialist societies/Department of Health or other government bodies etc	Local agreement with trust

References

1. McCormick A, Fleming D, Charlton J. *Morbidity statistics from general practice, fourth national study 1991–1992.* RCGP 1991 statistics applied to year 2000 population. London: HMSO, 1995.

2. Arthritis Research Campaign. *Arthritis: the big picture.* Derbyshire: arc, 2002.

3. NHS Modernisation Agency. *Improving orthopedic services: a guide for clinicians, managers and service commissioners.* London: Action on orthopedics and the orthopedic services collaborative, December 2002. www.modern.nhs.uk/action-on

4. Data from the British Society for Rheumatology/Arthritis Research Campaign consultant workforce register, 2003.

5. Department of Health. *The expert patient: a new approach to chronic disease management for the 21st century.* London: DH, 2001.

6. Arthritis and Musculoskeletal Alliance. *Standards of care for people with back pain; Standards of care for people with inflammatory arthritis; Standards of care for people with osteoarthritis.* London: ARMA, 2004.

7. National institute for Clinical Excellence. *Guidance on the use of etanercept and infliximab for the treatment of rheumatoid arthritis,* March 2002. www.nice.org.uk/page.aspx?o=35993

8. Symmons D, Asten P, McNally R, Webb R. *Healthcare needs assessment for the musculoskeletal diseases.* 2nd edition. Derbyshire: Arthritis Research Campaign, 2002.

9. Office for National Statistics. *Health statistics quarterly.* Winter 2003. London: TSO, 2003.

10. Turner G, Symmons D, Bamji A, Palferman T. Consultant rheumatology workforce in the UK: changing patterns of provision 1997–2001. *Rheumatology* 2002;41(6):680–684.

Stroke medicine

i   Description of the specialty and clinical needs of patients

Stroke has a major impact on people's lives. It is caused by a disturbance of blood supply to the brain and may be ischaemic or haemorrhagic. It starts as an acute medical emergency, presents complex care needs, may result in long-term disability and can lead to admission to long-term care. Each year, 110,000 people in England and Wales have their first stroke, and 30,000 people go on to have further strokes. It is the single biggest cause of severe disability and the third most common cause of death in the UK. Over 5% of NHS resources and significant social care resources are devoted to the immediate and continuing care of people with stroke. In an average general hospital at any one time there are 25–35 patients with stroke as their primary diagnosis. The National Service Framework (NSF) for Older People Standard Five: Stroke requires every general hospital which cares for stroke patients to have a specialist stroke service.[1]

Patients with subarachnoid haemorrhage may have requirements similar to those of stroke patients (eg for rehabilitation and other services) but have differing needs for acute care and are not specifically included in the following paragraphs.

Despite recent improvements, stroke care remains suboptimal in many health districts. The *National sentinel stroke audit* 2004 found that 82% of hospitals in England but only 45% in Wales now have a stroke unit.[2] The standard and organisation of stroke services varies widely. There is a consultant physician with special responsibility for stroke in 90% of hospitals but physicians only have a median of three weekly sessions for stroke and training opportunities are limited.

There is a firm evidence base for stroke treatment. Organised stroke care improves patient outcome regardless of age or stroke severity. The NSF, the *National clinical guidelines for stroke*, and the Scottish Intercollegiate Guidelines Network (SIGN) (**www.sign.ac.uk**) have set out clear and explicit standards of care for all people suffering from stroke illness irrespective of age.[1,3,4]

Stroke medicine was recognised as a subspecialty of acute medicine by the specialist training authority of the Joint Committee on Higher Medical Training (JCHMT) in April 2004. Consultant physicians currently specialising in stroke are based within a number of parent specialties including geriatric medicine, neurology, rehabilitation medicine, clinical pharmacology and therapeutics, and cardiology. An increasing number of consultants are being appointed with a special interest in stroke medicine. The British Association of Stroke Physicians (BASP) (**www.basp.ac.uk**) was formed in 1998 to bring together physicians involved in the care of stroke patients and to promote high quality stroke services.

ii   Organisation of the service and patterns of referral

There are four main components of integrated stroke services:

- *Primary and secondary prevention*   In most cases stroke is part of a spectrum of vascular disorders closely linked to cardiac and peripheral vascular disease and sharing key risk factors such as hypertension, diabetes and smoking.

■ *Immediate care*   Admission to a stroke unit reduces death and disability. Thrombolysis is likely to become an accepted treatment for acute cerebral infarction, needing rapid access to a stroke physician and neuroradiology services at all times.

■ *Early and continuing rehabilitation*   This should be provided by an appropriately skilled multidisciplinary team (MDT).

■ *Long-term support*   This is needed during recovery and adaptation, which may continue for many years.

Primary, secondary and tertiary levels

Primary care   The primary care team is central to the primary and secondary prevention of stroke, the recognition of symptoms requiring urgent admission to a stroke unit or referral to a neurovascular transient ischaemic attack (TIA) clinic, and to the long-term support of people with stroke. Stroke service planning teams should include primary care trusts (PCTs), general practice, community nursing services, crisis care organisations, social services departments and the ambulance service, as well as user and carer representatives.

Effective and systematic programmes of prevention can identify those at risk and reduce the incidence of stroke. Previous stroke or TIA, high blood pressure, atrial fibrillation, carotid stenosis and diabetes are key risk factors. Modification of lifestyle, especially smoking cessation, reduced alcohol consumption, improved diet and increased physical activity are also important. Practices should build on registers being developed for the prevention of coronary heart disease.[1]

In the treatment of acute stroke, GPs, ambulance teams and other frontline staff need to play an increasing role in educating and advising people with stroke symptoms about the urgency of hospital assessment, and in implementing rapid admission protocols.

The role of primary care is further emphasised by the inclusion of indicators related to stroke in the quality and outcomes framework of the general medical services (GMS) contract.[5]

Secondary care   The *National sentinel stroke audit* found that stroke units provide better care for stroke patients than general medical or geriatric wards.[6] The components of a comprehensive stroke service are:

■ An *acute stroke unit* (ASU)   ASUs have two main service models: a geographically defined area with dedicated staff caring predominantly for stroke patients, or a ward area without specific resources in an elderly care, general medical, neurology, combined stroke and head injury, or rehabilitation ward. They must be capable of admitting patients within three hours of onset of symptoms and provide specialist medical, nursing and therapy input. Stroke patients need rapid and accurate diagnosis, careful monitoring and control of physiological variables, and treatment of medical complications. The thrombolytic agent r-tpa was licensed in the UK for use in acute ischaemic stroke in April 2003. It must be given within three hours of symptom onset, after assessment by a stroke specialist and brain imaging (computed tomography (CT) scan), and in a unit where appropriate monitoring can take place.

■ A *rehabilitation stroke unit* (RSU)   Different models of care are effective as long as certain standards of care are maintained. There may be integration with the acute unit, or separate units in the acute hospital, or in rehabilitation, community or specialist hospitals. All include specialist physician input. The proportion of patients with stroke in an RSU varies.

- A *neurovascular clinic* (TIA)   All patients with suspected TIA should be seen and investigated within one week of the neurological event and treated immediately.[3]

- *Outreach rehabilitation and community liaison*   After the acute phase, rehabilitation can be provided equally effectively either in hospital or at home.[3] A community stroke team should include therapists specialising in stroke.[3] Models of early supported discharge with specialist medical input have been shown to be effective in randomised controlled trials.

- *Secondary prevention and stroke follow up*   Specialist clinics are required for the initiation of secondary prevention treatment and to provide advice to primary care for difficult management problems.

- *Longer-term management of disability*   The NSF requires review of patients six months after the stroke to assess whether further treatment would be beneficial. This should be by a specialist MDT.[1]

Tertiary care   Reasons for referral to a tertiary centre might include:

- specialised diagnostic or therapeutic input, for example by a vascular neurologist or neurosurgeon, or neuroradiological investigations not available in a general radiology department

- assessment and treatment of carotid stenosis by a vascular surgeon, where this is not available locally

- specialist rehabilitation, particularly for complex disability including management of spasticity and neuropsychological problems; provision of equipment such as specialist seating; or techniques such as functional electrical stimulation.

Clinical networks and community arrangements

Clinical networks will become established as stroke services continue to evolve. These would typically serve a number of PCTs and secondary care trusts and one or two tertiary providers. They will help to ensure consistency of provision of all parts of the stroke service, equality of access for service users, education of all staff and sharing of good practice and experience. Early templates include regional stroke coordinators' forums, stroke research groups and professional forums, which are already active in parts of the UK. Stroke networks and local services should work closely with user and carer groups and the voluntary sector, and should seek patients' views from as many sources as possible.

Relationship with other services/agencies

Stroke medicine has key relationships with the parent specialties whose skills benefit the patient at different times during their journey through care, and also with radiology, neurosurgery, vascular surgery, general practice, intermediate care and community services. Districts will differ in the approach taken to provide stroke services. Some consultants may provide stroke services exclusively, others may have other clinical responsibilities, for example in geriatrics, neurology or general medicine.

iii Working with patients: patient-centred care

Patient choice and involving patients in decisions about their treatment

The Stroke Association (**www.stroke.org**) and other organisations have played a key role in working with patients, carers and health professionals to develop stroke services.

Focus groups, conducted by the College of Health in 1998, were used to inform the *National clinical guidelines for stroke*.[3] Patient and carer views should be obtained when developing guidelines. Patients and their carers want timely access to appropriate quality services and to be looked after by knowledgeable staff who understand the full range of their needs.

All interventions, including drug treatment and therapeutic interventions, should be discussed with the patient. Despite time constraints, the use of thrombolysis for the treatment of acute ischaemic stroke must be fully explained to the patient or, when this is not possible, to their next-of-kin in view of the potentially serious side effects of this treatment.

Successful recovery from stroke depends upon full and equal involvement of the patient. All members of the healthcare team should work together with the patient, carer and family using a shared philosophy and common goals.[3] Rehabilitation goals should be functional and relevant. Where possible, choice should be offered regarding location and style of rehabilitation.

Younger stroke patients may have different medical, rehabilitative, psychological and social needs, which must be recognised. Services should be provided in an environment suited to their personal needs. A separate set of guidelines covering stroke in children has been produced by the Royal College of Physicians and the Royal College of Paediatrics and Child Health.[7]

Given the higher prevalence of stroke in some minority ethnic communities, integrated stroke services and stroke prevention advice should consider the need for language interpretation or advocacy support, especially for those patients and carers whose first language is not English.[1] People in lower socioeconomic groups are at higher risk of stroke and may be less likely to receive the best treatment.

Opportunities for education and promoting self-care

There is a lack of awareness about the risk factors, warning signs and early symptoms of stroke. Continuing efforts to address these are necessary. Specific education of people at high risk and after a stroke episode can be undertaken by both primary and secondary care teams. Stroke services should have educational programmes for staff, patients and carers.[3]

Stroke rehabilitation aims, directly or indirectly, to increase independence and ability. Organised rehabilitation directly improves activities of daily living. The NSF and the *National clinical guidelines for stroke* give clear guidance on appropriate rehabilitation and on the provision of equipment and adaptation needed to alleviate the impact of a stroke-related impairment.[1,3] Patients and their families should be given information about statutory and voluntary organisations offering services specific to their long-term needs with the aim of maximising independence and participation.

Patients with chronic conditions

Recovery from stroke can continue over a long period, and rehabilitation should continue until it is clear that maximum recovery has been achieved. Of stroke patients surviving at one year, 35% are significantly disabled and approximately 5% are admitted to long-term care.[1] Some patients will need ongoing support, possibly for many years. These people and their carers should have access to a stroke coordinator.[1,2]

Any patient reporting a significant disability at six months should be reassessed and offered further targeted rehabilitation if this can help them to recover further function.[1] Multidisciplinary stroke clinics with a network of available therapy options can deliver this care. Treatment of spasticity, provision of aids and equipment, and psychological care are all key elements in the management of stroke-related disability.

All stroke patients should undergo monitoring of long-term treatment. Anticoagulants such as warfarin should be monitored by a specialist anticoagulant service.

The role of the carer

Stroke is a family illness. Initially, as in any other acute illness, relatives need information and support through the crisis, but they will usually need long-term practical, emotional, social and financial support to cope with the many residual problems.[3] Families provide much of the long-term care and support for stroke patients, often finding their own lives radically altered. Emotional distress is seen in 55% of caregivers at six months after stroke.[8] The needs of carers must be considered at each stage of the stroke patient's journey. Education and training for the carer role is needed. Family support workers help to reduce carer distress.[3]

Access to information, patient support groups and the role of the expert patient

Patients and carers need to be offered relevant user-friendly information at each stage of their care and to have access to contacts for further questions and problems that arise later. They need the diagnosis and management plan to be explained in a manner that they can comprehend and recall, to be treated as responsible adults, and to be involved in shared decision making. Carers want to know what is being done or planned for their relative. Patients and carers should know what care they may expect. This can be helped by providing patient/carer-friendly versions of guidelines.[3] A patient and carer guide to the *National clinical guidelines* is available from the College.[9]

The Stroke Association and other organisations, for example Different Strokes (**www. differentstrokes.co.uk**) and Speakability (**www.speakability.org.uk**), provide information, both written and on their websites, and give telephone advice. Most areas have local patient and carer support groups, often affiliated to the national organisations. Stroke teams must work closely with local groups to get feedback on local service provision and to inform and support group leaders and members. All patients should be provided with a list of local groups on hospital discharge or during rehabilitation at home.

Expert patients play a key role in stroke service planning teams and can offer other support to services, for example collecting information on current patient experience and participating in education for staff and users.

Availability of clinical records/results

The availability of clinical records and results is important to the provision of effective care. Brain imaging results must be available to the stroke physician at the time of consultation and need to be shared with tertiary centres when issues of diagnosis or therapeutic intervention arise. Digital image servers have vastly improved the accessibility of radiological investigations and images can now often be linked to tertiary centres.

The use of a stroke clerking proforma and integrated patient record (shared by all members of the MDT) is good practice and improves management and communication. Information must be available to all those working with the stroke patient in hospital and the community. This is particularly important when the patient moves from one area of care to another. Accurate and timely hospital discharge summaries improve the quality of care, and time for accurate record keeping and communication must be allowed for. Patient-held records may be useful.

iv Interspecialty and interdisciplinary liaison

Multidisciplinary team working

Stroke care is dependent upon multidisciplinary working and stroke physicians will expect to have particularly close working relationships with rehabilitation and therapy services, including nursing, physiotherapy, occupational therapy, speech and language therapy, dietetics, clinical and neuropsychology and social work services, both in hospital and the community. The stroke coordinator is a key member of the team and can liaise between disciplines and localities.

Working with other specialists

Stroke physicians work closely with general physicians, geriatricians, neurologists, vascular surgeons, neurosurgeons, and radiology and A&E departments. Local guidelines for assessment and management of people with acute stroke, for imaging for acute stroke and TIA patients, and for referral for rehabilitation are needed. Stroke physicians may need to refer complex patients for a neurological opinion, and to work with other colleagues to provide a full spectrum of stroke care.

A large number of stroke patients develop cognitive impairment in addition to significant anxiety and depression so liaison with departments of psychiatry is important. Complex feeding issues, often leading to consideration of artificial feeding and placement of gastrostomy tubes, necessitates liaison with the gastroenterology and nutrition team. Severely ill patients need high quality care and often pose considerable management challenges. Palliative care and pain management teams contribute to patient care.

Working with GP specialists

The prevalence of stroke disease and its association with other common medical problems, together with the often long-term nature of the illness, makes stroke medicine a strong contender for developing the concept of GP specialists.

v Delivering a high quality service

Characteristics of a high quality service:

There is strong evidence that people who have a stroke are more likely to survive and to recover more function if admitted promptly to a hospital-based stroke unit with treatment and care provided by a specialist-coordinated stroke team within an integrated stroke service.

The *National clinical guidelines for stroke* and the NSF make the following recommendations:[3]

1. Stroke services should be organised so that patients are admitted under the care of a specialist team for their acute care and rehabilitation.

2. Stroke services should satisfy the following criteria by having:
    -   a geographically identified unit as part of the inpatient service
    -   a coordinated MDT that meets at least once a week for the interchange of information about individual patients
    -   staff with specialist expertise in stroke and rehabilitation
    -   educational programmes for staff, patients and carers
    -   agreed protocols for common problems
    -   access to brain and vascular imaging services.

3. Each service should conduct a needs assessment exercise to determine the level of service so that all stroke patients in the area have access to the same standards of care.

4. Any patient with persistent/continuing symptoms should be rapidly referred to hospital with the expectation of admission to a stroke unit. Exceptions may include those relatively few patients for whom the diagnosis will make no difference to management.

5. A neurovascular clinic for the rapid assessment of TIA and minor stroke should be available. Patients should be seen within one week of symptoms and started on secondary prevention immediately.

6. Services for TIA should have rapid access to imaging for patients who need it.

7. Hospitals offering thrombolysis to patients after ischaemic stroke, outside of a trial, should only do so after specialist staff training and registration with the UK Safe Implementation of Thrombolysis in Stroke Monitoring Study (SITS-MOST) programme.

8. Specialist stroke services should be available in the community as part of an integrated system of care to facilitate early supported discharge.

9. Specialist day hospital rehabilitation or specialist domiciliary rehabilitation can be offered to outpatients with equal effect.

10. There should be access to services supplying orthotics, specialist seating and assistive devices.

11. There should be an in-house programme of education for all staff involved in providing the stroke service.

Resources required for a high quality service

Specialised facilities

Acute stroke units are based within district or specialist hospitals and must have good functional relationships with A&E, acute assessment and radiology departments. There should be access to continuous physiological monitoring (currently available in 54% of acute stroke units).[2]

Rehabilitation stroke units can be effective in a number of different settings. The environment must permit rehabilitation, including the practice of functional tasks at varying levels of ability, for example getting in and out of bed and chairs, bathing, use of the toilet and stairs, and meal preparation. A gymnasium and specialised rehabilitation equipment must be provided. Rooms for therapists from a number of disciplines to work with patients in private and in groups must be available. Patients must be able to take their meals in a dining area and must have adequate space in which to relax (including quiet areas). This is particularly important because the length of stay for stroke patients may be longer than for those with other conditions.

Neurovascular (TIA) clinics need access to timely brain imaging and carotid ultrasound services. This needs to be radically improved to meet the targets for management of patients with TIA.[2]

Workforce requirements: clinical and support staff

The specialist stroke team should include specific staff with specialist knowledge of stroke:[1,2]

■ consultant physician specialising in stroke medicine

■ nurses

■ physiotherapist

■ occupational therapist

■ speech and language therapist

■ neuroradiologist

■ dietitian

■ clinical psychologist

■ pharmacist

■ social worker

■ stroke coordinator.

The team should be supported adequately by staff in training.

There are wide variations in the staffing levels between units, and in most units is below that of those in the randomised controlled trials. Some elements of the team, for example clinical psychology, are rarely present. Currently, much of the nursing care of stroke patients is delivered by care assistants.[2] Current staffing levels may not permit the early and intensive rehabilitation identified in the NSF.[10]

There are no specific recommendations for staffing numbers on a stroke unit. However, the median numbers nationally per 10 beds are:

Nursing staff (trained and untrained on duty)	3.3 WTEs
Physiotherapists	1.3 WTEs
Occupational therapists	1.0 WTEs
Speech and language therapists	0.3 WTEs

WTE = whole time equivalent

vi Quality standards and measure of the quality of specialist services

Specialist society guidelines

The BASP supports the *National clinical guidelines for stroke* and the NSF for Older People Standard Five: Stroke.[1,3]

The European Stroke Council (**www.eurostrokecouncil.org**) is an organisation of professionals in a number of specialties focused on advancement and promotion of knowledge, treatment and prevention of stroke. It supports the annual European Stroke Conference, together with the

European Stroke Initiative (EUSI) (**www.eusi-stroke.org**). The International Stroke Society (**www.internationalstroke.org**) aims to provide access to stroke care and to promote research and teaching. It sponsors the annual World Stroke Conference.

National Institute for Clinical Excellence (NICE) guidelines and clinical governance

The *National sentinel stroke audit* is now in its fourth cycle.[2] It examines both organisational and clinical aspects of the management of stroke. All applicable hospitals that admit patients for stroke in England, Wales, Northern Ireland, the Isle of Man and the Channel Islands took part in the 2004 audit. This is the first time that 100% participation has been achieved for a national audit of this kind.

The *National clinical guidelines* recommend the following indicators for audit of stroke:[3]

- the proportion of patients spending more than 50% of their stay on a stroke unit
- the 'top ten' process indicators of stroke from the *National sentinel audit of stroke* which include standards relating to investigation, MDT assessment and treatment.

The quality and outcomes framework of the GMS contract includes 31 quality points relating to stroke indicators.[5]

Many NICE guidelines are relevant to stroke medicine, including those relating to the treatment of vascular disorders in general. Specific areas of guidance, either produced or in development, include:

- ximelagatran in patients with stroke and other thromboembolic complications associated with atrial fibrillation
- clopidogrel and modified-release dipyridamole in the prevention of occlusive vascular events
- ramipril and other ACE inhibitors for the prevention of cardiovascular disease and stroke
- closure of the patent foramen ovale for prevention of cerebral embolic stroke
- embolisation of intracranial aneurysms.

CLINICAL WORK AND/OR LABORATORY WORK OF CONSULTANTS IN STROKE MEDICINE

Contributions made to acute medicine

The extent of contribution to acute medicine will depend on the parent specialty of the stroke physician. Most consultants participate in acute medical, elderly care or integrated on-call rotas. The specialty of acute medicine is developing but is unlikely to obviate the need for this participation soon.

Direct clinical care

Inpatient work

Stroke patients are currently cared for in a wide variety of settings including general medical and elderly care wards in addition to stroke units. In an average district of 250,000 people there are approximately 400 first strokes and 150 recurrent strokes per year, with 25–35 stroke patients in a district hospital at one time. The number of stroke patients looked after by an individual consultant will vary depending on their work programme, but should not generally exceed 10 acute and 20 rehabilitation patients. Work includes ward rounds, MDT meetings and meetings with carers and relatives.

Outpatient work

Neurovascular clinics   The number of patients referred by primary care and emergency departments for evaluation could be expected to be between 300–500. It can be extremely difficult to diagnose TIA. Most neurovascular clinics operate as one-stop shops. Adequate time for assessment of the patient, formulating a management plan, and for discussion and information giving are required. The number of patients who can be seen will depend on the support available and may be reduced if junior staff are being supervised. Consultants might expect to see four to five new patients and one to two follow-up patients personally in this model.

Outreach rehabilitation and community liaison   This may involve work with a community stroke team or in day hospitals, community hospitals, intermediate care or primary care.

Secondary prevention   Specialist clinics for early review of stroke patients, especially those not admitted or discharged early from hospital, and for initiation of secondary prevention. A consultant might expect to see two to three new patients and six to seven follow-up patients in this model.

Longer-term management of disability   The NSF requires six-monthly multidisciplinary review and specialist management of complex disability.

Specialist investigative and therapeutic procedures

Time allocated for these will depend on the service model and work programme of the consultant. Specialised procedures, such as use of botulinum toxin for the management of spasticity, often require joint clinics, for example with a neurophysiotherapist.

Specialist on call

For a trust to implement thrombolysis for acute ischaemic stroke, 24-hour availability of a physician experienced in stroke, together with immediate access to brain imaging, is needed. It is desirable for ASUs to have 24-hour stroke physician cover, which would require a minimum of three consultants. Most trusts have only one stroke physician at present so a large increase in consultant resources is necessary before a 24-hour service for stroke can be implemented. Few hospitals will have sufficient experienced consultants within the stroke/neurology service to provide cover within European Working Time Directive criteria. Clinical networks, telemedicine and nurse consultant posts are possible methods of achieving a 24-hour service.

Clinically related administration

Administration duties include:

■ communicating by letter and telephone with patients, GPs and other clinicians
■ processing new referrals, arranging investigations and reviewing results
■ writing reports, for example for social services departments
■ assisting patients with legal and administrative activities, for example meeting with other professionals over such issues as mental incapacity.

Time must be allowed for this when planning the work programme. A four-hour outpatient clinic generates one to two hours of immediate administration followed by additional administration time as results and correspondence are generated. Adequate secretarial, administrative and IT resources are required.

with NHS consultant colleagues. Academic stroke physicians contribute to the education of professions allied to medicine involved in stroke services.

Research

See section on research in work to maintain and improve the quality of care, and above. The Stroke Association and Chest, Heart and Stroke (**www.chss.org.uk**) provide important financial support for project and programme grants, and junior training fellowships.

WORKFORCE REQUIREMENTS FOR STROKE MEDICINE

Due to the evolving nature of stroke medicine it is difficult to make accurate estimations of the resources allocated to specialist stroke services. Many consultants have taken a lead role in stroke but there are often little additional resources allocated. In parallel, many districts have developed hospital and community stroke teams, often by reorganising existing staff.

A benchmarking survey for the BASP estimated that, if it identified all inpatient services in the UK, 187 new ASUs, 158 new RSUs and 186 new neurovascular clinics would be required.[10] If only 50% of existing service were identified then 147 ASUs, 89 RSUs and 145 neurovascular clinics would be required. The survey also found that many services are run by a single consultant. There was no SpR in 37% of ASUs and 82% of RSUs.

The *National sentinel stroke audit* reported an increase in the number of stroke units to 82% of hospitals in England but found that only 50% of stroke patients were in a stroke unit. Only two-thirds of hospitals have a neurovascular clinic and only just over half of these are able to see and investigate patients within 14 days.[2]

The BASP Executive produced a position paper in June 2002 detailing the requirements for a specialist-led stroke service for England and Wales for an average district of 250,000 people:[11]

ASU	Ward rounds and daytime emergency cover	3 sessions/week
	Night time emergency cover	2 sessions/week
RSU	Ward rounds, MDT meetings and meetings with carers and relatives	3 sessions/week
Neurovascular clinic		2 sessions/week
Outreach rehabilitation and community liaison		1 session/week
Secondary prevention		1 session/week
Longer term management of disability		1 session/week
Training of other staff, CPD, management of the service, audit, research		3 sessions/week

The total number of sessions per district per week should therefore be approximately 16.

When clinical commitments in the parent specialty and cover for leave are taken into account, two WTEs will be required per district. There are approximately 209 districts (193 in England and 16 in Wales). This would mean a long-term target of 418 stroke physicians for the UK.

In the consultant Census, 102 consultants recorded some stroke-related work, of which the majority were geriatricians.[12] There were some specialist stroke sessions in 90% of districts.[2] The median number of sessions in districts where there is a stroke physician is three, equivalent nationally to 0.27 of a stroke physician (equivalent to 63 WTE) per district. The shortfall in terms of WTE is approximately 287.

It will be impossible to train and fund these posts within the timescale allowed by the NSF, but the BASP believes that the DH should set a target date. Given sufficient commitment, the profession could train enough stroke physicians to provide two per district by 2010. To achieve this, postgraduate deans would need to be given sufficient resources to fund the one-year training recently accepted by the JCHMT, and districts would be required to create additional consultant posts or convert existing posts from other specialties to stroke. It is reasonable to expect that every district would have at least one WTE stroke physician during the next three to five years, that is an increase of approximately 152 WTEs.

A small number of hospitals in the UK are already providing, or are in a position to provide, one-year stroke medicine training fellowships following the proposed curriculum but only a handful of such posts are currently available. The Stroke Association has funded 15 such posts over the last seven years. Trainees from any of the five parent specialties will now be able to spend a minimum of one year training in stroke. The Joint Committee for Higher Medical Training carried out a postal survey of all SpRs enrolled in the parent specialties in January and February 2003 on behalf of the stroke subspecialty advisory committee, and 218 trainees expressed an interest in spending an additional year of subspecialty training in stroke medicine. This may have a knock on effect on other doctors with a certificate of completion of specialist training (CCST), particularly those in geriatric medicine, neurology and rehabilitation. It has been agreed that SACs will be able to approve some of the subspecialty training in stroke medicine towards the parent CCST. This will need to be taken into account when determining the required number of training posts in the parent specialties.

CONSULTANT WORK PROGRAMME/SPECIMEN JOB PLAN

Activity	Workload	Programmed activities (PAs)
Direct clinical care		
Rehabilitation stroke unit (RSU) including rounds, MDT meetings, meetings with carers/relatives		1–2
Neurovascular clinic		1
Follow up clinic/secondary prevention		1
Outreach rehabilitation and community liaison/secondary prevention/long-term management of disability		1–2
General medicine on-call/ward work		1–2
Specialist on-call (minimum three physicians required) Acute stroke unit (ASU) day including emergency cover		1–2
ASU night emergency cover		1
Total number of direct clinical care PAs		**7.5 on average**
Supporting professional activities (SPA)		
Work to maintain and improve the quality of healthcare	Education and training, appraisal, departmental management and service development, audit and clinical governance, CPD and revalidation, research	**2.5 on average**
Other NHS responsibilities	eg medical director/clinical director/lead consultant in specialty/clinical tutor	**Local agreement with trust**
External duties	eg work for deaneries/Royal Colleges/specialist societies/Department of Health or other government bodies etc	**Local agreement with trust**

References

1. Department of Health. *National Service Framework for Older People.* London: The Stationery Office, 2001.

2. Intercollegiate Stroke Working Party. *National sentinel stroke audit: organisational audit 2004 (Concise report). A blueprint for better patient care,* August 2004. www.rcplondon.ac.uk/pubs/books/strokeaudit/strokeaudit2004.pdf

3. Royal College of Physicians. *National clinical guideline for stroke.* Report of an intercollegiate working party. London: RCP, 2000 (revised 2004).

4. Scottish Intercollegiate Guidelines Network (SIGN). *Management of patients with stroke.* Edinburgh: Royal College of Physicians, 1998.

5. Department of Health. *General Medical Services contract.* London: The Stationery Office, 2003.

6. Royal College of Physicians Clinical Effectiveness and Evaluation Unit. *National sentinel audit for stroke 2001/2.* London: RCP, 2002.

7. Paediatric Stroke Working Party. *Stroke in childhood: clinical guidelines for diagnosis, management and rehabilitation.* London: Royal College of Physicians, 2004.

8. Dennis M, O'Rourke S, Lewis, et al. A quantitative study of the emotional outcome of people caring for stroke survivors. *Stroke* 1998;**29**:1867–72.

9. Intercollegiate Stroke Working Party. *Care after stroke and transient ischaemic attack. Information for patients and their carers.* London: Royal College of Physicians, 2004.

10. Rodgers H, Dennis M, Cohen D, Rudd A. British Association of Stroke Physicians: Benchmarking survey of stroke services. *Age Ageing* 2003;**32**:211–7.

11. British Association of Stroke Physicians. *Requirements for a specialist led stroke service (for England & Wales)*, June 2002. www.basp.ac.uk/basp2003staffingastroke.htm

12. The Federation of the Royal Colleges of the United Kingdom. *Census of consultant physicians in the UK, 2003. Data and commentary.* London: The Federation of the Royal Colleges of the United Kingdom, 2003.